Cutaneous Lymphoma
Diagnosis and Treatment

Editors:

John C. Hall, MD
Associate Staff, Department of Medicine and Dermatology
University of Missouri—Kansas City School of Medicine
Primary Staff, St. Luke's Hospital
Kansas City Free Health Clinic
Kansas City, Missouri

Brian J. Hall, MD
University of Utah
Department of Pathology
Salt Lake City, Utah

2012
PEOPLE'S MEDICAL PUBLISHING HOUSE—USA
SHELTON, CONNECTICUT

People's Medical Publishing House-USA

2 Enterprise Drive, Suite 509
Shelton, CT 06484
Tel: 203-402-0646
Fax: 203-402-0854
E-mail: info@pmph-usa.com

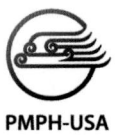

PMPH-USA

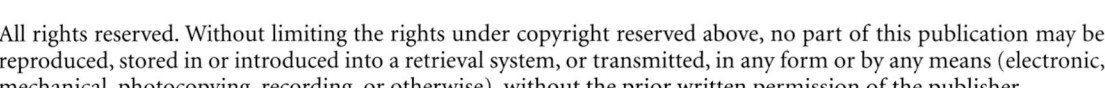

11 12 13 14/PMPH/9 8 7 6 5 4 3 2 1

ISBN-13: 978-1-60795-170-4
ISBN-10: 1-60795-170-3

Printed in China by People's Medical Publishing House
Copyeditor/Typesetter: Spearhead Global, Inc.

Library of Congress Cataloging-in-Publication Data
Cutaneous lymphoma : diagnosis and treatment / editors, John C. Hall, Brian J. Hall.
   p. ; cm.
  Includes bibliographical references and index.
  ISBN-13: 978-1-60795-170-4
  ISBN-10: 1-60795-170-3
  I. Hall, John C., 1947- II. Hall, Brian J. (Brian John), 1981-
  [DNLM: 1. Lymphoma, T-Cell, Cutaneous—diagnosis. 2. Lymphoma, T-Cell, Cutaneous—therapy. WR 500]
  616.99'446—dc23

                  2012005641

Sales and Distribution

Canada
McGraw-Hill Ryerson Education
Customer Care
300 Water St
Whitby, Ontario L1N 9B6
Canada
Tel: 1-800-565-5758
Fax: 1-800-463-5885
www.mcgrawhill.ca

Foreign Rights
John Scott & Company
International Publisher's Agency
P.O. Box 878
Kimberton, PA 19442
USA
Tel: 1-610-827-1640
Fax: 1-610-827-1671

Japan
United Publishers Services Limited
1-32-5 Higashi-Shinagawa
Shinagawa-ku, Tokyo 140-0002
Japan
Tel: 03-5479-7251
Fax: 03-5479-7307
Email: hayashi@ups.co.jp

United Kingdom, Europe, Middle East, Africa
McGraw Hill Education
Shoppenhangers Road
Maidenhead
Berkshire, SL6 2QL
England
Tel: 44-0-1628-502500
Fax: 44-0-1628-635895
www.mcgraw-hill.co.uk

Singapore, Thailand, Philippines, Indonesia
Vietnam, Pacific Rim, Korea
McGraw-Hill Education
60 Tuas Basin Link
Singapore 638775
Tel: 65-6863-1580
Fax: 65-6862-3354
www.mcgraw-hill.com.sg

Australia, New Zealand, Papua New Guinea, Fiji, Tonga, Solomon Islands, Cook Islands
Woodslane Pty Limited
Unit 7/5 Vuko Place
Warriewood NSW 2102
Australia
Tel: 61-2-9970-5111
Fax: 61-2-9970-5002
www.woodslane.com.au

Brazil
SuperPedido Tecmedd
Beatriz Alves, Foreign Trade
Department
R. Sansao Alves dos Santos, 102 | 7th floor
Brooklin Novo
Sao Paolo 04571-090
Brazil
Tel: 55-16-3512-5539
www.superpedidotecmedd.com.br

India, Bangladesh, Pakistan, Sri Lanka, Malaysia
CBS Publishers
4819/X1 Prahlad Street 24
Ansari Road, Darya Ganj,
New Delhi-110002
India
Tel: 91-11-23266861/67
Fax: 91-11-23266818
Email:cbspubs@vsnl.com

People's Republic of China
People's Medical Publishing House
International Trade Department
No. 19, Pan Jia Yuan Nan Li
Chaoyang District
Beijing 100021
P.R. China
Tel: 8610-67653342
Fax: 8610-67691034
www.pmph.com/en/

CONTRIBUTORS

Derek Thomas Bernstein, BS [15]
Department of Dermatology
Baylor College of Medicine
Houston, Texas

Kara Braudis, MD [12]
Department of Dermatology
University of Missouri
Columbia, Missouri

Lauren C. Pinter Brown, MD [19]
Hematology/Oncology
Oncology Treatment Center
UCLA School of Medicine
Los Angeles, California

Derek V. Chan, MD, PhD [18]
Division of Dermatology
Department of Internal Medicine
The Ohio State University
Columbus, Ohio

Abhinav B. Chandra, MD, MSc, FACP [10]
Fellow, Hematology/Oncology
Department of Medicine
Maimonides Medical Center
Brooklyn, New York

Wang L. Cheung, MD, PhD [4]
Assistant Professor
Dermatopathology Division
Department of Pathology and Department of
    Biochemistry and Molecular Biology
University of Arkansas for Medical Sciences
Little Rock, Arkansas

Katherine L. Craven, MD [9]
Department of Dermatology
University of Virginia School of Medicine
Charlottesville, Virginia

Mark D. P. Davis, MD [7]
Professor of Dermatology
Mayo Clinic Rochester
Rochester, Minnesota

Francine M. Foss, MD [17]
Professor of Medicine
Hematology and Bone Marrow Transplantation
Yale University School of Medicine
New Haven, Connecticut

John P. Galvin, MD, MPH [8]
Fellow, Division of Hematology/Oncology
Department of Medicine
Feinberg School of Medicine
Northwestern University
Chicago, Illinois

John C. Hall, MD [3]
Associate Staff
Department of Medicine and Dermatology
University of Missouri—Kansas City
    School of Medicine
Primary Staff
St. Luke's Hospital
Kansas City Free Health Clinic
Kansas City, Missouri

Mai P. Hoang, MD [13]
Associate Professor of Pathology
Massachusetts General Hospital
Boston, Massachusetts

Maura Jane Holcomb, MD [15]
Department of Dermatology
Baylor College of Medicine
Houston, Texas

Yiwu Jim Huang MD, PhD [10]
Assistant Professor of Medicine
State University of New York Downstate
    School of Medicine
Brooklyn, New York

Jacqueline M. Junkins-Hopkins, MD [1]
Dermpath Diagnostics Institute for
    Dermatopathology
Bryn Mawr, Pennsylvania

Jennifer R. Kaley, MD [4]
University of Arkansas for Medical Sciences
Department of Pathology
Little Rock, Arkansas

William A. Kanner, MD [9]
Fellow, Dermatopathology
University of Virginia Health System
Charlottesville, Virginia

Ellen J. Kim, MD [5]
Department of Dermatology
University of Pennsylvania
Philadelphia, Pennsylvania

Won Seog Kim, MD [11]
Professor, Division of Hematology-Oncology
Department of Medicine
Sungkyunkwan University School of Medicine
Samsung Medical Center
Seoul, Korea

Young-Hyeh Ko, MD [11]
Professor, Department of Pathology
Sungkyunkwan University School of Medicine
Samsung Medical Center
Seoul, Korea

Agnieszka W. Kubica, MD [7]
Mayo Medical School
Mayo Clinic
Rochester, Minnesota

Timothy M. Kuzel, MD [8]
Professor, Division of Hematology/Oncology
Department of Medicine
Feinberg School of Medicine
Northwestern University
Chicago, Illinois

Jo-Ann Latkowski, MD [6]
Assistant Professor of Dermatology
Associate Director of Residency Training
New York University School of Medicine
New York City, New York

Agustin Llopis-Gonzalez, PhD [2]
Assistant Professor of Preventive Medicine and
    Public Health
Unit of Public Health and Environmental Care
Department of Preventative Medicine
University of Valencia
CIBER Epidemiology and Public Health
    (CIBERESP)
Spain Center for Public Health Research (CSISP)
Valencia, Spain

Maria M. Morales Suárez-Varela, MD, PhD [2]
Assistant Professor of Preventive Medicine and
    Public Health
Unit of Public Health and Environmental Care
Department of Preventative Medicine
University of Valencia
CIBER Epidemiology and Public Health
    (CIBERESP)
Spain Center for Public Health Research (CSISP)
 Valencia, Spain

Maria Teresa Morales-Suárez-Varela, PhD [2]
Cordoba South Health District
Department of Health
District of Andalucia
 Cordoba, Spain

Amy Musiek, MD [5]
Department of Dermatology
The Raymond and Ruth Perelman School of
    Medicine at the University of Pennsylvania
Philadelphia, Pennsylvania

James W. Patterson, MD [9]
Professor of Pathology and Dermatology
 University of Virginia Health System
 Charlottesville, Virginia

Mark R. Pittelkow, MD [7]
Professor, Department of Dermatology,
    Biochemistry and Molecular Biology
Mayo Clinic College of Medicine
Mayo Medical School
Rochester, Minnesota

Ted Rosen, MD [15]
Professor of Dermatology
Baylor College of Medicine
Chief of Dermatology
Michael E. DeBakery VA Medical College
Houston, Texas

Maria Angelica Selim, MD [13]
Associate Professor of Pathology and
    Dermatology
Duke University Medical Center
Durham, North Carolina

Antonio Subtil, MD, MBA [16]
Associate Professor
Dermatology and Pathology
Yale University School of Medicine
New Haven, Connecticut

Neelam Vashi, MD [6]
Dermatology Resident
The Ronald O. Perelman Department of
    Dermatology
New York University Langone Medical Center
New York City, New York

Dana S. Ward, MD [12]
Department of Dermatology
University of Missouri
Columbia, Missouri

Henry K. Wong, MD, PhD [18]
Associate Professor of Internam Medicine
Department of Internal Medicine
Division of Dermatology
The Ohio State University
Columbus, Ohio

Yiqing Xu, MD, PhD [10]
Attending Physician
Division of Hematology/Oncology
Maimonides Medical Center
Brooklyn, New York

John Alan Zic, MD [14]
Associate Dean for Admissions; Associate
    Professor of Medicine/Dermatology
Vanderbilt University Cutaneous Lymphoma
    Clinic
Vanderbilt University School of Medicine
Nashville, Tennessee

CONTENTS

CHAPTER 5
MYCOSIS FUNGOIDES (CUTANEOUS T-CELL LYMPHOMA)

Amy Musiek, MD, and Ellen J. Kim, MD

CHAPTER 6
MYCOSIS FUNGOIDES VARIANTS

Jo-Ann Latkowski, MD, and Neelam Vashi, MD

CHAPTER 7
SÉZARY SYNDROME

Agnieszka W. Kubica, MD, Mark D. P. Davis, MD, and Mark R. Pittelkow, MD

INTRODUCTION

The study of cutaneous lymphoma has evolved dramatically over the last 50 years.

This evolution has led to cutaneous lymphoma clinically replacing syphilis as the great imitator of skin disease. From a classification standpoint, the disease has been dramatically reorganized. From a histopathology standpoint, a revolution of revised standard techniques and new sophisticated techniques has changed lymphomatous disease and dermatopathology forever. Scientifically, an explosion of information on the molecular and genetic understanding of the malignant cutaneous cancerous lymphocyte and its association with the immune system has occurred. And, possibly most important of all, therapeutic frontiers have been breached that have led to advancements in the care of the cancer patient specifically with skin lymphoma as well as the cancer patient in general.

To explore these advancements, we have assembled world leaders on this ever-changing topic. We first discuss the new classifications of cutaneous lymphoma. Epidemiology is then reviewed. A general approach to the patient suspected of having a cutaneous lymphoma is outlined. Discussion of diagnosis, histopathology, molecular genetics, and treatment of each subgroup is discussed. Precursors and mimics, which make this such a fascinating group of diseases, are reviewed. Systemic considerations of this primarily cutaneous disease are also covered. Molecular genetics of cutaneous lymphomas that have helped advance all of medicine are discussed, and finally, the future of this dynamic area of medicine is detailed.

Dermatology, oncology, pathology, and internal medicine have used this disease, as only scientists can, to advance our understanding of the human lymphocyte and its aberrant malignant state in that most accessible of all organs, the skin. If mimicry is the master of deceit, cutaneous T-cell lymphoma is indeed the king of confusion on the skin and under the microscope. Let us see if we can clear the murky waters that often lead to overdiagnosis or underdiagnosis and misdirected therapy to match them both.

An affordable summary of this dynamic branch of medicine is long overdue. This is it.

CUTANEOUS LYMPHOMA: DEFINITION, CLASSIFICATION, AND STAGING

Jacqueline M. Junkins-Hopkins, MD

INTRODUCTION

Primary cutaneous lymphoma is a subtype of non-Hodgkin's lymphoma that is restricted to the skin at the time of diagnosis and frequently remains skin-limited for long periods of time. These tumors are heterogeneous and subtyped based on clinical, microscopic, and immunophenotypic features. The diagnosis may be apparent on clinical or histopathologic grounds alone but should be confirmed by clinicopathologic correlation. The features often overlap with benign inflammatory dermatoses, and in these instances, immunohistochemistry and/or molecular confirmation may be required to make a diagnosis of cutaneous lymphoma with certainty. Moreover, immunophenotypic features have been incorporated into diagnostic criteria for selective subtypes of T- and B-cell lymphomas. Once a diagnosis of cutaneous lymphoma is rendered, staging should be performed in order to exclude secondary cutaneous lymphoma and establish the extent of disease burden. Management of the lymphoma will be dictated by the degree of skin, node, and peripheral blood involvement; the presence or absence of visceral tumor; and the subtype of lymphoma. Socioeconomic and comorbidity status also may factor into management options.

Immunophenotypic, molecular, and genetic investigations have contributed greatly to the nosology of cutaneous lymphomas, and the classification of these tumors will continue to evolve through further research and the accumulation of longitudinal prognostic data. Currently, primary cutaneous lymphomas are recognized under the classification put forth initially by the European Organization for Research and Treatment of Cancer (EORTC) in 1997. This scheme recognized the unique qualities of primary cutaneous lymphomas, stressing the need to incorporate the anatomic site and clinical context to avoid overtreatment for indolent cutaneous lymphomas

that are histologically identical to their aggressive nodal counterparts. This scheme was adopted by the World Health Organization (WHO) in 2005 as the WHO/EORTC classification of cutaneous lymphomas, and with minor modifications, published in the 4th edition of the WHO classification in 2008. The WHO/EORTC classification includes a distinct set of cutaneous T- and B-cell lymphomas that preferentially involve the skin and, with a few exceptions, are limited to the skin at the time of diagnosis (Table 1-1). It distinguishes cutaneous lymphomas with indolent, intermediate, and aggressive behavior and includes provisional entities (Table 1-2). The clinical utility has been validated by large clinical studies and is now recognized by dermatologists, dermatopathologists, pathologists, and oncologists worldwide. The entities are briefly discussed later and are detailed in subsequent chapters.

CUTANEOUS T-CELL LYMPHOMA

Mycosis Fungoides

Cutaneous T-cell lymphoma (CTCL) represents approximately 65% of primary cutaneous lymphomas and includes a variety of clinical, pathologic, and immunophenotypic presentations and subtypes. The most common presentation is that of patch/plaque disease, known as *mycosis fungoides* (MF), a tumor composed of an expanded clone of memory T-helper (CD45RO+, CD4+) lymphocytes, representing approximately 44% of CTCLs. MF is the prototype from which most other CTCLs are distinguished as separate entities. This indolent lymphoma typically presents as variably erythematous or dyschromic (hyper- or hypopigmented, poikilodermatous) patches with scaly or wrinkled (atrophic) surfaces that arise initially on double-covered sites, such as the breast, buttock, inner thighs, upper inner

TABLE 1-1   World Health Organization/European Organization for Research and Treatment of Cancer Classification of Cutaneous Lymphomas with Primary Cutaneous Manifestations

Cutaneous T-cell and NK-cell Lymphomas
MF
MF variants and subtypes
    Folliculotropic MF
    Pagetoid reticulosis
    Granulomatous slack skin
SS
ATLL
Primary cutaneous CD30+ lymphoproliferative disorders
    Primary cutaneous ALCL
    LyP
Subcutaneous panniculitis-like T-cell lymphoma (restricted to α/β TCR phenotype)
Extranodal NK/T-cell lymphoma, nasal type
Primary cutaneous peripheral T-cell lymphoma, unspecified
    Primary cutaneous aggressive epidermotropic CD8+ T-cell lymphoma, provisional
        (Primary cutaneous aggressive CD8+ epidermotropic cytotoxic T-cell lymphoma)[*]
    (Primary)[*] Cutaneous γ/δ T-cell lymphoma, provisional
    Primary cutaneous CD4+ small/medium-sized pleomorphic T-cell lymphoma (provisional)
        (Primary cutaneous CD4+ small/medium-sized T-cell lymphoma)[*]

Cutaneous B-cell Lymphomas
Primary cutaneous marginal zone B-cell lymphoma[†]
    Includes primary cutaneous immunocytoma, primary cutaneous plasmacytoma, follicular
    hyperplasia with monotypic plasma cells
Primary cutaneous follicle center lymphoma
    Includes follicular, follicular and diffuse, and diffuse growth patterns
Primary cutaneous diffuse large B-cell lymphoma, leg type
Primary cutaneous diffuse large B-cell lymphoma, other
    (Diffuse large B-cell lymphoma, NOS)[*]
    Primary cutaneous intravascular large B-cell lymphoma
        (Intravascular large B-cell lymphoma)[*]

Precursor Hematologic Neoplasm
CD4+/CD56+ hematodermic neoplasm (formerly blastic NK-cell lymphoma)
(Blastic plasmacytoid dendritic cell neoplasm)[*]

[*]Classification terminology in the WHO classification for lymphoid tissue (4th edition).

Willemze R, Jaffe ES, Burg G et al. WHO-EORTC classification for cutaneous lymphomas. Blood 2005; 105: 3768–3785

Swerdlow A, Campo E, Harris NL et al. World Health Organization Classification of Tumours of Hematopoietic and Lymphoid Tissue. Lyon: IARC Press, 2008.

[†]WHO classification of this subtype of B-cell lymphoma is extranodal marginal zone lymphoma of MALT lymphoma.

ALCL, anaplastic large cell lymphoma; ATLL, adult T-cell leukemia/lymphoma; LyP, lymphomatoid papulosis; MALT, mucosa-associated lymphoid tissue; MF, mycosis fungoides; NK, natural killer; NOS, not otherwise specified; SS, Sézary syndrome; TCR, T-cell receptor; WHO, World Health Organization.

Adapted from Kempf W, Sander CA. Classification of cutaneous lymphomas—an update. *Histopathology*. 2010;56:57–70.

TABLE 1-2   Clinical Behavior of Cutaneous Lymphomas

Cutaneous T-cell Lymphoma with *Indolent* Clinical Behavior
MF
Folliculotropic MF*
Pagetoid reticulosis
Granulomatous slack skin
Primary cutaneous anaplastic large cell lymphoma
Lymphomatoid papulosis
Subcutaneous panniculitis-like T-cell lymphoma
Primary cutaneous CD4+ small/medium-sized pleomorphic T-cell lymphoma (provisional)

Cutaneous T-cell Lymphoma with *Aggressive* Clinical Behavior
SS
Extranodal NK/T-cell lymphoma, nasal type
Primary cutaneous aggressive epidermotropic CD8+ T-cell lymphoma, provisional
Cutaneous γ/δ T-cell lymphoma, provisional
Primary cutaneous peripheral T-cell lymphoma, unspecified

Cutaneous B-cell Lymphomas with *Indolent* Behavior
Primary cutaneous marginal zone B-cell lymphoma
Primary cutaneous follicle center lymphoma

Cutaneous B-cell Lymphoma with *Aggressive* Clinical Behavior
Primary cutaneous diffuse large B-cell lymphoma, leg type
Primary cutaneous diffuse large B-cell lymphoma, other
Primary cutaneous intravascular large B-cell lymphoma

*Folliculotropic MF was initially considered indolent in the WHO-EORTC 2005 classification, but this may have a 5-year survival rate ranging from 60% to 70%.
EORTC, European Organization for Research and Treatment of Cancer; MF, mycosis fungoides; NK, natural killer; SS, Sézary syndrome; WHO, World Health Organization.

arms, and hips (Figure 1-1). With disease progression, lesions become more generalized and indurated. The patch/plaque stage may last indefinitely or may progress to tumors, such that a patient with advanced disease will typically have a combination of morphologies (see Figure 1-1).

Microscopically, MF is characterized by a constellation of histopathologic features, which may vary depending on the evolutionary stage and morphology biopsied (Table 1-3). In patch stage MF, there is a mild to moderate infiltrate of atypical lymphocytes that preferentially involve the epidermis (epidermotropism) and/or adnexal epithelium (adnexotropism) (Figure 1-2). Intraepidermal collections of four or more atypical lymphocytes (Pautrier microabscesses) are classic, but these are usually absent in early disease. Collections of atypical lymphocytes in

the dermal papillae may be a clue to the diagnosis (see Figure 1-2). The malignant cells have hyperchromatic and variably enlarged nuclei, with hyperconvoluted nuclear contours, imparting a cerebriform appearance on routine histology (see Figure 1-2). The atypia may be inconspicuous in early disease (Figure 1-3). Frequently, there are perinuclear halos. The papillary dermis becomes altered by thickened collagen bundles that entrap lymphocytes (Figure 1-4). Nonmalignant reactive lymphocytes accompany the malignant cells in the dermis and initially may predominate. The epidermis shows variable atrophy and/or psoriasiform hyperplasia (Figure 1-5) and typically is devoid of significant spongiosis or lichenoid tissue reaction, although exceptions exist, making the diagnosis of MF more challenging. In fact, diagnosing early MF is difficult for several reasons: (1) diagnostic

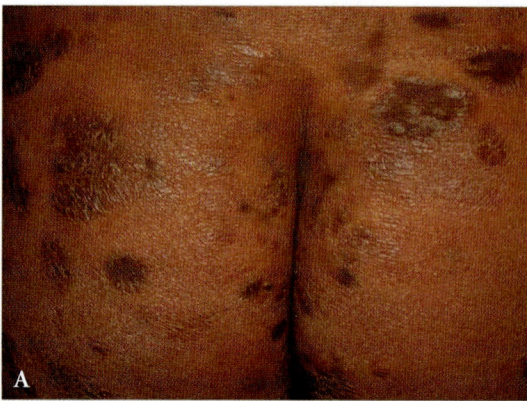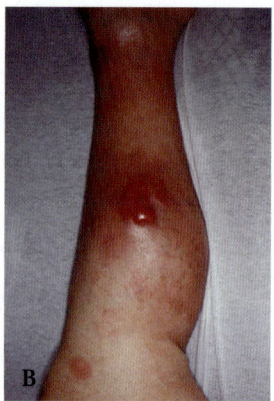

Figure 1-1 A, Patch/early plaque stage mycosis fungoides (MF). There are scaly hyperpigmented patches and thin plaques with xerotic patches on the buttock. **B,** MF, advanced stage. There are erythematous tumors, plaques, and patches.

features, such as nuclear atypia and epidermotropism may be subtle or focal, especially in early disease when there may be a prominent host response, (2) cutaneous lymphoid hyperplasia (CLH; pseudolymphoma) shows overlapping histologic features with CTCL, (3) MF may have overlapping features with some inflammatory diseases, including lichenoid keratosis, medication-induced infiltrates, and allergic contact dermatitis,

and (4) unawareness of the MF variants may result in erroneously excluding MF from the differential diagnosis. Incorporating treatment history is important (including even mild topical steroid application) because topical therapy may eliminate some of the diagnostic features. Review of previous biopsies may provide enough additional histologic data to comfortably render a diagnosis of MF. Correlation of the histology with

TABLE 1-3   Histopathologic Features of Patch/Early Plaque Mycosis Fungoides

Epidermotropism: preferential involvement of epidermis (or adnexal epithelium—adnexotropism)
> Peppering of rete, beading, pagetoid patterns; Pautrier microabscess formation.

Patchy to band-like lymphocytic infiltrate in papillary dermis
> Atypical cells often aggregate in dermal papillae; the papillary dermis may show admixture of nonatypical lymphocytes.

Lymphocyte atypia
> Hyperchromatic and cerebriform nuclei, nuclear enlargement; atypia may be inconspicuous.

Epidermal atrophy
> Basal cells not effaced by an interface dermatitis.

Rete hyperplasia
> Atrophic rete juxtaposed with atrophic epidermis; may be psoriasiform.

Papillary dermal fibroplasia
> "Wiry collagen bundles"; fettuccine-like.
> May be absent if recurrent or early onset lesions.

Hyperkeratosis: Compaction of stratum corneum, variable parakeratosis.

Variable nonlymphocytic inflammatory cells
> Eosinophils, histiocytes/multinucleated giant cells forming granulomas, plasma cells.

Absence of significant epidermal alteration
> Lichenoid and spongiotic changes *typically* not more prominent than epidermotropism.

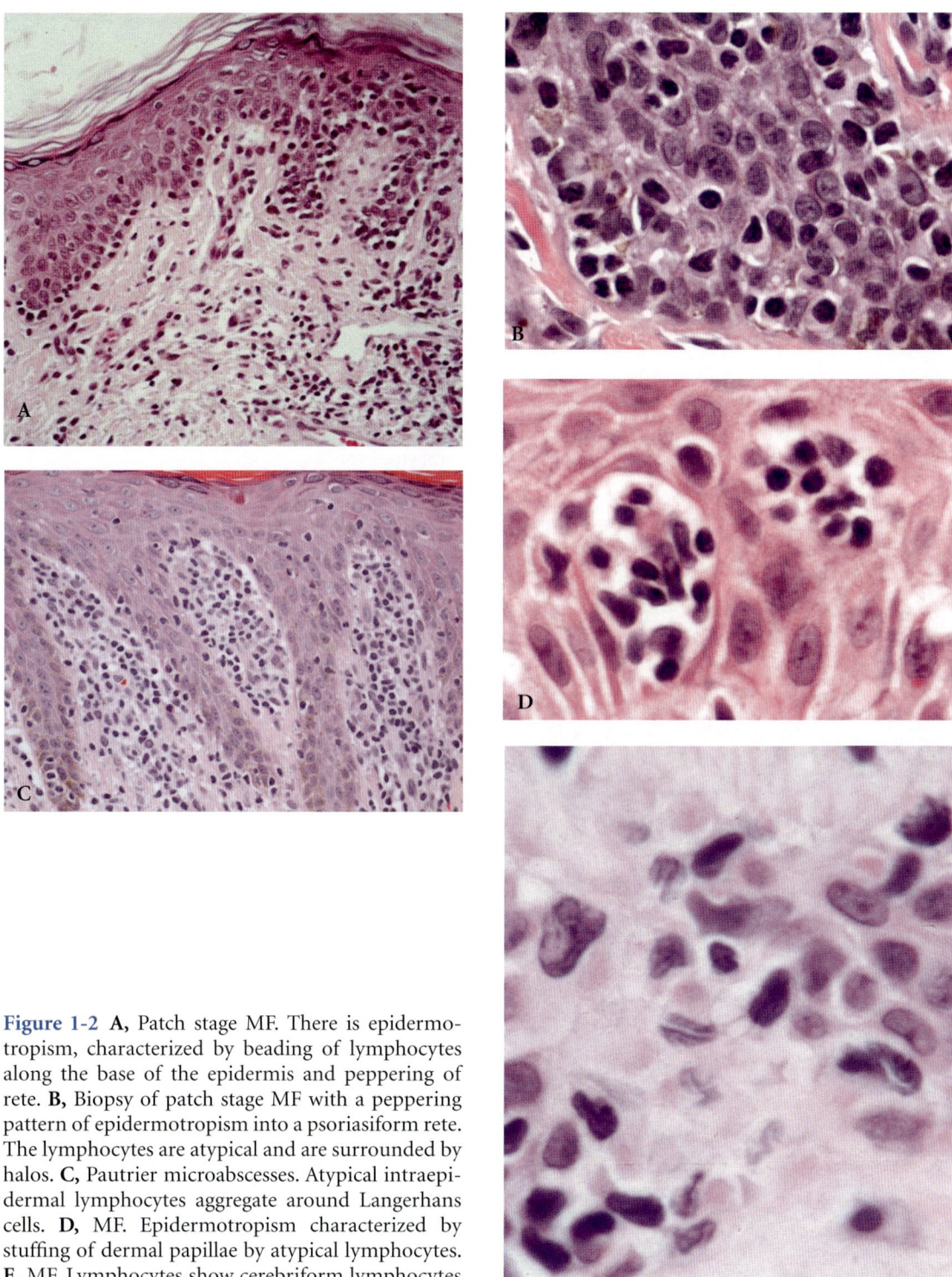

Figure 1-2 A, Patch stage MF. There is epidermotropism, characterized by beading of lymphocytes along the base of the epidermis and peppering of rete. **B,** Biopsy of patch stage MF with a peppering pattern of epidermotropism into a psoriasiform rete. The lymphocytes are atypical and are surrounded by halos. **C,** Pautrier microabscesses. Atypical intraepidermal lymphocytes aggregate around Langerhans cells. **D,** MF. Epidermotropism characterized by stuffing of dermal papillae by atypical lymphocytes. **E,** MF. Lymphocytes show cerebriform lymphocytes with nuclear slits and irregularities.

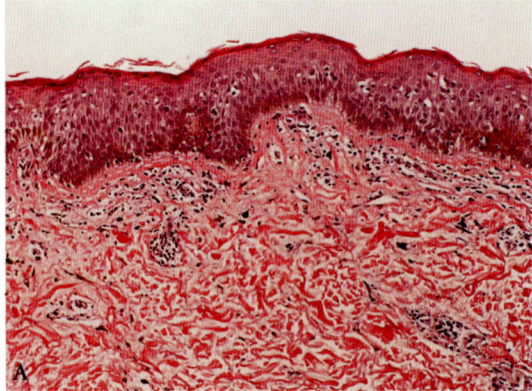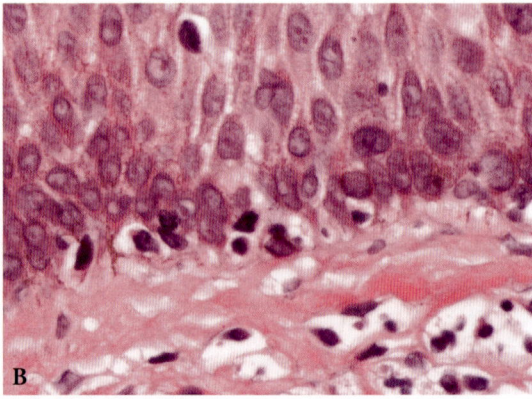

Figure 1-3 A, Patch MF with subtle epidermotropism of small lymphocytes with perinuclear halos. The epidermis shows compaction of the stratum corneum, without significant spongiosis. There is papillary dermal fibroplasia. **B,** Patch MF. High-power view demonstrates small but hyperconvoluted lymphocytes with irregular nuclei with halos collecting along the basal keratinocytes.

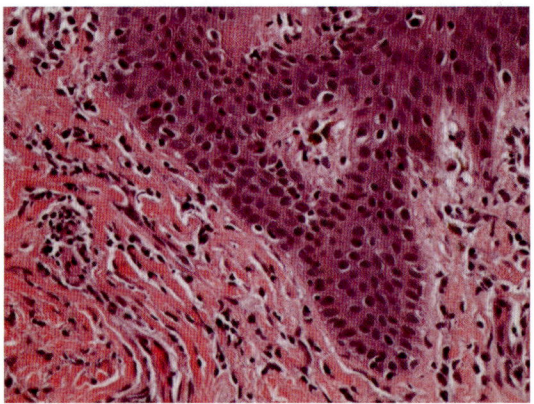

Figure 1-4 MF. Papillary dermal fibroplasia.

the clinical distribution (e.g., generalized lesions or persistent lesions on buttocks or hips) and course of the lesions (e.g., recurrence of the *same* lesion following treatment with topical steroids) may help confirm a diagnosis of MF if the biopsy shows borderline histology. Review of slides by an experienced pathologist may be required for borderline cases. The International Society for Cutaneous Lymphoma (ISCL) has proposed an algorithm for a diagnosis of early MF, which incorporates clinical, histopathologic, molecular, and immunophenotypic data. Assessment of leveled sections is crucial to making a more accurate diagnosis, especially with the MF subtypes

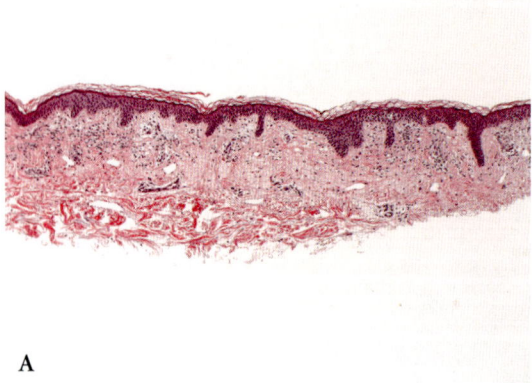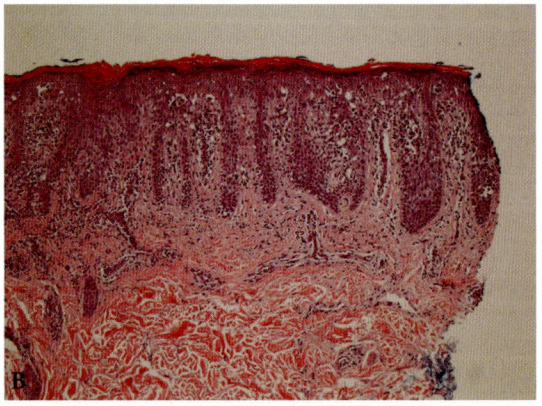

Figure 1-5 A, Epidermal changes of MF. There is epidermal atrophy with an irregular proliferation of atrophic rete. **B,** Epidermal changes of MF. There is psoriasiform rete hyperplasia with an epidermotropic lymphocytic infiltrate collecting beneath and within the epidermis.

TABLE 1-4 Predominantly Clinical Variants of Mycosis Fungoides

Erythrodermic
Hypopigmented
Palmar-plantar
Syringotropic
Bullous
Ichthyotic
Papuloerythroderma of Ofuji
Papular
Pustular
Unilesional
Verrucous
Poikilodermatous
Invisible
Atrophoderma
Acanthosis nigricans–like
Zosteriform

TABLE 1-5 Predominantly Histologic Variants of Mycosis Fungoides

Lichenoid
Interstitial
Pigmented purpura*
Spongiotic
Bullous*
Syringotropic*
Syringolymphoid hyperplasia
Granulomatous
CD20+

*May be associated with corresponding clinical variants of MF.

that involve adnexae. Clinical-pathologic correlation is also important in order to avoid missing an MF variant. These variants are listed in Tables 1-4 and 1-5, and many are discussed in detail in Chapter 6.

With disease progression into tumor stage, the infiltrate becomes more prominent in the reticular dermis and around the vascular plexi (Figure 1-6).

The malignant T cells may become large and transformed (see Figure 1-6) and can eventually be detected in the peripheral blood, lymph nodes, and viscera. MF typically demonstrates an immunophenotype that is CD2+, CD3+, CD4+, CD45RO+, T-cell receptor-beta–positive (TCR-β+), CD8–, but the neoplastic lymphocytes may exhibit immunophenotypic variations including CD8+/CD4–, CD4–/CD8– (double negative), CD56+, and TIA-1 or granzyme B (cytotoxic)–positive MF. Some of these immunophenotypes define aggressive variants of CTCL, but this is not the case when associated with an MF *clinical*

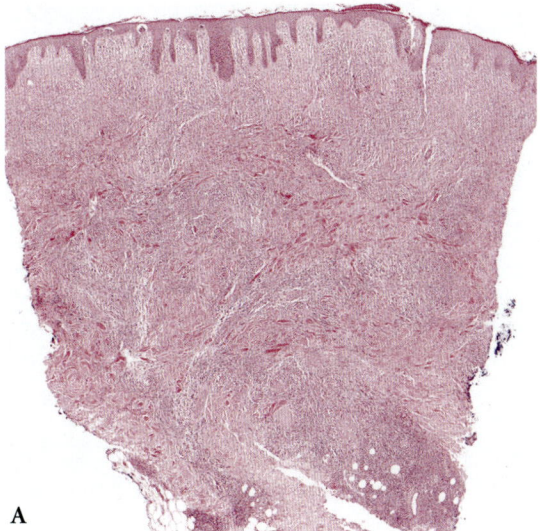

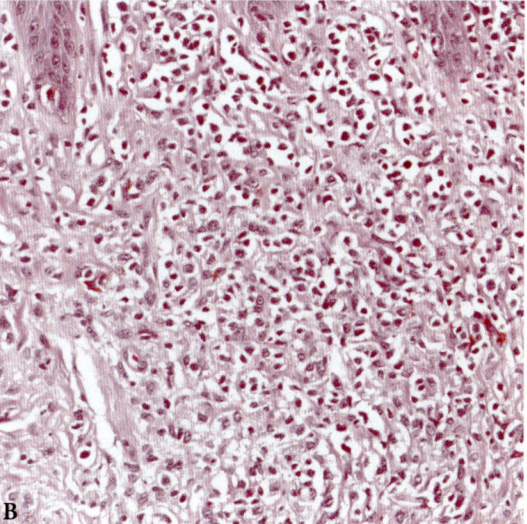

Figure 1-6 A, Plaque or early tumor stage MF. There is a dense pandermal lymphocytic infiltrate extending to the subcutis. The epidermis shows a proliferation of atrophic rete. **B,** High-power view of MF with early large cell transformation.

phenotype. CD30 positivity in blast-like cells may indicate progression of MF with large cell transformation (defined as lymphocytes four or more times the size of a small lymphocyte, exceeding 25% of the infiltrate, or forming small micronodules). There may be loss of CD7, CD3, CD2, and/or CD5 with disease progression. Immunophenotyping may help distinguish MF from benign inflammatory simulators. Diminished staining or loss of CD7 may also be seen in eczematous dermatoses, but in the context of other microscopic and immunophenotypic abnormalities, such as an increased CD4/CD8 ratio indicating a helper T-cell infiltrate (Figure 1-7), CD7 loss may be used to favor MF. Documenting a monoclonal rearrangement of the TCR also helps to support a diagnosis of CTCL. However, T-cell dyscrasias such as pityriasis lichenoides may be clonal, or there may be false-positive and false-negative

polymerase chain reaction (PCR) results, so one should not rely on this test to confirm malignancy. Dual TCR-PCR, using two specimens from the patient to document identical clones, has been found to have high specificity in distinguishing MF from inflammatory dermatoses. These adjunctive tests can especially be helpful in diagnosing non-MF subtypes of CTCL. These are discussed briefly in this chapter and are detailed in Chapters 7 to 12.

Mycosis Fungoides Variants

MF may have clinical or histopathologic presentations that vary from that described previously. Clinically, the lesions may be hypopigmented, purpuric, bullous, pustular, papular, ichthyotic, verrucous, pigmented purpura-like, poikilodermatous, unilateral/zosteriform, volar-restricted,

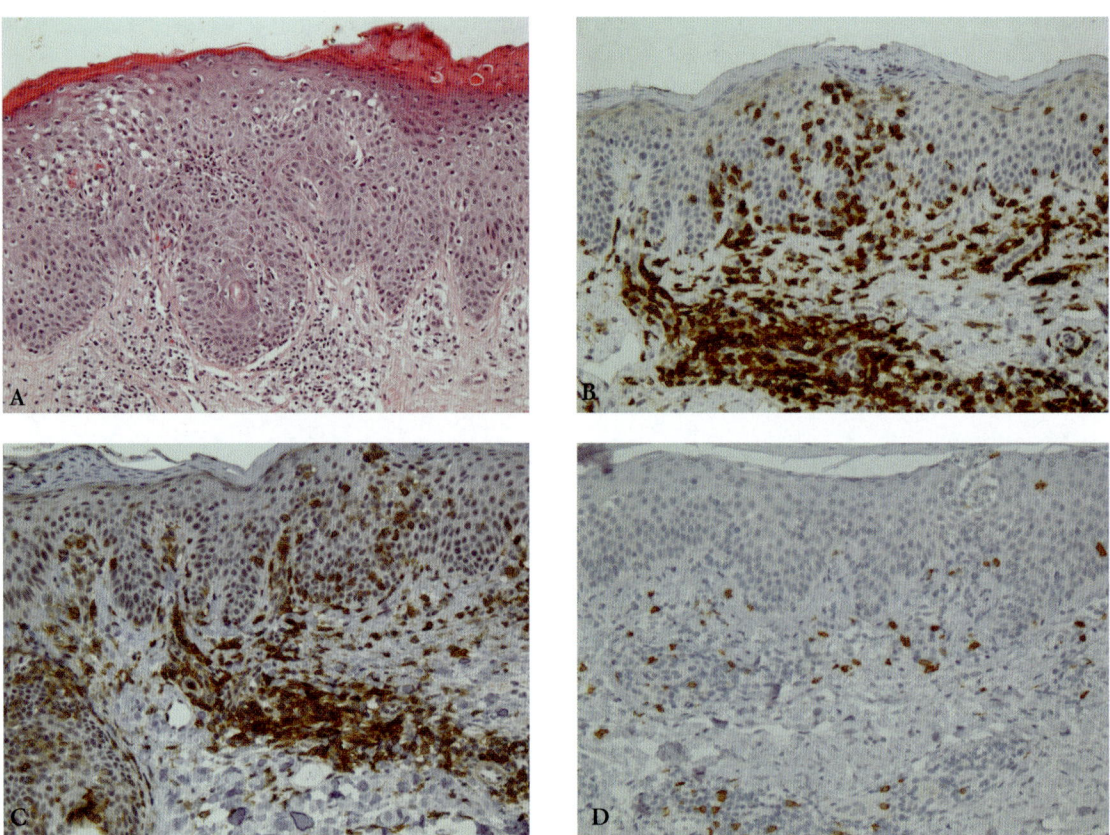

Figure 1-7 **A,** Biopsy of MF with spongiosis and borderline diagnostic features. **B,** CD3 stain of biopsy in part A demonstrates an epidermotropic T-cell infiltrate. **C,** CD4 stain of biopsy in **A** demonstrates an epidermotropic T-helper infiltrate. **D,** CD8 stain of biopsy in **A** demonstrates negative staining of epidermotropic T-cell infiltrate consistent with CD4 immunophenotype in MF with spongiosis.

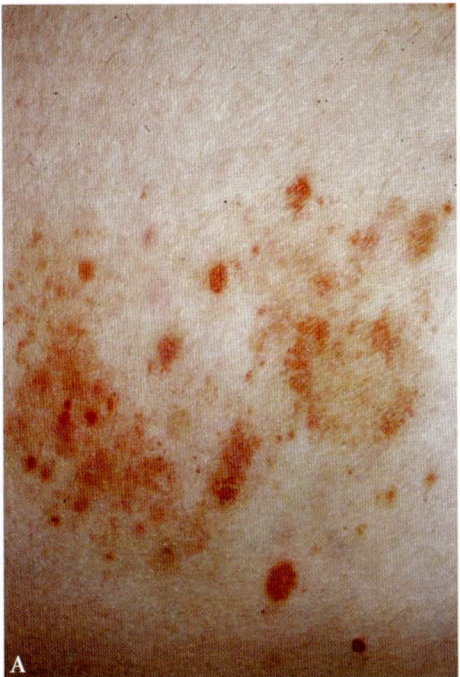
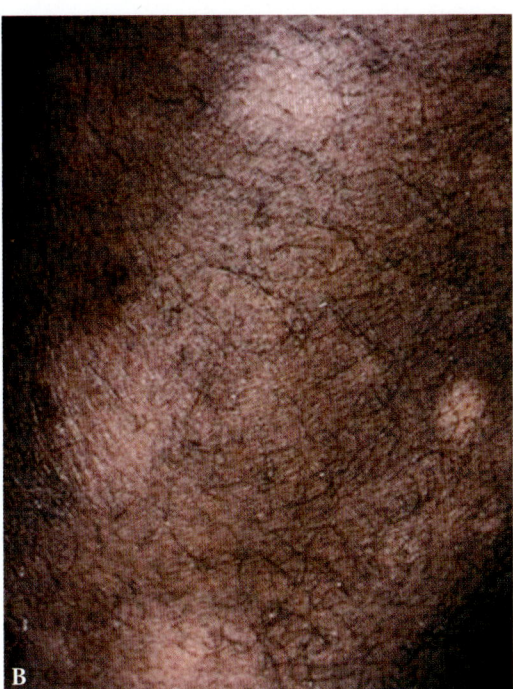

Figure 1-8 A, Pigmented purpura variant of MF. The location on the trunk is unusual for benign pigmented purpura. **B,** Hypopigmented variant of MF. This frequently arises in dark-skinned patients.

or atrophodermic (Figure 1-8). Histologic variations include cases with secondary epidermal changes, such as spongiosis, bullae, or lichenoid tissue reaction. Some cases may be associated with sarcoidal or granuloma annulare–like changes. These histologic variations may be seen in biopsies of classic patch/plaque MF. However, some histologic variants such as atrophoderma/elastolysis or pigmented purpura may be associated with clinical lesions similar to their benign counterparts. Syringotropic MF, characterized by epitheliotropism involving eccrine epithelium, may be associated with a unique glandular alteration, termed *syringolymphoid hyperplasia* (Figure 1-9). Patients with this histology often have characteristic small red-brown papules or macules (see Figure 1-9). However, syringotropic MF has not been formally designated as a subtype of MF in the WHO/EORTC classification scheme. This is in contrast to folliculotropic mycosis fungoides (FMF), granulomatous slack skin (GSS), and pagetoid reticulosis (PR), all of which have a distinct clinicopathologic presentation worthy of inclusion in the WHO/EORTC classification of primary cutaneous

lymphoma. These are discussed briefly later and detailed in Chapters 5 and 6.

Folliculotropic Mycosis Fungoides

FMF is characterized clinically by alopecic patches and plaques, the surface of which may be studded with comedones, milia, and/or follicular spines (Figure 1-10). In contrast to classic MF, FMF frequently involves the head and neck and is concentrated in other hair-bearing sites, such as the groin, axilla, and extremities. Moreover, whereas in classic MF, lymphocytes may extend into hair follicles in addition to the epidermis, in FMF, the T-helper lymphocytes *preferentially* involve hair follicles. The follicles often exhibit comedonal alteration with keratin plugging (see Figure 1-10). There may be mucinous degeneration of follicle epithelium with histopathologic changes of alopecia mucinosa (Figure 1-11), a solitary or oligolesional clonal plaque that may or may not progress to generalized FMF. There may be concomitant syringotropic MF. The clinical presentation of FMF may simulate an

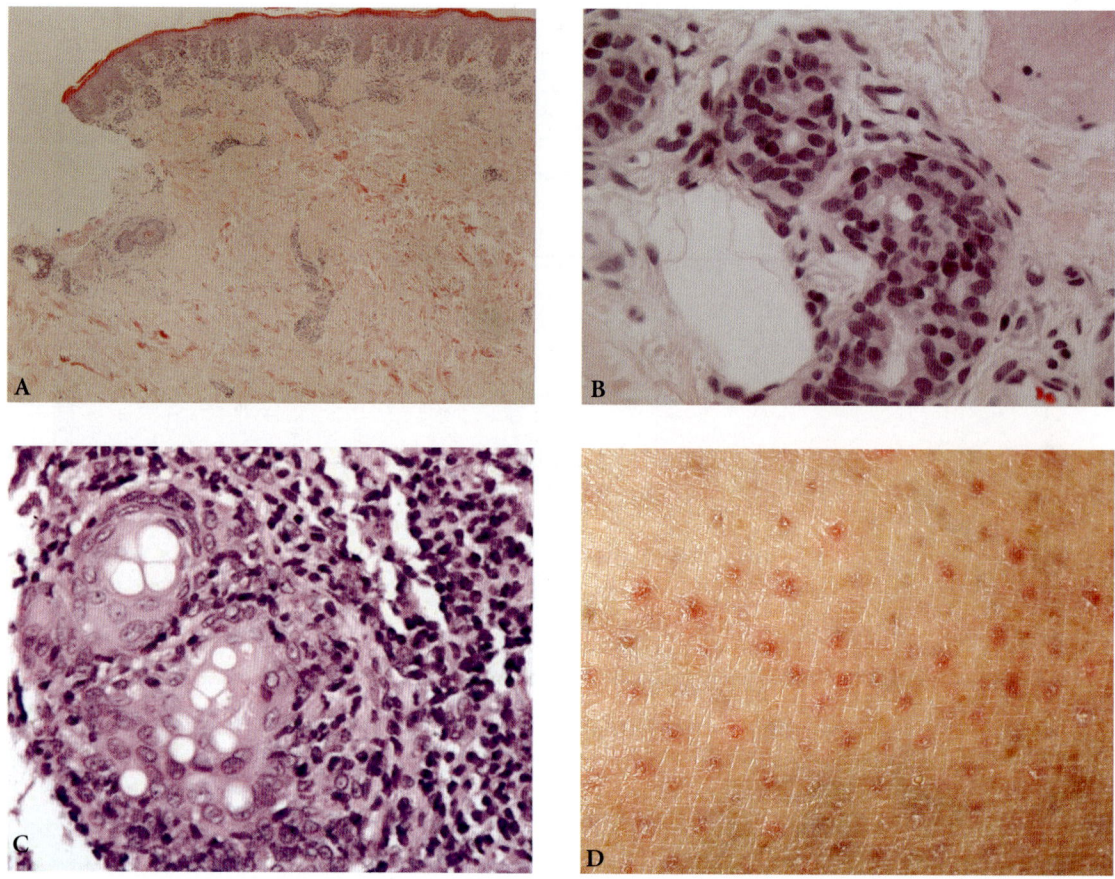

Figure 1-9 A, Biopsy of syringotropic MF. Lymphocytes are deep in the dermis around and within the eccrine glands. **B,** High-power view of syringotropic MF. Lymphocytes are deep in the dermis around and within the eccrine glands. **C,** Syringolymphoid hyperplasia. There is hyperplasia of eccrine glands and ductules with adnexotropic lymphocytes. **D,** Syringotropic MF. Small red-brown scaly macules and papules at the ostia of the eccrine duct.

allergic contact or nummular dermatitis owing to pruritic eczematous patches and spongiotic biopsy findings, causing a delay in the diagnosis. Granulomatous reactions to ruptured comedonal follicles may also elicit an erroneous diagnosis of CLH. Recognition of FMF as a distinct subset of MF is critical because the disease often requires systemic therapy, and the prognosis may be worse than classic MF, despite a clinical presentation of "patches."

Granulomatous Slack Skin

GSS is a distinct clinicopathologic subtype of MF affecting adults and pediatric populations, characterized by indurated plaques arising on intertriginous sites, with histologic features of an atypical dermal non- or minimally epidermotropic T-helper lymphocytic infiltrate admixed with multinucleated giant cells engulfing elastic fibers and lymphocytes (Figure 1-12). As a result of extensive elastolysis, the plaques become wrinkled and slack. GSS should be distinguished from classic MF or Sézary syndrome (SS) with a granulomatous component because the prognosis of GSS tends to be better, despite clinical plaques. It is also important to recognize GSS as a separate clinicopathologic entity because there may be an increased risk of developing systemic Hodgkin's or non-Hodgkin's lymphoma.

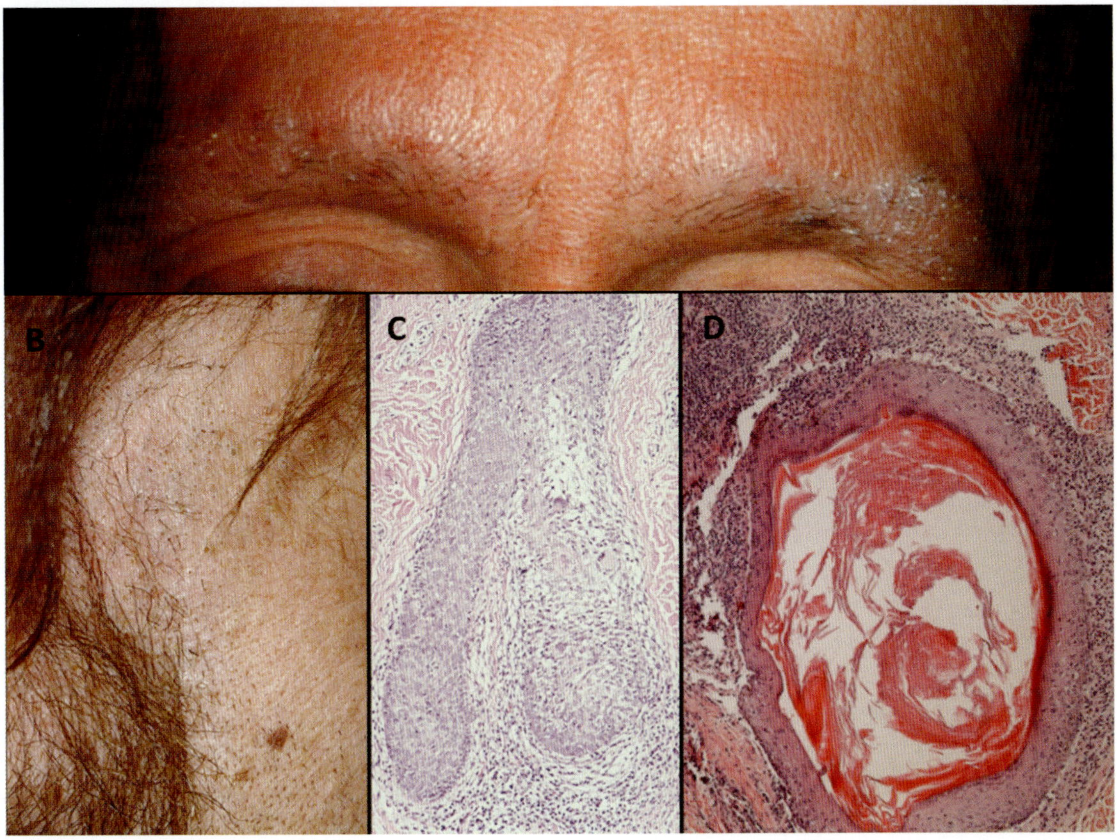

Figure 1-10 **A,** Folliculotropic mycosis fungoides (FMF). There is loss of eyebrow hair with fine follicular spines. **B,** FMF. There are comedones and early alopecia. **C,** FMF. Biopsy shows folliculocentric, folliculotropic lymphocytes. **D,** FMF. Follicles with comedonal plugs and folliculotropic lymphocytic infiltrate.

Pagetoid Reticulosis

PR is defined by the histopathologic findings of a markedly epidermotropic infiltrate of

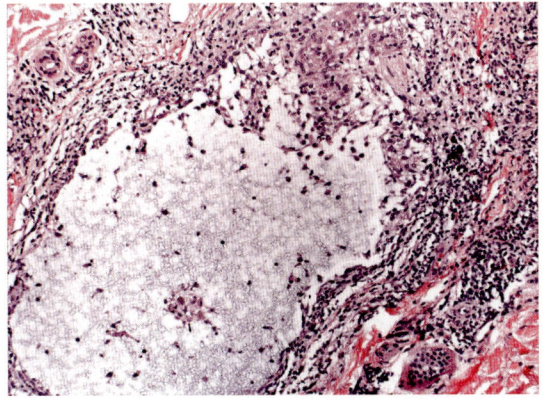

Figure 1-11 Follicular mucinosis in lesion of FMF.

T lymphocytes with perinuclear halos, arising in the clinical context of indolent acrally accentuated psoriasiform hyperkeratotic plaques. Palmarplantar MF may represent a form of PR restricted to the volar surface. The lymphocytes are CD2+, CD3+, βF1+, TIA-1+, and CD45RO+, and may have either a CD4+, a CD8+, or a CD30+ immunophenotype. PR is also referred to as Woringer-Kolopp disease, and it should be distinguished from primary cutaneous aggressive epidermotropic CD8+ T-cell lymphoma, which has similar striking epidermotropism but presents with generalized mucocutaneous nodules, associated with an aggressive course and poor prognosis.

Sézary Syndrome

Patients with SS present with erythroderma involving greater than 80% of the body surface

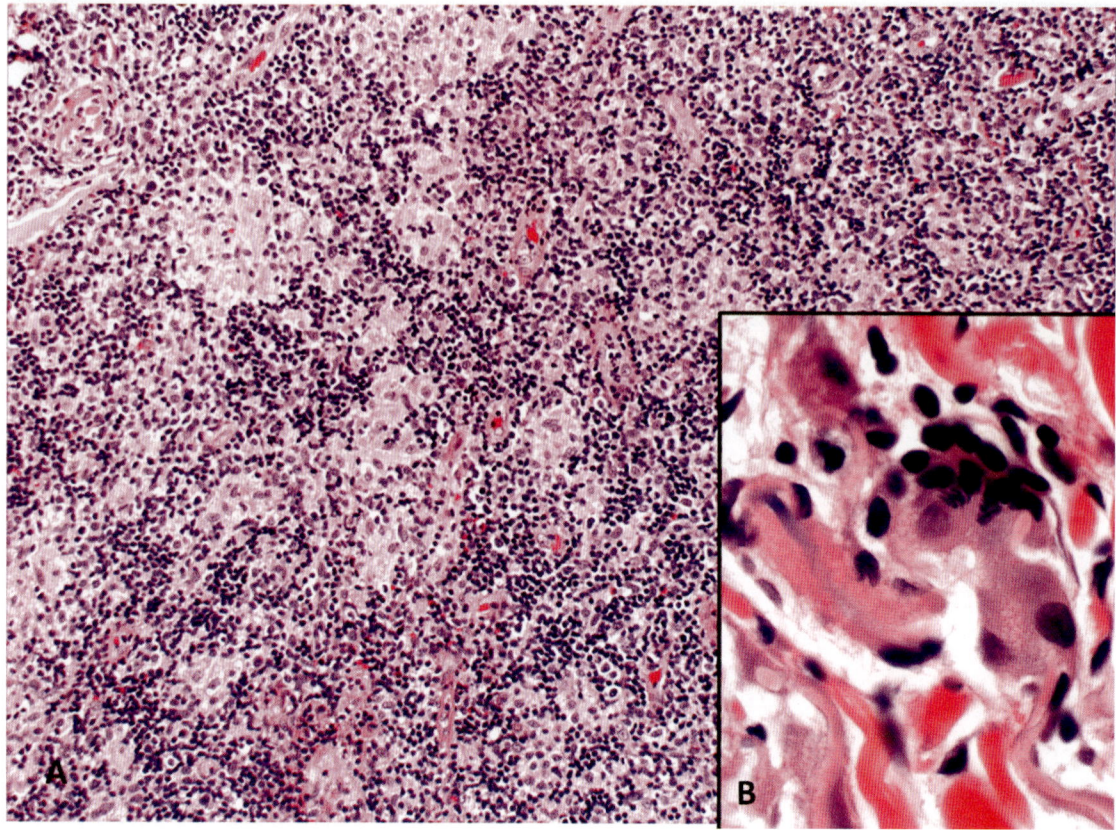

Figure 1-12 A, Granulomatous slack skin (GSS). There is a dermal infiltrate of atypical lymphocytes and multi-nucleated giant cells with emperipolesis. **B,** GSS. Emperipolesis of cerebriform lymphocytes and elastophagia.

area (BSA), with significant tumor burden in the peripheral blood and lymph nodes (Figure 1-13). Frequently, biopsies will be devoid of epidermotropism (see Figure 1-13) or significant lymphocyte atypia. Thus, the possibility of SS should not be excluded without evaluation of the peripheral blood. A spectrum of blood involvement may be seen in patients with erythroderma, but not all of these patients will fulfill criteria for SS. SS, or B2 stage erythroderma, requires documenting a dominant T-cell clone by PCR analysis or Southern blot and either an absolute Sézary count of 1. 0 K/μL or greater by Sézary preparation or one of the following: (1) expanded CD3+ CD4+ cells or CD4/CD8 ratio of 10 or higher; (2) expanded CD4+ T cells with abnormal immunophenotype (such as loss of CD7 ≥ 40% or CD26 ≥ 30%) by flow cytometry. B0 is defined as having 5% or fewer Sézary cells. B1 is defined as greater than 5% but less than 1.0 K/μL Sézary

cells, or negative TCR clone, or both. Patients with SS have a poor prognosis if left untreated and, in fact, represents stage IV disease. Pruritus, keratoderma, ectropion, and increased risk for infection contribute to morbidity.

As MF progresses, tumor burden in the peripheral blood may reach clinically relevant levels. This may arise in the context of extensive skin involvement covering over 80% of BSA. This leukemic presentation of MF (cases that meet criteria for SS but are preceded by MF) is distinct from SS. Both are malignancies of T-helper lymphocytes, but MF is a malignancy of skin resident effector memory T cells and SS is a malignancy of central memory T cells.

Adult T-cell Leukemia/Lymphoma

Adult T-cell leukemia/lymphoma (ATLL) is a peripheral T-cell malignancy associated with the

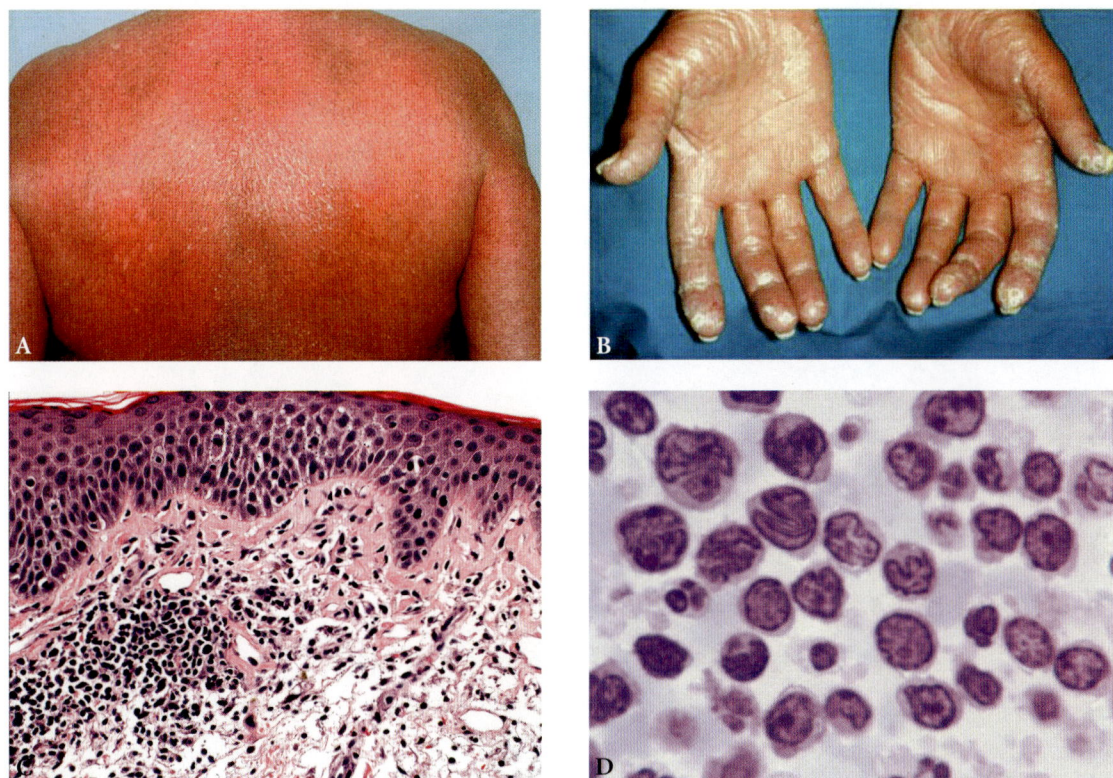

Figure 1-13 A, Sézary syndrome (SS). Diffuse erythroderma involves more than 80% of the body surface area (BSA). **B,** SS in a patient with typical keratoderma. **C,** SS. The biopsy shows spongiosis with no epidermotropism. There are atypical lymphocytes in the dermis. **D,** SS. Buffy coat preparation of peripheral blood demonstrates cerebriform Sézary cells in the peripheral blood.

retrovirus human T-cell leukemia virus type 1 or human T-cell lymphotropic virus type 1 (HTLV-1). This virus is endemic in Japan, the Caribbean islands, South and Central America, southeastern United States, and some regions in Africa; however, only about 1% to 5% of seropositive individuals will develop ATLL. There is a broad spectrum of clinical subtypes: acute, chronic, smoldering, and lymphoma. Acute ATLL is the most common and is characterized by high peripheral blood tumor burden, lymphadenopathy, hepatosplenomegaly, fever, cough, hypercalcemia associated with lytic bone lesions, and cutaneous nodules and tumors. The chronic and smoldering variants may simulate MF, with minimal circulating cells. Histologic features are also similar to MF and SS, with either an epidermotropic or a mild dermal infiltrate of atypical CD4+ CD3+ CD25+ lymphocytes (Figure 1-14). The lymphocytes in ATLL have hyperlobated cloverleaf-like nuclei, but this is less

obvious in skin biopsies (see Figure 1-14). ATLL is an aggressive lymphoma that should be differentiated from MF/SS. The presentation of rapidly evolving papules, nodules, and tumors in the characteristic demographic context, especially in the setting of hepatomegaly or liver dysfunction, should prompt evaluation for clonally integrated HTLV-1 provirus in the host genome to diagnose ATLL. Proposed diagnostic criteria for the subtypes are as follows:

1. Smoldering type: 5% or more circulating abnormal T cells; normal lymphocyte and calcium levels; lactate dehydrogenase (LDH) value of up to 1.5 times the normal upper limit; no lymphadenopathy; no involvement of liver, spleen, central nervous system, bone, and gastrointestinal tract; and neither ascites nor pleural effusion. Skin and pulmonary lesions may be present. If less than 5%

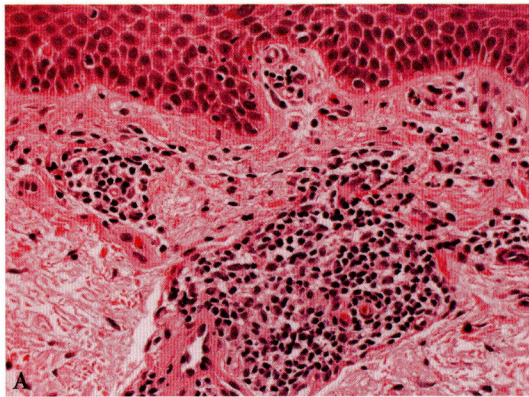

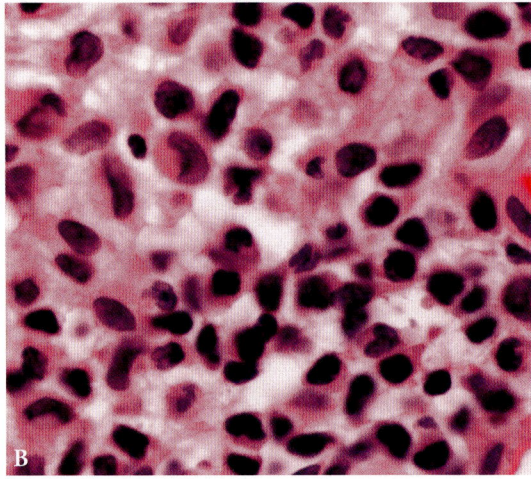

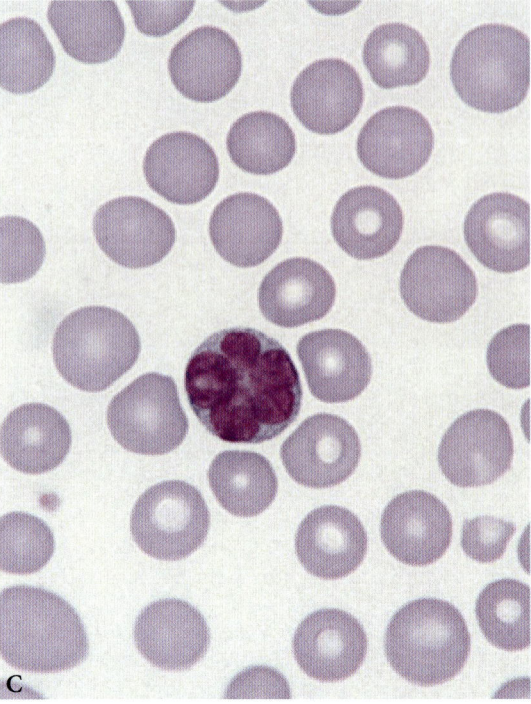

Figure 1-14 A, Adult T-cell leukemia/lymphoma (ATLL). Biopsy of a papule shows perivascular lymphocytes without epidermotropism. **B,** ATLL. High power view of atypical dermal lymphocytes. **C,** ATLL. Peripheral blood lymphocyte with a clover-leaf multilobated nucleus.

abnormal circulating T lymphocytes are present, biopsy confirmation of skin or lung involvement is required.

2. Chronic type: Absolute lymphocytosis (≥4 × 10(9)/L) with T lymphocytosis (>3.5 × 10(9)/L); LDH up to twice the normal upper limit; no hypercalcemia; no involvement of central nervous system, bone, and gastrointestinal tract; and neither ascites nor pleural effusion. Lymphadenopathy and involvement of liver, spleen, skin, and lung may be present; 5% or greater circulating abnormal T lymphocytes usually present.

3. Lymphoma type: Histologically proven lymphadenopathy with or without extranodal lesions. No lymphocytosis, 1% or fewer circulating abnormal T lymphocytes.

4. Acute type: Leukemic manifestation and tumor lesions are usually present, and the patients do not fulfill criteria for the other subtypes. ATLL is discussed in detail in Chapter 8.

CD30+ Lymphoproliferative Disorder

CD30 lymphoproliferative disorder (LPD) includes lymphomatoid papulosis (LyP), anaplastic large cell lymphoma (ALCL), and borderline CD30+ tumors that have overlapping features of LyP and ALCL. These tumors are defined histologically by the presence of variable numbers of atypical CD30+ lymphocytes. The diagnosis ultimately requires correlating the histologic findings with the clinical presentation. LyP presents as recurring crops of papules and nodules that self-resolve, whereas patients with ALCL present with ulcerated and necrotic tumors and plaques (Figure 1-15).

In LyP, the infiltrate is perivascular and interstitial to band-like, imparting a "wedge-shape" (Figure 1-16). There is variable epidermotropism, which may be quite striking in some cases. The epidermis shows variable acanthosis, scale-crust, and necrosis that are determined by the

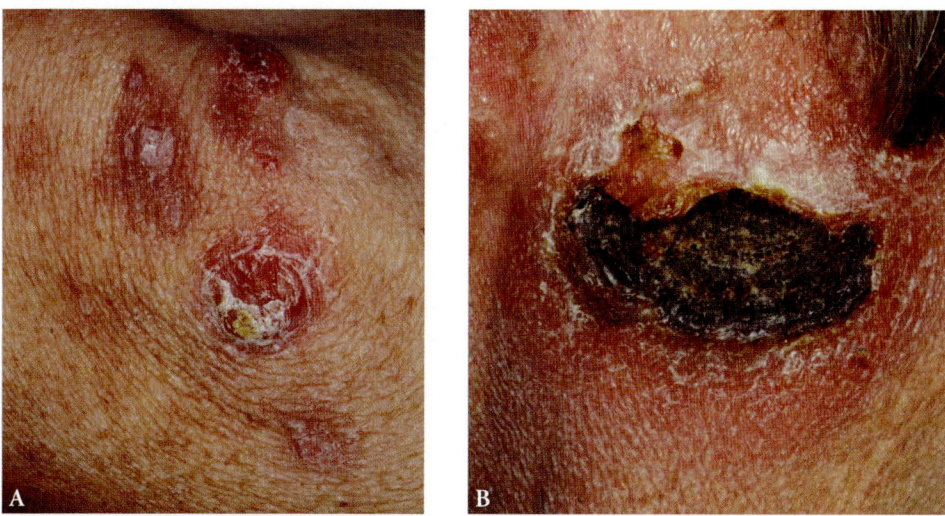

Figure 1-15 A, Lymphomatoid papulosis (LyP). Necrotic and scaly papules in various stages of evolution with evidence of scarring. **B,** Anaplastic large cell lymphoma (ALCL). Ulcerated necrotic plaque surrounded by indurated erythema.

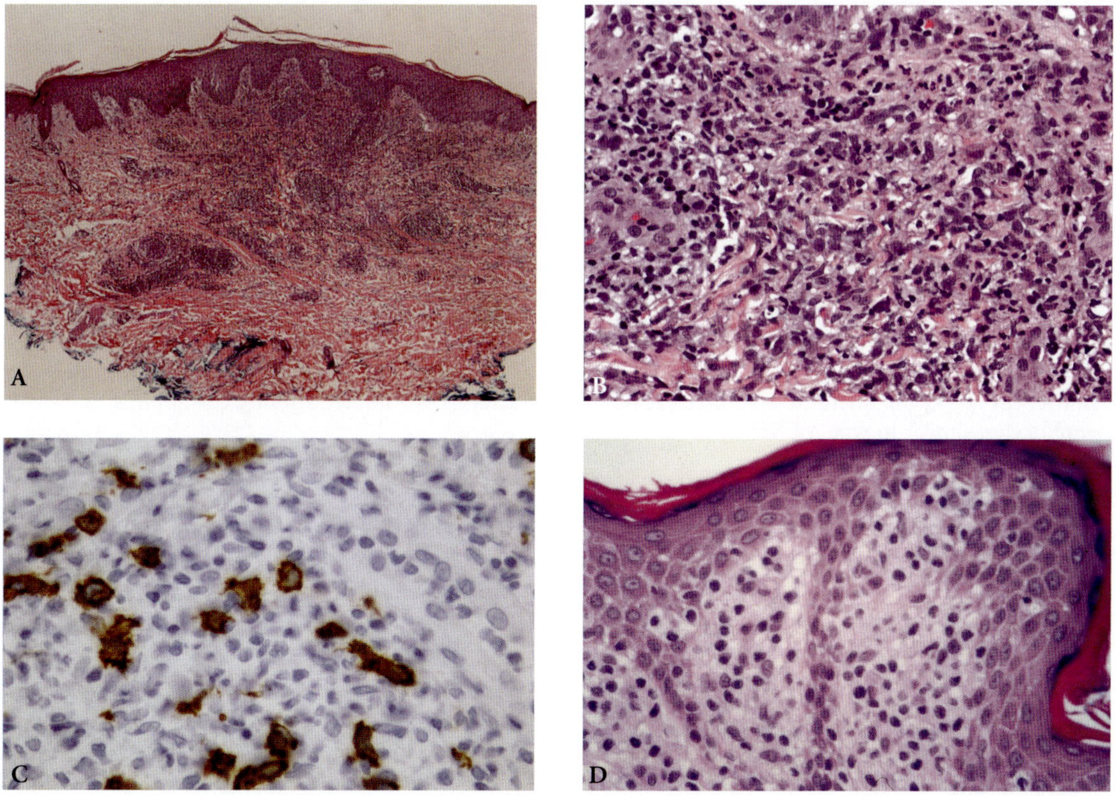

Figure 1-16 A, LyP. Biopsy shows a wedge-shaped lymphocytic infiltrate in the dermis with acanthosis, exocytosis, and scale. **B,** LyP. High-power view shows a mixed dermal infiltrate of atypical lymphocytes with nucleoli, small lymphocytes, and neutrophils. **C,** LyP. CD30 immunohistochemical stain shows scattered atypical CD30+ cells. **D,** LyP. Type B variant composed of small cerebriform lymphocytes, simulating MF.

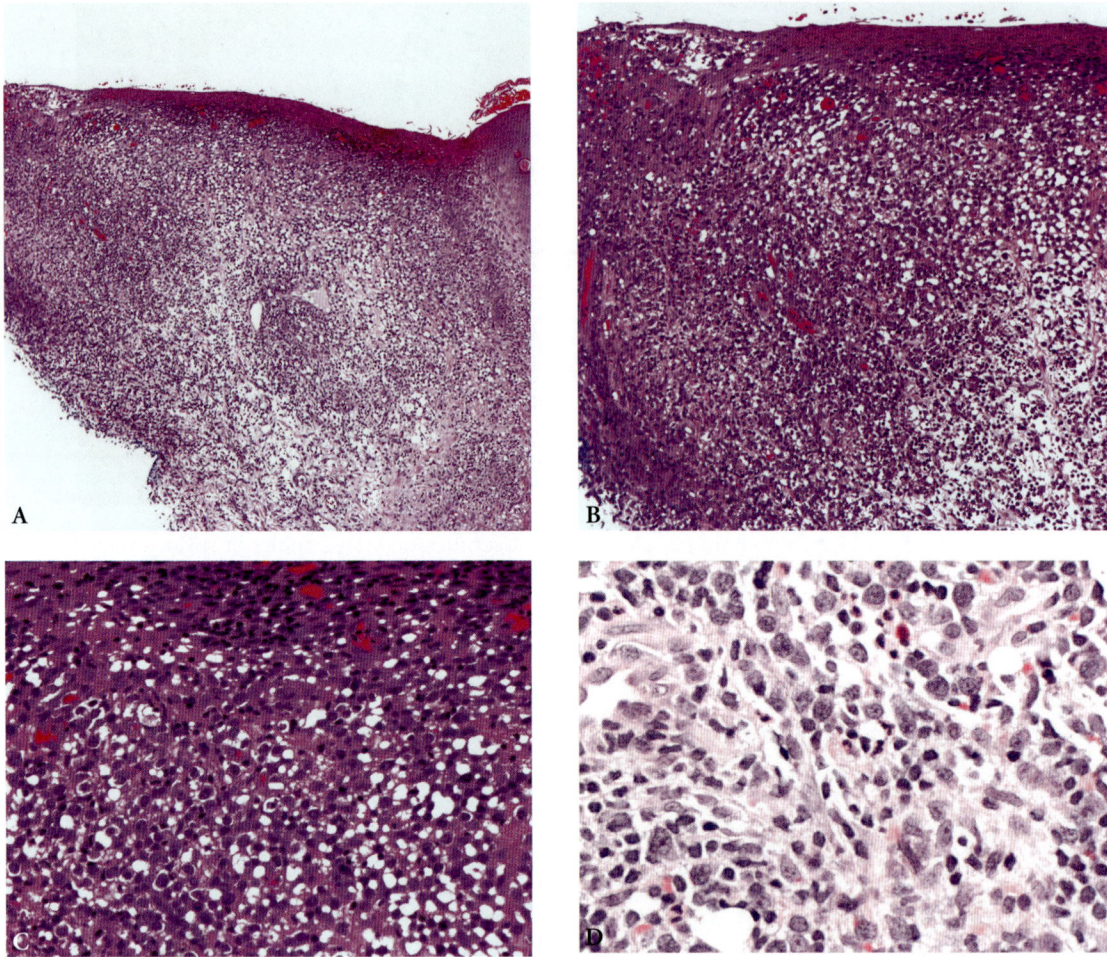

Figure 1-17 A, LyP. Epidermotropic wedge-shaped infiltrate of atypical lymphocytes with epidermal necrosis. **B,** LyP. Markedly epidermotropic atypical lymphocytes with epidermal necrosis and scale crust. **C,** LyP. High-power view shows sheets of atypical lymphocytes with nucleoli, similar to ALCL. **D,** CD30 lymphoproliferative disorder (LPD), ALCL. There are atypical large lymphocytes admixed with neutrophils, eosinophils, and small lymphocytes, similar to type A LyP.

morphology of the lesion biopsied. There are three histologic subtypes: A, B, and C, which may coexist in the patient and bear no prognostic significance. In type A, scattered large CD30+ lymphocytes with prominent nucleoli are immersed in a background of small lymphocytes, neutrophils, and eosinophils (see Figure 1-16). Cerebriform lymphocytes that may be CD30–, simulating MF, characterize type B (see Figure 1-16), and type C LyP presents with sheets of atypical CD30+ lymphocytes, indistinguishable from ALCL (Figure 1-17). ALCL also has a spectrum of cellular composition, similar to LyP, but the infiltrate is more extensive and dense, often extending into

the subcutis. The CD30+ cells may be anaplastic, immunoblastic, or pleomorphic, and represent greater than 75% of the infiltrate. Associated pseudocarcinomatous changes and small/medium cell, neutrophil-rich, and eosinophil-rich variants may simulate other malignancies or infectious processes. The immunophenotype of the lymphocytes in CD30 LPDs may be CD4+, CD8+, CD4–/CD8–, or TIA-1+. Differentiating CD30 LPD from transformed MF may be challenging, at times requiring correlation with the clinical course. CD30 expression may also be seen in other T- and B-cell lymphomas and in nonmalignant infiltrates, such as herpesvirus infections, ruptured molluscum

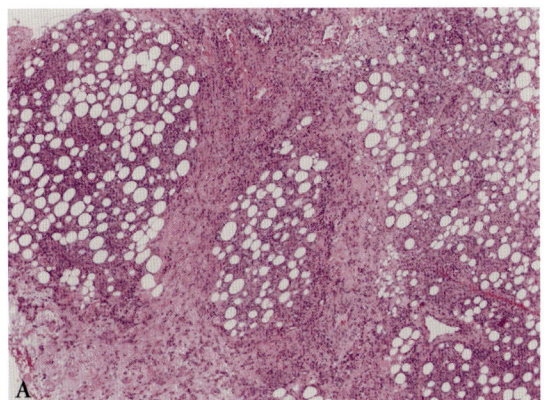

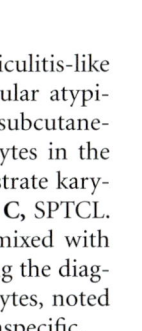

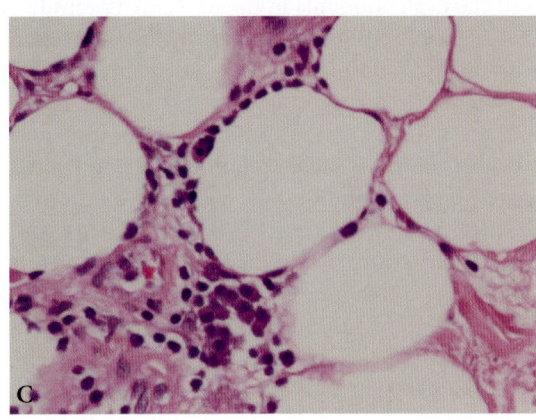

Figure 1-18 A, Subcutaneous panniculitis-like T-cell lymphoma (SPTCL). A dense lobular atypical lymphocytic infiltrate replaces the subcutaneous tissue. **B,** SPTCL. Atypical lymphocytes in the subcutaneous fat rim adipocytes demonstrate karyorrhexis. Erythrocytophagia is also seen. **C,** SPTCL. The lymphocytes may be small and admixed with plasma cells, as seen in this image, making the diagnosis more difficult. Rimming of adipocytes, noted in the biopsy, is a diagnostic clue, but nonspecific.

contagiosum, and nodular scabies. LyP may be associated with MF concomitantly, preceding, or following a diagnosis of this CD30 LPD. There is a small risk of developing Hodgkin's or non-Hodgkin's lymphoma (including cutaneous ALCL) in patients with LyP. CD30 LPDs are discussed in further detail in a Chapter 9.

Subcutaneous Panniculitis T-cell Lymphoma

Subcutaneous panniculitis T-cell lymphoma (SPTCL) is characterized by a subcutaneous infiltrate of malignant T cells that typically arises on the trunk and proximal extremities, resulting in indurated and atrophic plaques. Both adult and pediatric populations may be affected. Characteristic histologic features include a predominantly lobular infiltrate of small to medium-sized atypical T cells with a CD8 immunophenotype, which express the α/β TCR, as documented by positive βF1 immunohistochemical staining. The

lymphocytes rim adipocytes and exhibit karyorrhexis and emperipolesis resulting in "beanbag cell" formation (Figure 1-18). The atypia may be subtle and/or not uniformly present in the specimen, making the diagnosis difficult (see Figure 1-18). Differentiation of SPTCL from lupus erythematosus is an important but frequently daunting task because the clinical and pathologic features overlap significantly in some cases. Lupus profundus is favored when there is prominent mucin, interface dermatitis, a prominent B-cell component, and hyalinization of the fat. The absence of these findings, in concert with cytologic atypia and TCR monoclonality, favors SPTCL. Rarely, lupus profundus and SPTCL may coexist. Compared with MF, SPTCL has an intermediate prognosis but a frequently indolent course. γ/δ lymphoma should be excluded because it is has similar histology but a more aggressive course. Extension into the dermis with negative βF1 staining usually implies a γ/δ lymphoma, but TCR gamma staining, when possible, is recommended.

Extranodal Natural Killer/T-cell Lymphoma, Nasal Type

Extranodal natural killer (NK)/T-cell lymphoma, nasal type, is an aggressive Ebstein-Barr virus (EBV)–positive cytotoxic lymphoma that typically presents in the nasal cavity or nasopharynx but may arise in extranasal sites. It is frequently disseminated at or near the time of diagnosis; thus, the distinction of primary from secondary cytotoxic lymphoma has little relevance. This subtype is more prevalent in Asian, South American, and Central American populations and classically presents in the nasal area as midfacial destructive tumors (previously termed "lethal midline granuloma"). It frequently presents in non-nasal areas, such as the skin of the trunk and extremities, as ulceronecrotic tumors and plaques, or as a facial cellulitis or nonhealing ulcer. Atypical lymphocytes infiltrate the dermis and subcutis, where necrosis, angiocentricity, and angiodestruction of dermal and subcutaneous vessels are often seen. The immunophenotype helps define this tumor and differentiates it from cutaneous γ/δ T-cell lymphoma (CGDTCL). The cells express CD2, CD56, CD4, cytotoxic markers (TIA-1, granzyme B, perforin) and cytoplasmic CD3ε (surface CD3 is negative). EBV is best documented by in situ hybridization (EBER) because latent membrane protein detection by immunohistochemistry may be unreliable. There are rare instances in which either CD56 or EBV may be negative. CD30 expression may be seen, possibly portending a better prognosis. The TCR is usually in germline configuration, so gene rearrangement testing will not be helpful if used to help confirm a malignant diagnosis. Recognition of extranodal NK/T-cell lymphoma, nasal type, is critical because these patients have a median survival of less than 12 months, especially if they present with extracutaneous disease.

PRIMARY CUTANEOUS PERIPHERAL T-CELL LYMPHOMA, UNSPECIFIED

This represents a group of non-MF cutaneous lymphomas delineated in the WHO/EORTC classification with clinicopathologic and prognostic features that show overlap with but are distinct from the MF and non-MF subtypes listed previously. These should be excluded by clinicopathologic correlation and immunophenotyping. These are discussed briefly later and more extensively in Chapter 12.

Primary Cutaneous Aggressive Epidermotropic CD8+ T-cell Lymphoma

These patients have disseminated or localized hyperkeratotic or ulceronecrotic nodules, plaques, and tumors, often in unusual locations such as the oral mucosa and genitalia (Figure 1-19). There is frequent dissemination to non-nodal sites such as testis, central nervous system, and lung. Histologically, there is striking epidermotropism by atypical lymphocytes with blastlike morphology and a characteristic immunophenotype in which the cells express CD8, CD3, CD45RA, cytotoxic markers (TIA-1, granzyme B, perforin), and variable CD7. There is loss of CD2 and CD5. It is critical to exclude γ/δ lymphoma by documenting βF1 positivity. This tumor carries a poor prognosis and should be differentiated from PR by the clinical presentation and immunophenotype.

Cutaneous γ/δ T-cell Lymphoma

CGDTCL is an aggressive cytotoxic lymphoma presenting with ulceronecrotic and indurated tumors, plaques, and nodules, similar to that which may be seen in the other cytotoxic lymphomas, or with panniculitic infiltrates that overlap clinically and histologically with SPTCL. Combined dermal and subcutaneous infiltrates with angiodestruction and necrosis are frequently seen on biopsy (Figure 1-20). CGDTCL is differentiated from extranodal NK/T-cell lymphoma, nasal type, and SPTCL by immunohistochemistry, documenting a γ/δ immunophenotype. Because this stain is difficult to perform on paraffin, the absence of βF1 (TCR-β) expression is usually sufficient to support this diagnosis. However, because there are rare cases of TCR-γ–lymphomas in which βF1 expression is also absent, documenting a γ/δ immunophenotype is advised. Absence of CD4, CD8, and sometimes CD5 should prompt further investigation for this lymphoma (Figure 1-21).

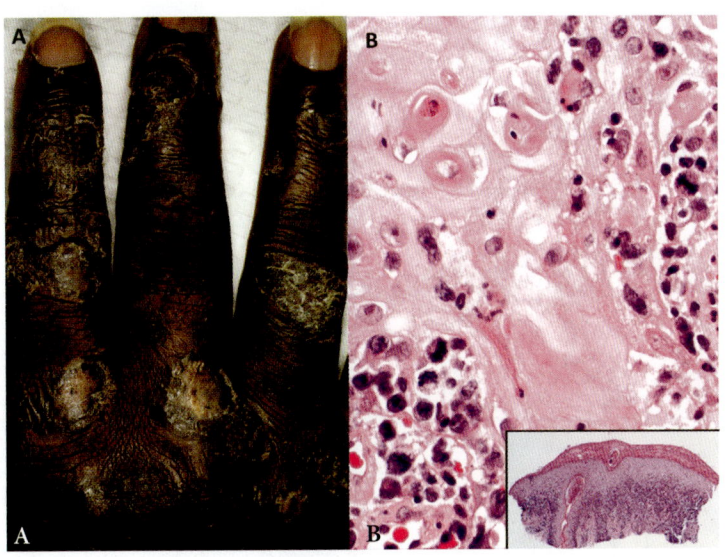

Figure 1-19 A, Primary cutaneous aggressive epidermotropic CD8+ T-cell lymphoma. Numerous hyperkeratotic nodules are seen on the digits. **B,** Primary cutaneous aggressive epidermotropic CD8+ T-cell lymphoma. Markedly atypical lymphocytes are present within an acanthotic epidermis with dyskeratosis. **Inset,** Acanthosis with scale crust and marked epidermotropism of atypical lymphocytes is seen.

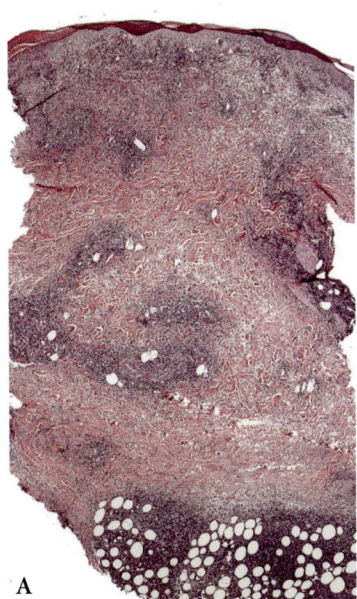

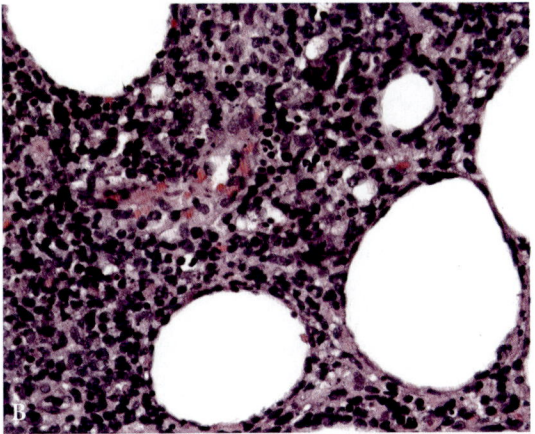

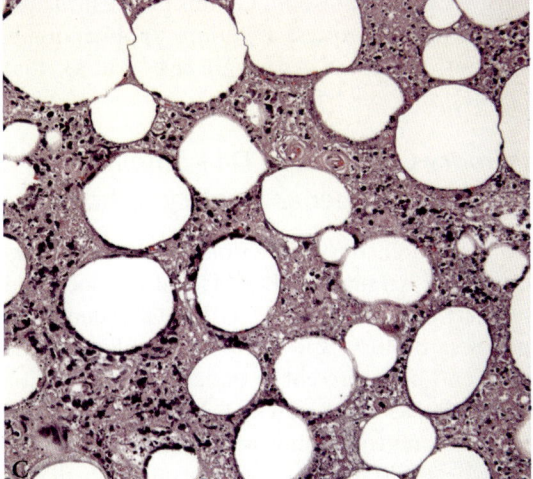

Figure 1-20 A, Cutaneous γ/δ lymphoma. A subcutaneous lobular lymphocytic infiltrate is seen, which also involves the dermis and epidermis. **B,** Cutaneous γ/δ lymphoma involving the fat. Karyorrhexis with erythrocytophagia and cytologic atypia is also present. **C,** Cutaneous γ/δ lymphoma demonstrates prominent necrosis.

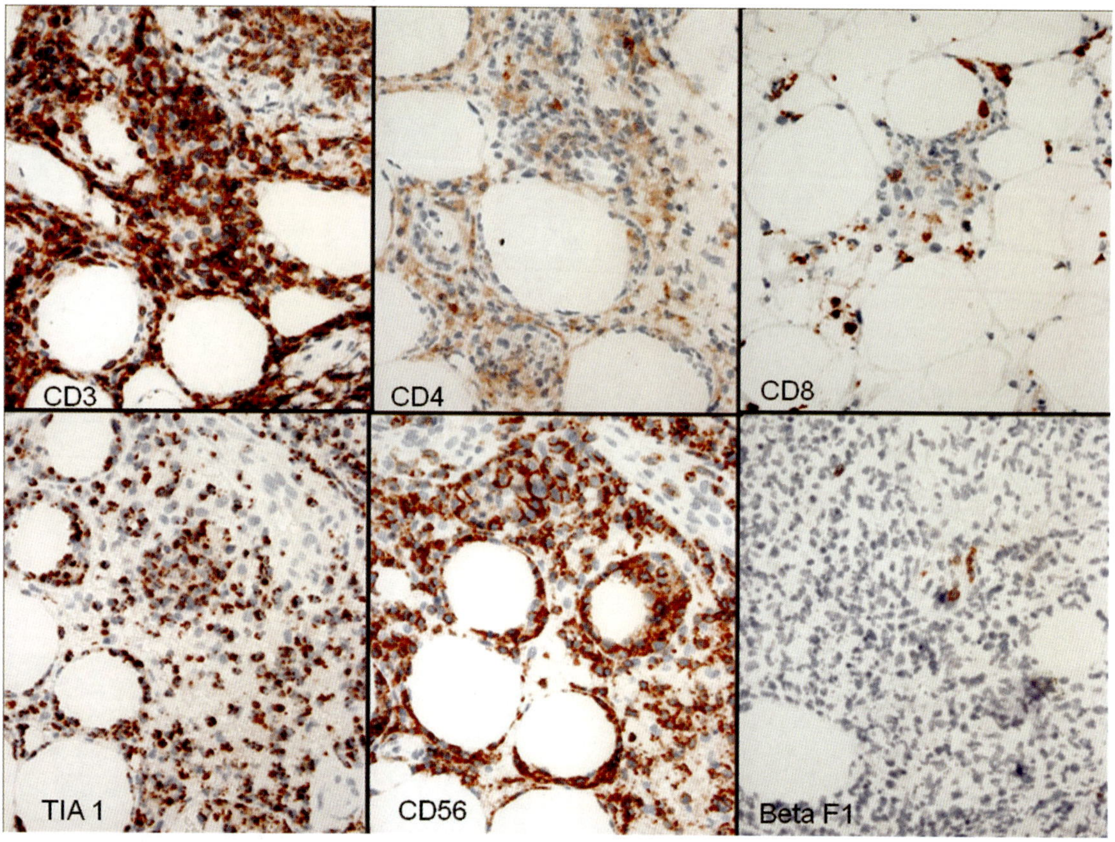

| CD3 | CD4 | CD8 |
| TIA 1 | CD56 | Beta F1 |

Figure1-21 Cutaneous γ/δ T-cell lymphoma (CGDTCL). Immunohistochemical stains demonstrate positive TIA-1, CD56, and CD3, and negative βF1, CD4, and CD8. Note positive internal control with T-cell receptor–beta (TCR-β).

CD56 is frequently positive, so extranodal NK/T-cell lymphoma, nasal type, should be excluded by documenting EBV negativity. SPTCL is excluded by demonstrating negative TCR-β and negative CD8 expression. Lesions of patch/plaque MF may rarely express a γ/δ immunophenotype, without an associated aggressive course that typifies γ/δ T-cell lymphoma.

Primary Cutaneous CD4+ Small/Medium Cutaneous T-cell Lymphoma

Primary cutaneous CD4+ small/medium cutaneous T-cell lymphoma (PCSMTCL) is a localized (solitary or oligolesional) CTCL in which nodules, papules, tumors, and plaques, usually on the head and neck, present in patients without prior patch/plaque MF (Figure 1-22). Histologically, there is a nonepidermotropic nodular to diffuse dermal infiltrate of pleomorphic small to

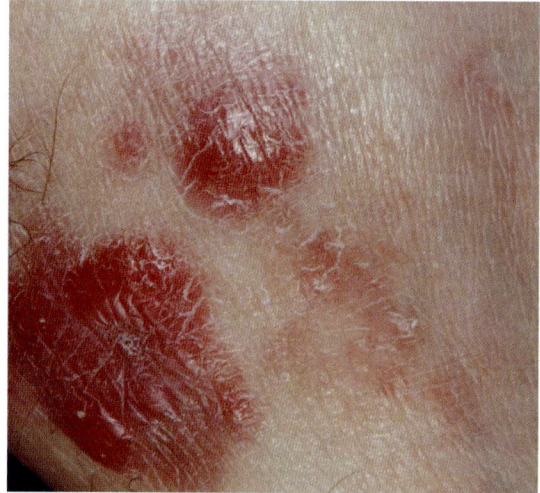

Figure 1-22 CD4+ small/medium pleomorphic cutaneous T-cell lymphoma. Plum-colored dermal nodules and plaques with surrounding erythema are present.

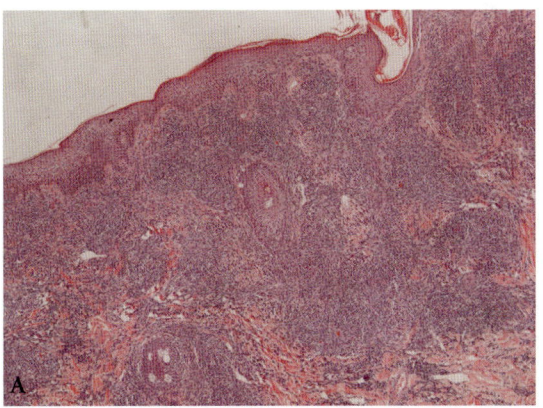

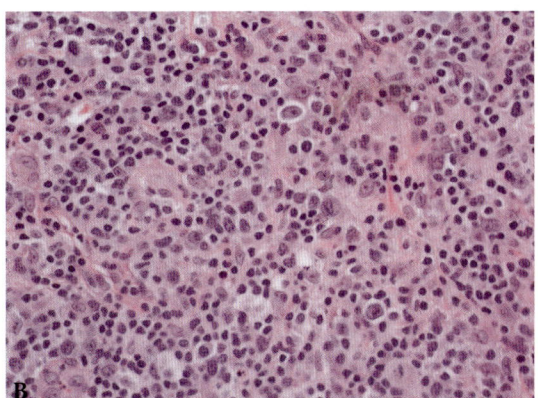

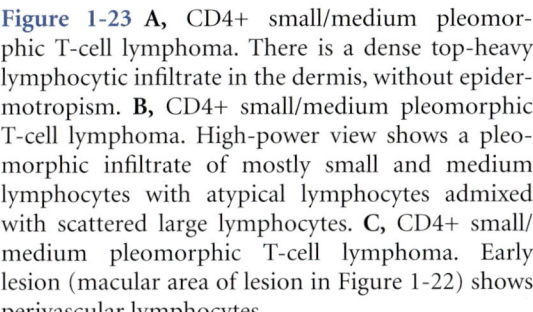

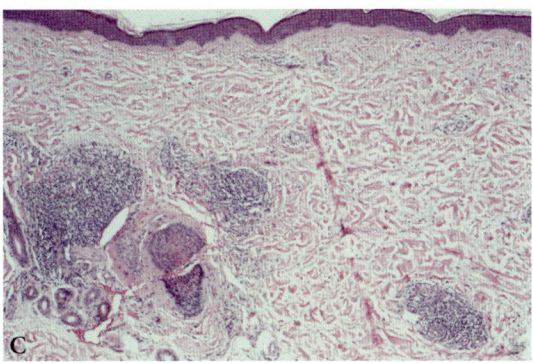

Figure 1-23 **A,** CD4+ small/medium pleomorphic T-cell lymphoma. There is a dense top-heavy lymphocytic infiltrate in the dermis, without epidermotropism. **B,** CD4+ small/medium pleomorphic T-cell lymphoma. High-power view shows a pleomorphic infiltrate of mostly small and medium lymphocytes with atypical lymphocytes admixed with scattered large lymphocytes. **C,** CD4+ small/ medium pleomorphic T-cell lymphoma. Early lesion (macular area of lesion in Figure 1-22) shows perivascular lymphocytes.

intermediate-sized CD4+ T lymphocytes (Figure 1-23). It is important to differentiate this subtype from tumor stage MF and the non-MF CTCL subtypes by lesion distribution and immunophenotype (e.g., exclude CD30 LPD). Aggressive fatal cases have been reported, but the majority of cases follow a more indolent course, requiring less aggressive treatment, compared with some of the other CTCL subtypes. This tumor may have diagnostic challenges. The lymphocytic infiltrate may be patchy, simulating other benign lymphocytic infiltrates (see Figure 1-23). The neoplastic CD4+ lymphocytes may be obscured by a prominent CD8 population, making it difficult to document an abnormal CD4/CD8 ratio. In addition, the tumor is frequently accompanied by B-cell hyperplasia, along with a mildly granulomatous component, simulating CLH. The B-cell association has been attributed to a possible follicular helper T-lymphocyte cell of origin, based on the characteristic profile of PD-1, CXCL-13, and bcl-6 positivity demonstrated in CD4+ small/medium pleomorphic T-cell lymphoma. If close inspection of the infiltrate for a predominance of

CD4-staining atypical cells does not confirm the diagnosis, a monoclonal TCR gene rearrangement may be supportive, but these tumors are not uniformly clonal. Because these tumors usually follow an indolent course, some advocate that PCSMTCL be reported as a borderline lymphocytic tumor with uncertain malignant potential. Additional longitudinal and immunohistochemical data will hopefully better define this heterogeneous group of lymphomas.

PRIMARY CUTANEOUS B-CELL LYMPHOMA

There are three main subtypes of primary cutaneous B-cell lymphoma (CBL), two of which are indolent—primary cutaneous marginal zone lymphoma (PCMZL) and primary cutaneous follicle center lymphoma (PCFCL), and the more aggressive primary cutaneous diffuse large B-cell lymphoma, leg type (PCDLBCL,LT). One should be familiar with the presentation and biopsy findings of the latter because the management and prognosis differ significantly from the indolent variants, with a 5-year survival of approximately 50%, in contrast to nearly 100% for the indolent variants. PCMZL and PCFCL have overlapping features, and although it is not as critical to differentiate these subtypes, certain clinical, histopathologic, and immunophenotypic features may distinguish one from the other. These are discussed briefly later and more in depth in Chapter 13.

Primary Cutaneous Marginal Zone Lymphoma

PCMZL is a tumor composed of small lymphocytes, marginal zone or centrocyte-like cells, plasma cells, and lymphoplasmacytoid cells and includes entities previously designated as "cutaneous immunocytoma" and "follicular lymphoid hyperplasia with monotypic plasma cells." PCMZL presents in adults and occasionally the pediatric population as red to plum-colored papules, nodules, tumors, and plaques, arising most frequently on the trunk and extremities (Figure 1-24). Cases in Europe may be associated with *Borrelia burgdorferi* infections. Multifocal disease and recurrences after complete remission are common, but extracutaneous spread is rare. Histologically, there is a dermal and occasionally subcutaneous nodular to diffuse infiltrate of small lymphocytes, marginal zone or centrocyte-like cells, plasma cells, and plasmacytoid cells, admixed with variable transformed cells. The infiltrate may be top-heavy, often with vertical columns along the adnexal regions, or may be more prominent in the reticular dermis with extension into the subcutis (bottom-heavy) (Figure 1-25). PCMZL cells express CD19, CD20, CD22, CD79a, and bcl-2. CD20 may miss portions of the tumor if it is rich in plasma cells. There may be a prominent T-cell component, making it difficult to make a diagnosis (Figure 1-26). In addition, reactive germinal centers and inflammatory cells, such as eosinophils, histiocytes, and multinucleated giant cells, may derail one from rendering a malignant diagnosis. Colonized germinal centers can be highlighted with CD21, showing a disrupted or nearly absent follicular network, supporting the diagnosis of PCMZL. Clusters of plasma cells with Dutcher bodies also favor PCMZL over CLH

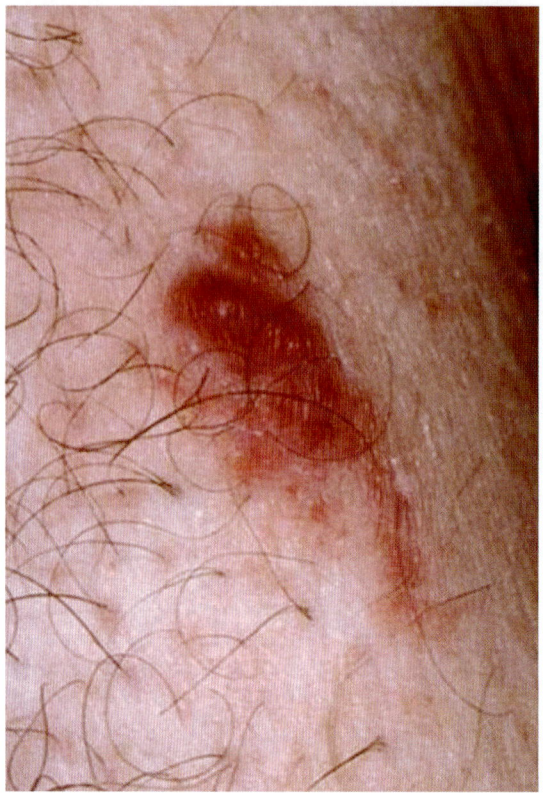

Figure 1-24 Cutaneous B-cell lymphoma (BCL). A plum-colored dermal nodule is present.

(see Figure 1-25). Documentation of a clonal plasma cell population by κ/λ/lambda immunohistochemistry (see Figure 1-26) or in situ hybridization or demonstrating monoclonality of the immunoglobulin H (IgH) receptor by PCR also will help differentiate from CLH. Fortunately, the 5-year survival is approximately 100%; thus, patients with borderline cases may be followed without significant consequence.

Primary Cutaneous Follicle Center Lymphoma

PCFCL is composed of malignant follicle center lymphocytes, which include a variable admixture of centrocytes (cleaved nuclei) and centroblasts (larger noncleaved cells with prominent nucleoli). In contrast to PCMZL, PCFCL arises on the head and trunk, frequently as nodules surrounded by a periphery of plaques or papules. Microscopically, PCFCL may present as a nodular to diffuse dermal

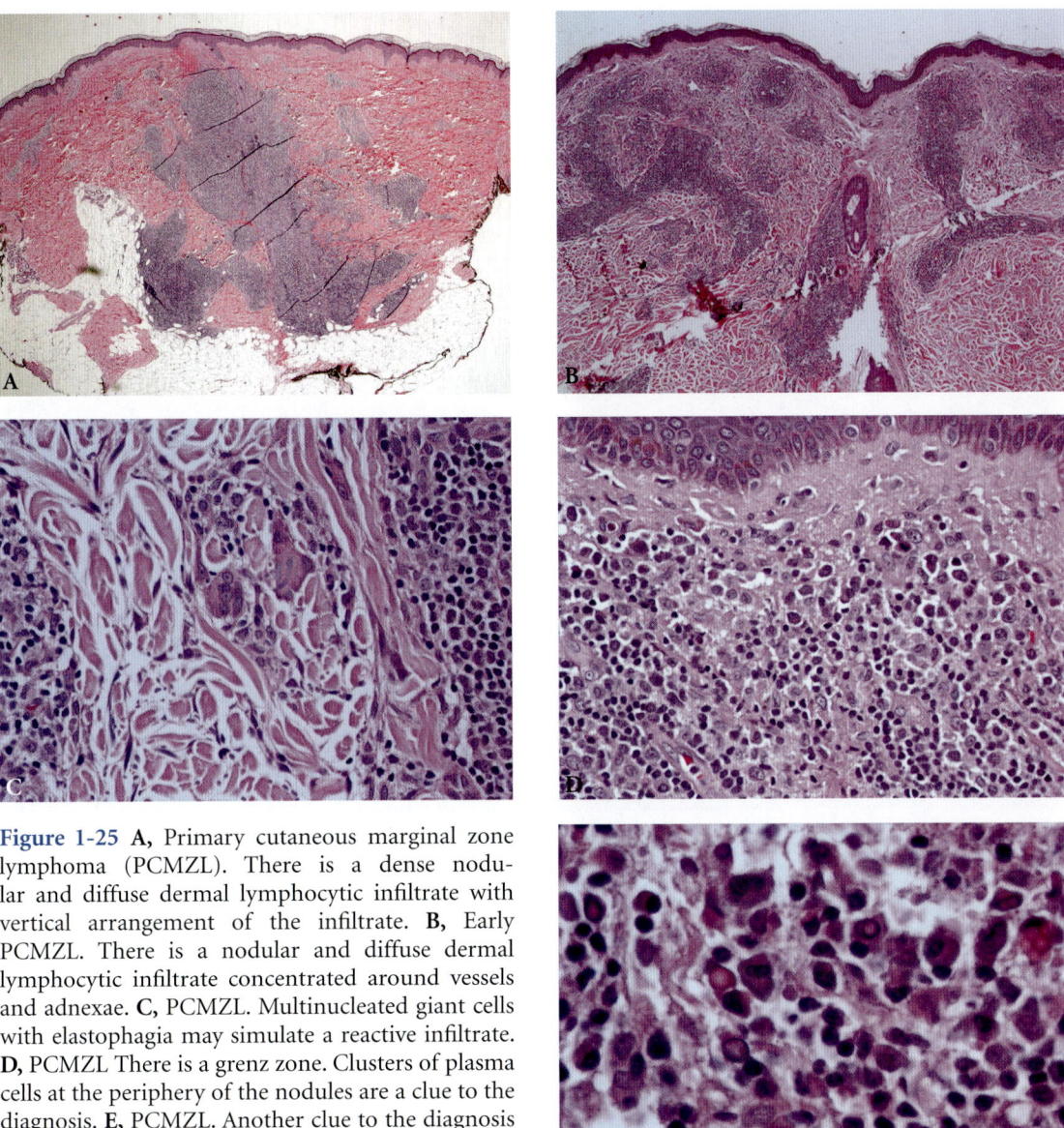

Figure 1-25 A, Primary cutaneous marginal zone lymphoma (PCMZL). There is a dense nodular and diffuse dermal lymphocytic infiltrate with vertical arrangement of the infiltrate. **B,** Early PCMZL. There is a nodular and diffuse dermal lymphocytic infiltrate concentrated around vessels and adnexae. **C,** PCMZL. Multinucleated giant cells with elastophagia may simulate a reactive infiltrate. **D,** PCMZL There is a grenz zone. Clusters of plasma cells at the periphery of the nodules are a clue to the diagnosis. **E,** PCMZL. Another clue to the diagnosis is numerous plasma cells with Dutcher bodies (pseudonuclear inclusions), shown here.

(and frequently subcutaneous) lymphocytic infiltrate that may exhibit either a follicular growth pattern, a diffuse pattern without follicles but composed of follicle center lymphocytes, or a combination of both (Figure 1-27). The follicular growth pattern is more common in the earlier lesions, especially from the head. The follicles are large, with an absent or thin mantle zone (Figures 1-28 and 1-29) lacking polarity and tingible body macrophages (macrophages containing karyorrhectic debris), differentiating them from reactive germinal centers. Early lesions may be T-cell–rich, with a predominance of centrocytes and minimal large cells, but with time, large cells with multilobated or occasionally spindled nuclei predominate, with less well-formed follicles. Stromal changes are common. Tumor cells express CD20, CD79a, CD19, CD22, bcl-6, and variable CD10 and are negative for CD5 and CD43 (see Figure 1-28). The malignant cells may

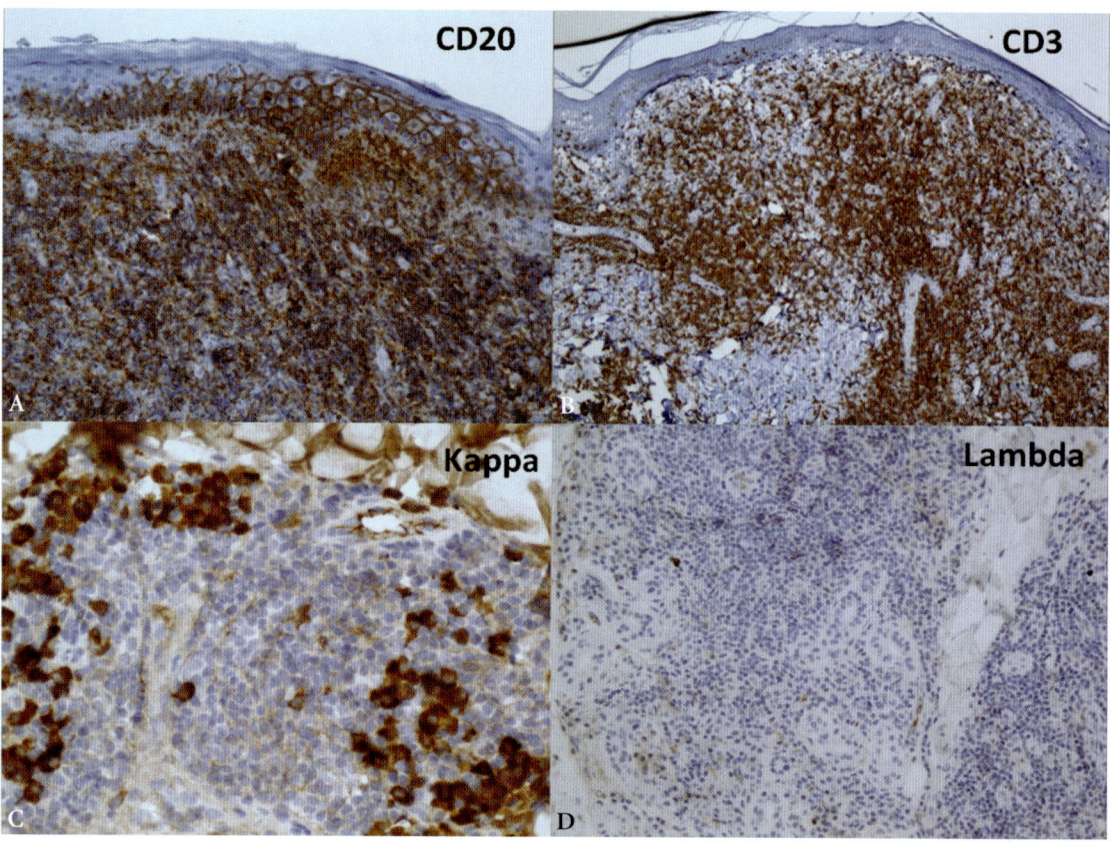

Figure 1-26 A, PCMZL. Immunohistochemical stain CD20 shows a diffuse infiltrate of B cells. **B,** PCMZL. Immunohistochemical stain CD3 shows a prominent T-cell infiltrate. **C,** PCMZL. Immunohistochemical stain kappa light chain shows numerous kappa-positive plasma cells at the periphery of a nodule. **D,** PCMZL. Immunohistochemical stain lambda light chain shows rare lambda-positive plasma cells.

be identified within a CD21+ or CD35+ follicular dendritic network as well as in the interfollicular components of the infiltrate. Ki-67 does not show a polarized pattern, in contrast to reactive germinal centers (Figure 1-29). CD10 expression is usually seen only if there is a follicular growth pattern. In PCFCL, the lymphocytes typically do not express bcl-2, in contrast to systemic follicle center lymphoma, in which bcl-2 expression is associated with the presence of t(14;18). As PCFCL progresses to tumors, there may be a diffuse infiltrate of large cells. In contrast to systemic follicle center lymphoma, in which a histologic grade based on the percentage of large centroblasts correlates with prognosis, the predominance of large cells does not negatively affect the prognosis

in PCFCL. The cells of PCFCL do not express MUM/IRF4, which is positive in PCDLBCL,LTs.

Primary Cutaneous Diffuse Large B-cell Lymphoma

Primary cutaneous diffuse large B-cell lymphomas (PCDLBCLs) are composed of large B cells with round cell morphology (centroblasts and immunoblasts). This category includes diffuse large B-cell lymphoma, leg type (DLBCL,LT) and diffuse large B-cell lymphoma (DLBCL), other, which includes T-cell–rich B-cell lymphoma, plasmablastic lymphoma, and other lymphomas with diffuse large cell morphology that do not fulfill criteria for DLBCL,LT.

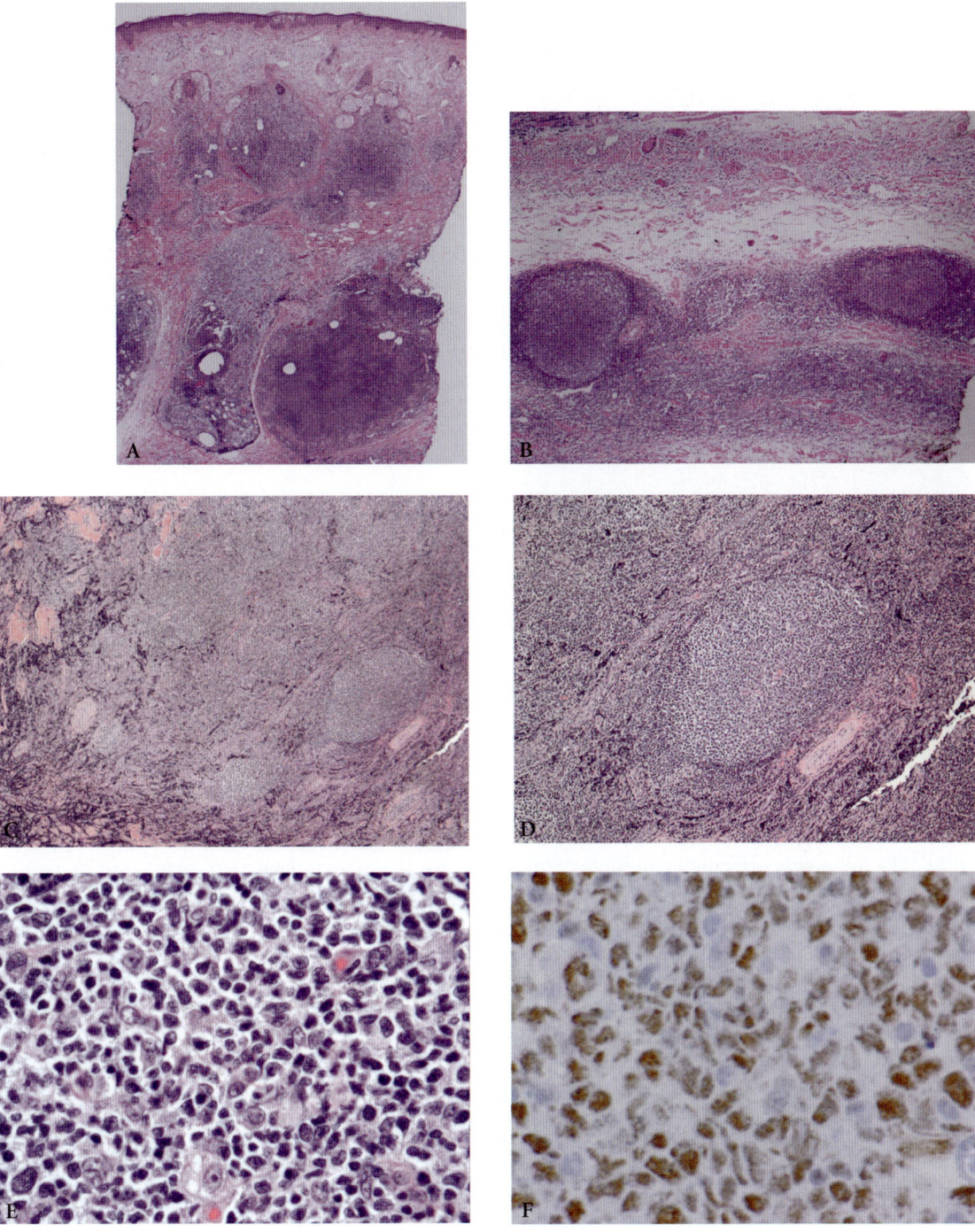

Figure 1-27 **A,** Primary cutaneous follicle center lymphoma (PCFCL). There is a nodular and diffuse bottom-heavy dermal lymphocytic infiltrate. **B,** PCFCL. The subcutis of biopsy shown in Figure 1-27A contains abnormal lymphoid follicles. **C,** PCFCL. There is a dense tumor of lymphocytes with diffuse patternless areas and areas of large abnormal lymphoid follicles. **D,** PCFCL. Medium-power view of an abnormal lymphoid follicle lacking a well-formed mantle zone. **E,** PCFCL. High-power view shows atypical lymphocytes with cleaved nuclei (centrocytes) and scattered larger cells with prominent central nucleoli (immunoblasts) and peripheral nucleoli (centroblasts). **F,** PCFCL. Bcl-6 positivity of diffuse B-cell infiltrate

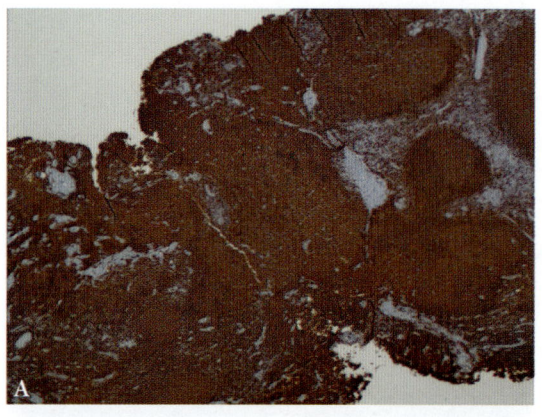

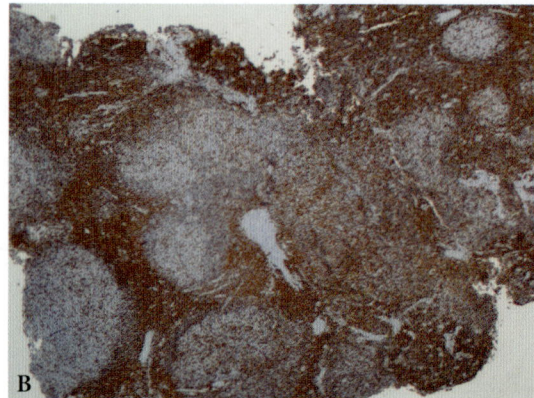

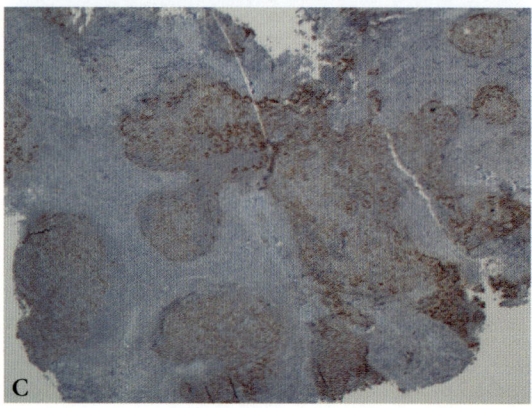

Figure 1-28 A, PCFCL. Immunohistochemical stain of biopsy shown in Figure 1-27C shows diffuse positivity with CD20. **B,** PCFCL. Immunohistochemical stain of biopsy shown in Figure 1-27C shows prominent positivity with CD3, highlighting negative staining malignant follicles. **C,** PCFCL. Immunohistochemical stain of biopsy shown in Figure 1-27C shows prominent positivity with CD21, highlighting malignant follicles.

Diffuse Large B-cell Lymphoma, Leg Type

DLBCL,LT frequently presents as multiple dermal nodules and tumors on the legs of elderly patients, but it is not restricted to this presentation. Histologically, there is a monotonous pandermal and occasionally subcutaneous infiltrate of medium and large round lymphocytes with nucleoli that are centrally placed (immunoblasts) or attached to the plasma membrane (centroblasts) (Figure 1-30). In contrast to PCMZL and PCFCL, there may not be a grenz zone, or stromal reaction, and mitoses are easily detected. The tumor cells are CD19+, CD20+, CD22+, and CD79a+. Bcl-6 is variable. Additional immunotypic features include expression of bcl-2 and MUM-1/IRF4, with negative staining for CD10 (see Figure 1-30). This staining pattern helps differentiate this tumor when it arises on nonleg sites from diffuse PCFCL with a prominent large cell component. IgM positivity has also been shown to favor

DLBCL,LT, over PCFCL. This distinction is critical because the 5-year survival rate with DLBCL,LT, is approximately 50% or less if multiple lesions arise on the legs versus approximately 95% for PCFCL.

Intravascular Large B-cell Lymphoma

Intravascular large B-cell lymphoma (IVBCL) is a rare lymphoma defined microscopically by the presence of intravascular tumor cells (Figure 1-31). Clinically, there are typically plaques simulating panniculitis, cellulitis, or livedo reticularis, but biopsies of seemingly uninvolved skin may reveal intravascular tumor. Histologically, small capillaries in the dermis and subcutis are occluded by atypical B lymphocytes with round to oval cell morphology exhibiting hyperchromatic or vesicular nuclei with prominent nucleoli. Reactive angiomatosis and/or extension of tumor cells into the surrounding dermis may be observed. The tumor

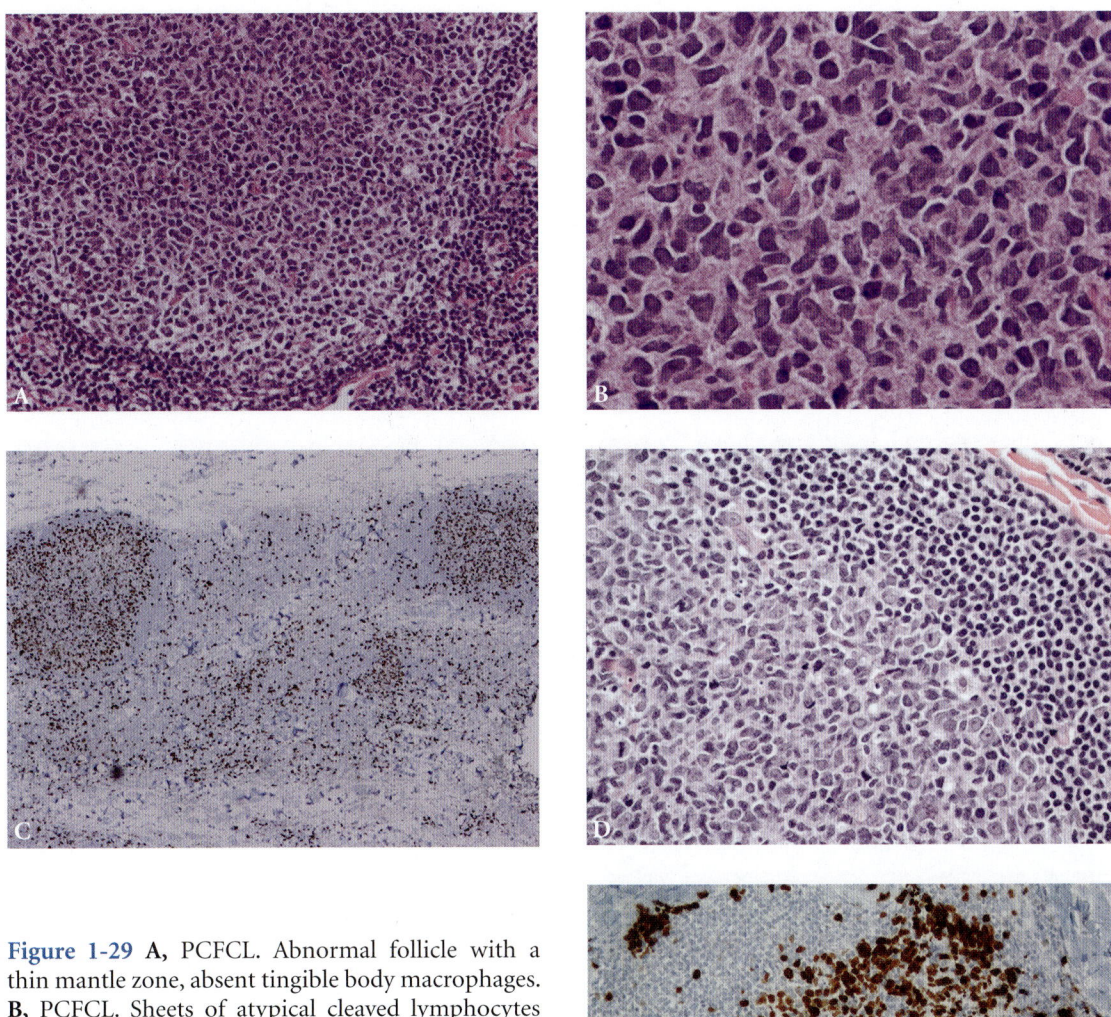

Figure 1-29 A, PCFCL. Abnormal follicle with a thin mantle zone, absent tingible body macrophages. **B,** PCFCL. Sheets of atypical cleaved lymphocytes (centroblasts). **C,** PCFCL. Immunohistochemical staining with Ki-67 shows diffuse staining of follicles and interfollicular lymphocytes without polarity. **D,** Germinal center from a biopsy of cutaneous lymphoid hyperplasia (CLH) demonstrates a well-developed mantle zone and tingible body macrophages. **E,** Germinal center from a biopsy of CLH demonstrates a polar staining pattern with immunohistochemical stain Ki-67.

cells may populate existing angiomas. The tumor cells express B-cell antigens such as CD20 or CD79a but may also co-express CD5. CD10 and bcl-2 are often positive. IVBCL is an aggressive lymphoma, frequently presenting with extracutaneous disease, in particular in the central nervous system, at the time of diagnosis.

T-cell–rich B-cell lymphomas are rare and include cases in which there are only few large CD30– pleomorphic Reed-Sternberg–like cells admixed in an infiltrate of greater than 75% small reactive T (and sometimes B) cells, histiocytes, and plasma cells. These tumors show overlapping features with PCMZL and PCFCL and perhaps

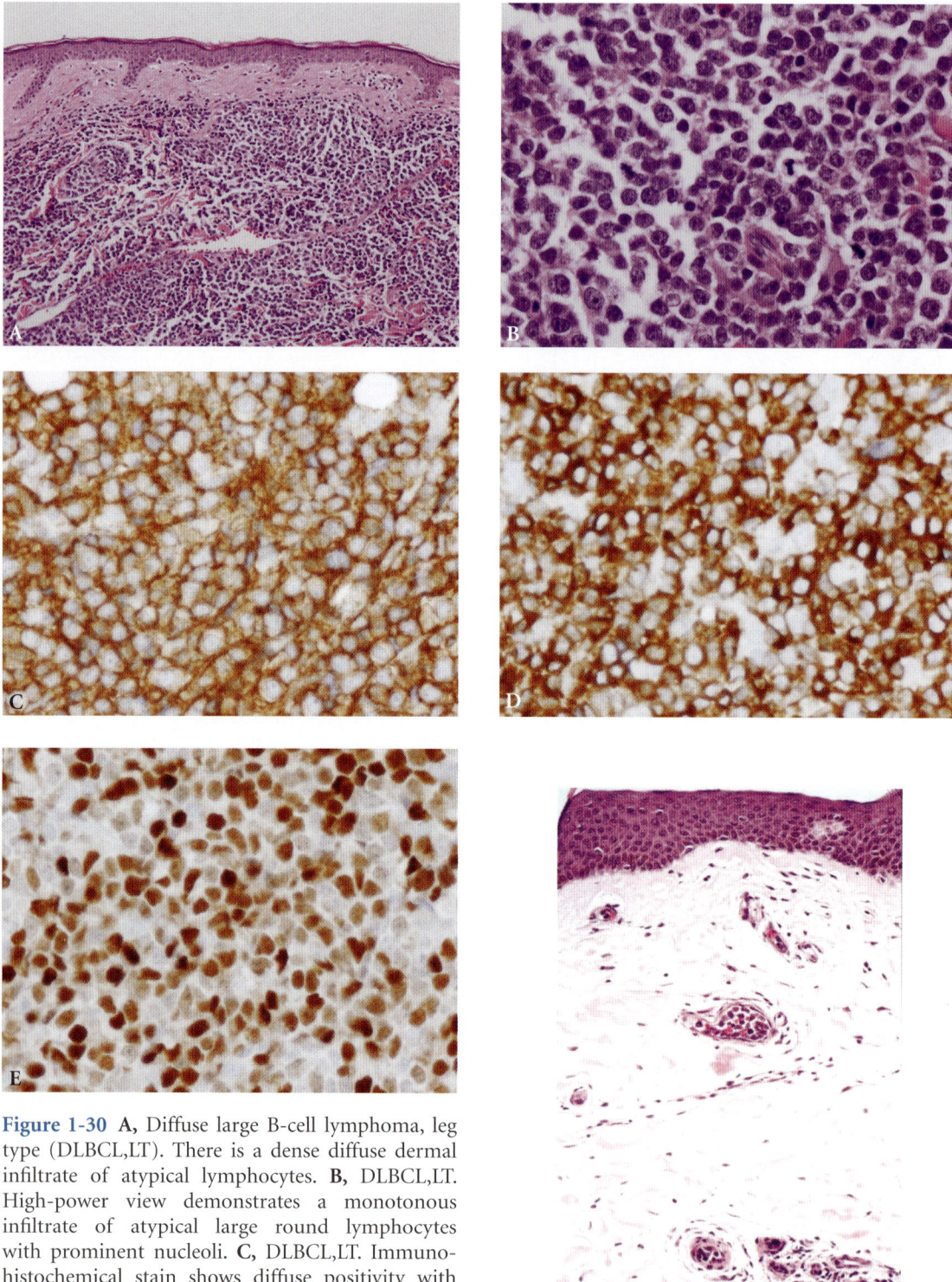

Figure 1-30 A, Diffuse large B-cell lymphoma, leg type (DLBCL,LT). There is a dense diffuse dermal infiltrate of atypical lymphocytes. **B,** DLBCL,LT. High-power view demonstrates a monotonous infiltrate of atypical large round lymphocytes with prominent nucleoli. **C,** DLBCL,LT. Immuno-histochemical stain shows diffuse positivity with CD20. **D,** DLBCL,LT. Immunohistochemical stain shows diffuse positivity with bcl2. **E,** DLBCL,LT. Immunohistochemical stain shows diffuse positivity with MUM-1.

Figure 1-31 Intravascular B-cell lymphoma. Atypical hyperchromatic lymphocytes occlude vessel lumina. There is reactive angiomatosis.

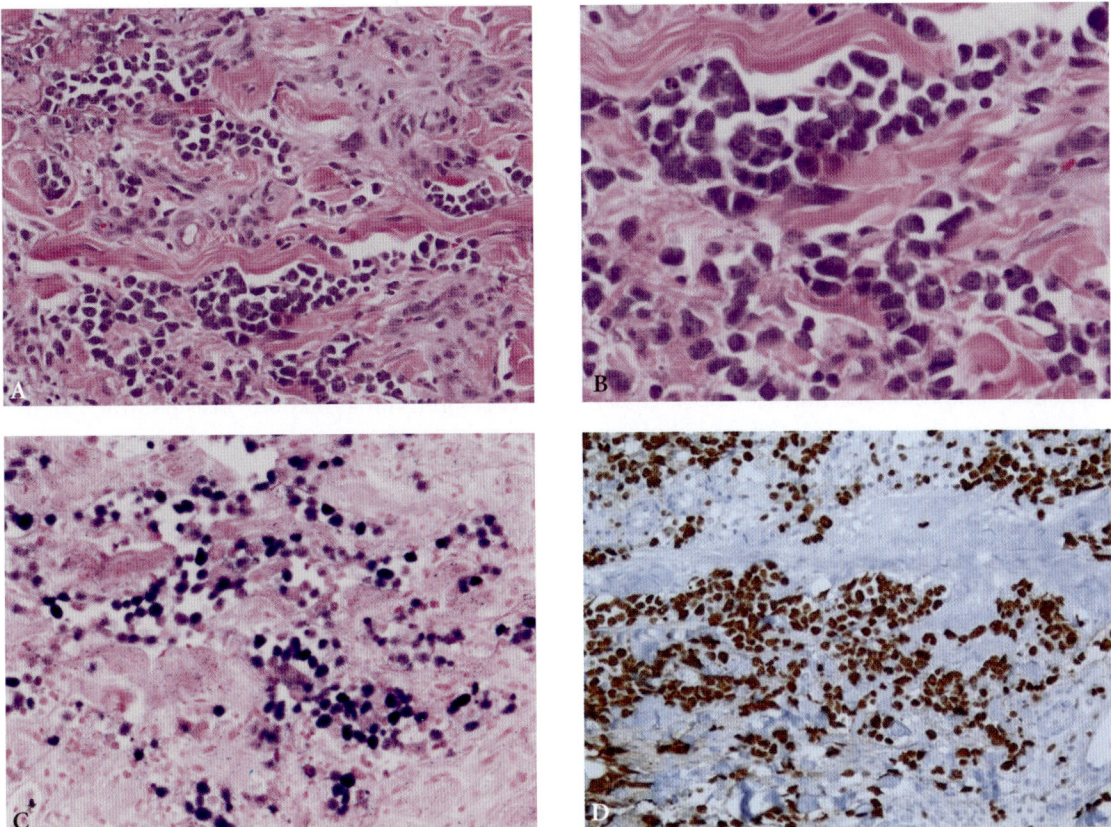

Figure 1-32 A, Plasmablastic lymphoma. The biopsy show an interstitial infiltrate of markedly atypical mononuclear cells with blastic and plasmacytoid nuclei. **B,** Plasmablastic lymphoma. High power view demonstrating markedly atypical cells with plasmacytic and plasmablastic morphology. **C,** Plasmablastic lymphoma. EBER in situ hybridization (Epstein-Barr virus [EBV]) shows diffuse positivity. **D,** Plasmablastic lymphoma. Ki-67 stain shows diffuse positivity.

may represent these entities with a brisk T-cell response because the tumors have a similar indolent course, unlike their nodal counterparts.

Plasmablastic lymphoma is an aggressive hematologic neoplasm that typically presents in patients who are immunocompromised, usually due to human immunodeficiency virus (HIV) infection. These typically arise in extracutaneous sites, especially the oral mucosa or gastrointestinal tract, but may rarely present in the skin as a monotonous dermal and sometimes subcutaneous infiltrate of atypical cells with plasmacytoid or plasmablastic morphology (Figure 1-32). This is considered a large B-cell lymphoma, but CD20 is usually negative. The tumor cells may be identified by plasma cell markers such as CD138, CD38, and sometimes CD79a, but the latter marker may be negative. CD45, and B cell markers such as CD20 and Pax 5 are negative or weakly positive. Most cases are positive for EBV by in situ hybridization (EBER) or less reliably by immunohistochemistry with latent membrane protein (LMP). The tumors also express MUM-1, EMA, and sometimes CD30 and have a high Ki-67 proliferative staining pattern. Expression of human herpes virus-8 (HHV-8) is seen with HHV-8 positive plasmablastic lymphoma, associated with multicentric Castleman disease, a large B cell lymphoma variant seen in HIV patients. Both entities are rare in the skin, but should be considered in patients with immunodeficiency states.

BLASTIC PLASMACYTOID DENDRITIC CELL NEOPLASM

Blastic plasmacytoid dendritic cell neoplasm (BPDCN) was previously known as "blastic NK-cell lymphoma and CD4+/CD56+ hematodermic neoplasm," but it is now designated in the WHO/EORTC classification scheme as a neoplasm of plasmacytoid dendritic cells. This is an aggressive tumor, with leukemic involvement in approximately 70% of patients. Some patients may have myelodysplastic syndrome. Mucocutaneous disease is common and characterized by bruise-like plaques affecting the head, trunk, and extremities (Figure 1-33). Histologically, there is a pandermal monotonous infiltrate of mononuclear cells with blastlike morphology (see Figure 1-33). A grenz zone and subcutaneous extension are also characteristic. These cells are positive for CD56, CD4, CD123, and TCL-1. This immunophenotype differentiates this tumor from other leukemias and lymphomas with similar nuclear morphology.

STAGING OF CUTANEOUS T-CELL LYMPHOMA (MYCOSIS FUNGOIDES/ SÉZARY SYNDROME)

Staging is the final step in securing the diagnosis of primary cutaneous lymphoma and is also critical in determining the prognosis and management of the disease. For instance, a diagnosis of primary cutaneous ALCLs and cutaneous CBLs requires exclusion of secondary cutaneous lymphoma from a systemic non-Hodgkin's lymphoma, or clinical-histologic findings may be consistent with MF, but staging workup may reveal a leukemic component, requiring a different management approach. Staging of cutaneous lymphoma incorporates the tumor-node-metastasis-blood (TNMB) stage into a clinical stage. This has recently been revised (Table 1-6). It is also important to note that this staging classification does not apply to non-MF/SS subtypes or CBL.

The T rating is determined by the lesion morphology and extent of BSA involved. Patches

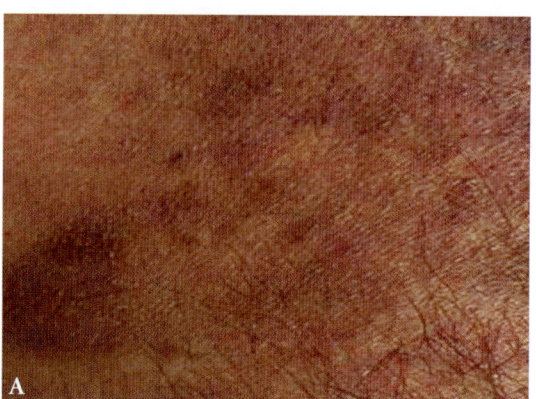

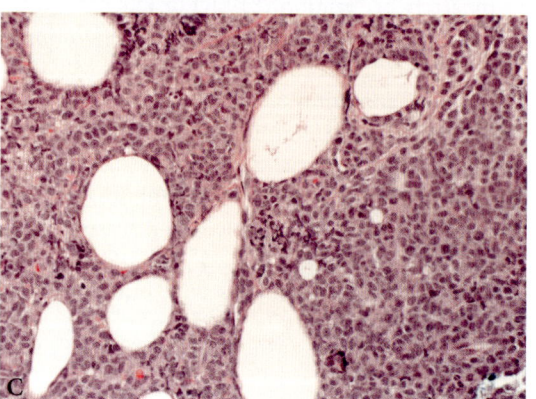

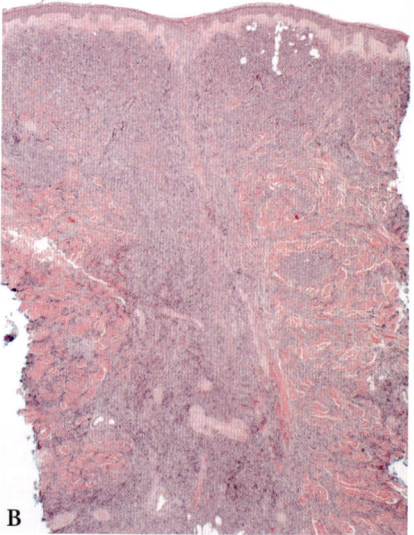

Figure 1-33 **A,** Blastoid plasmacytoid dendritic cell neoplasm (BPDCN). Bruise-like plaques are seen on the trunk. **B,** BPDCN. A dense pandermal infiltrate of atypical mononuclear cells is seen, sparing the epidermis with a grenz zone. **C,** BPDCN. High-power view of the subcutis shows a monotonous infiltrate of atypical mononuclear cells with blastlike morphology.

TABLE 1-6 International Society for Cutaneous Lymphoma/European Organization for Research and Treatment of Cancer Revision to the Tumor-Node-Metastasis-Blood Classification of Mycosis Fungoides and Sézary Syndrome[3]

Skin		
T1	Limited patches, papules, and/or plaques less than 10% of the BSA	May further stratify into T1a (patch only) vs. T1b (plaque ± patch)
T2	Patches, papules, or plaques covering 10% or more of the skin BSA	May further stratify into T2a (patch only) vs. T2b (plaque ± patch)
T3	One or more tumors (≥1 cm diameter)	Note total number and volume of lesions, largest size lesion, and body region
T4	Confluence of erythema over 80% or more of the BSA	
Node		Document all palpable peripheral nodes that are firm, irregular, clustered, fixed, or 1.5 cm or larger diameter
N_0	No clinically abnormal peripheral lymph nodes	Biopsy not required
N_1	Clinically abnormal peripheral lymph nodes; histopathology Dutch grade 1 or NCI LN_{0-2}	N_{1a} Clone negative N_{1b} Clone positive
N_2	Clinically abnormal peripheral lymph nodes; histopathology Dutch grade 2 or NCI LN_3	N_{2a} Clone negative N_{2b} Clone positive
N_3	Clinically abnormal peripheral lymph nodes; histopathology Dutch grades 3-4 or NCI LN_4	Clone positive or negative
Nx	Clinically abnormal peripheral lymph nodes; no histologic confirmation	
Visceral		
M_0	No visceral organ involvement	
M_1	Visceral involvement	Must specify organ involved, and confirm with pathology (splenomegaly and multifocal liver tumor excluded)
Blood		
B0	Absence of significant blood involvement: 5% or less of peripheral blood lymphocytes are atypical (Sézary) cells (defined as lymphocytes with cerebriform nuclei)	B_{0a} Clone negative B_{0b} Clone positive
B1	Low blood tumor burden: greater than 5% of peripheral blood lymphocytes are atypical (Sézary) cells but does not meet the criteria of B2	B_{1a} Clone negative B_{1b} Clone positive
B2	High blood tumor burden: 1000/µL or more Sézary cells with positive clone	If unable to determine Sézary cells, one of the following criteria along with (+) clonal rearrangement of the TCR may be used instead: 1. Expanded CD4+ or CD3+ cells with CD4/CD8 ratio of 10 or more 2. Expanded CD4+ cells with abnormal immunophenotype including loss of CD7 or CD26

B, blood; BSA, body surface area; M, metastasis; N, node; NCI, National Cancer Institute; T, tumor; TCR, T-cell receptor.
Adapted from Olsen E, Vonderheid E, Pimpinelli N, Willemze R, Kim Y, Knobler R, et al. Revisions to the staging and classification of mycosis fungoides and Sézary syndrome: a proposal of the International Society for Cutaneous Lymphomas (ISCL) and the cutaneous lymphoma task force of the European Organization for Research and Treatment of Cancer (EORTC). *Blood.* 2007;110:1713–1722.

are defined as nonelevated, nonindurated areas of involvement. Plaques are elevated and indurated. These may be T1 or T2, depending on whether there is less than 10% (T1) or 10% or greater (T2) skin involvement. A provisional designation a or b will hopefully allow accumulation of longitudinal data for prognostication (patch-only disease = T_{1a} or T_{2a}; plaque ± patch disease = T_{1b} or T_{2b}). T3 (tumor stage) is defined as having at least one nodular lesion of 1 cm or larger diameter, with evidence of depth (or vertical growth). T4 (erythrodermic) is defined as 80% or greater of BSA of skin involvement. The BSA may be calculated by using the palm, which is estimated to represent 0. 5% BSA. Alternatively, in a proposed revision of the tumor-node-metastasis (TNM) staging system, 12 regions of the body are assigned a specific BSA designation, and calculations are based on the total of the regions involved (Figure 1-34). Presence or absence of alopecia, hypo- or hyerpigmentation, poikiloderma, erosion, crusting, and ulceration are additional clinical features worth noting. Documentation of papular lesions also may add valuable diagnostic or prognostic information, especially concerning the differential diagnosis of LyP, papular MF, or adnexotropic MF.

Additional prognostic information should be extracted from the biopsy. For instance, in patch/plaque lesions, preferential involvement of hair follicles should be noted. This histologic feature of folliculotropic MF may be associated with more aggressive disease, with a 10 year survival that is similar to or worse than tumor stage MF. Thus, it is important to document on the pathology report. It is also important to indicate whether there is large cell transformation (LCT) in plaques and tumors of MF or in erythrodermic biopsies of SS patients because this has been associated with a poor prognosis. LCT may not alter the prognosis if noted in patch/plaque disease but should be documented. LCT has been defined as lymphocytes four or more times the size of a normal small lymphocyte representing 25% or more of the infiltrate or as micronodules. T-cell markers and CD30 may help identify these cells and distinguish them from histiocytes and B cells; however, not all transformed lymphocytes will be positive for CD30. Moreover, LyP and ALCL may show similar CD30 staining and need to be distinguished from LCT by clinical presentation and course. It has not been determined that LCT and changes of FMF warrant upstaging of CTCL, but documentation of these additional histologic features is recommended to guide management.

The N classification designates the peripheral nodal status in patients with MF and SS. Blind

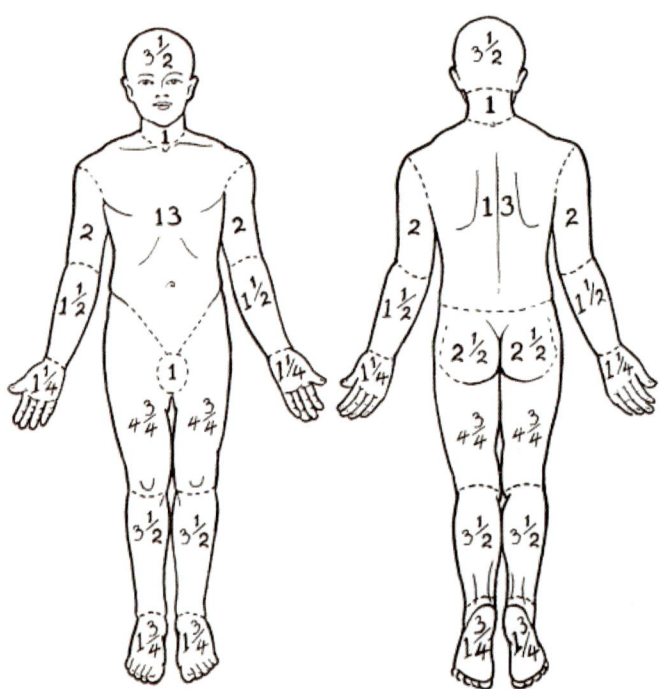

Figure 1-34 Regional percent BSA in the adult. (Adapted from, originally adapted from Lund CC, Browder NC. The estimation of areas of burns. Surg Gynecol Obstet. 1944;79:352–358. Olsen E, Vonderheid E, Pimpinelli N, Willemze R, Kim Y, Knobler R, et al. Revisions to the staging and classification of mycosis fungoides and Sézary syndrome: a proposal of the International Society for Cutaneous Lymphomas (ISCL) and the cutaneous lymphoma task force of the European Organization of Research and Treatment of Cancer (EORTC). *Blood.* 2007;110:1713–1722.

biopsies of nonenlarged nodes are not required in the revised classification. Clinically abnormal nodes are defined as being 1.5 cm or larger in diameter in the longest transverse diameter or any palpable peripheral node that is firm, irregular, clustered, or fixed. The abnormality should be documented by imaging studies, such as computed tomography (CT), with or without fluorodeoxyglucose–positron emission tomography (FDG-PET) scan, or magnetic resonance imaging (MRI). Assessment of architecture is required for grading; therefore, excision and not needle aspiration or core biopsy is the recommended method of lymph node sampling. The microscopic findings may be classified according to two different classification schemes (Dutch system and National Cancer Institute/Veterans Administration [NCI/VA] classification) (Table 1-7), which differ mainly in their definition of

abnormal lymphocytes: (Dutch requires > 7.5-μm cerebriform cells; NCI-VA defines involvement by relative number of cerebriform cells in the paracortex). N1 includes nodes with dermatopathic histology (according to the Dutch System); or nodes with no (LN_0), isolated (LN_1), or many/three to six cell clusters (LN_2) of atypical lymphocytes (according to the NCI-VA Classification). Nodes with an N2 grade have variable degrees of infiltration by atypical lymphocytes, with preservation of nodal architecture, and N3 nodes show partial to complete (grades 3-4 Dutch, respectively; LN4 NCI-VA) effacement by the malignant lymphocytes. In general, it is not imperative to incorporate results of molecular analysis into nodal grading. However, for uneffaced nodes with grade 2 (Dutch) or LN3 (NCI/VA), division into clone-negative (N_{2a}) and clone-positive (N_{2b}) categories is encouraged in order to capture

TABLE 1-7 Histopathologic Staging of Lymph Nodes in Mycosis Fungoides and Sézary Syndrome

Updated International Society for Cutaneous Lymphomas/European Organization for Research and Treatment of Cancer Classification	Dutch System	National Cancer Institute–Veterans Administration Classification
N_1	Grade 1: DL	LN_0: no atypical lymphocytes LN_1: occasional and isolated atypical lymphocytes (not arranged in clusters) LN_2: many atypical lymphocytes or in three- to six-cell clusters
N_2	Grade 2: early involvement by MF (presence of cerebriform cells with nuclei > 7.5 μm)	LN_3: aggregates of atypical lymphocytes; nodal architecture preserved
N_3	Grade 3: partial effacement of LN architecture; many atypical cerebriform mononuclear cells Grade 4: complete effacement	LN_4: partial/complete effacement of nodal architecture by atypical/neoplastic lymphocytes

DL, dermatopathic lymphadenopathy; LN, lymph node; MF, mycosis fungoides; N, node.
Adapted from Olsen E, Vonderheid E, Pimpinelli N, Willemze R, Kim Y, Knobler R, et al. Revisions to the staging and classification of mycosis fungoides and Sézary syndrome: a proposal of the International Society for Cutaneous Lymphomas (ISCL) and the cutaneous lymphoma task force of the European Organization of Research and Treatment of Cancer (EORTC). *Blood.* 2007;110:1713–1722.

potential prognostic longitudinal data. The decision as to which node to sample is determined by the size and/or number of enlarged nodes. If there is generalized lymphadenopathy, the cervical lymph node will have the highest yield of diagnostic findings, followed by the axillary and inguinal nodes. Otherwise, the largest node draining the involved skin or the node with the most uptake on FDG-PET scanning should be chosen. If the clinically abnormal node is not biopsied at the time of initial staging, an Nx rating is submitted to acknowledge the clinical abnormality. Regarding N staging, it is important to know that there is some histopathologic overlap with benign lymphadenopathy and criteria for N2 nodes. In addition, there may be sampling error, but this possibility does not require multiple node sampling.

The M classification indicates the status of visceral organs. M1 is designated as stage IVB disease and is associated with a poor prognosis. With the exception of splenomegaly (documented by imaging or unequivocal physical examination findings) and focal hepatic defects (cystic and vascular lesions excluded) noted on at least two imaging studies, biopsy confirmation is recommended to document the M1 status. Bone marrow evaluation should be performed in all MF/SS

patients with a significant peripheral blood tumor burden or B2 status or unexplained abnormalities on their complete blood count. Bone marrow evaluation of MF patients who do not meet these criteria is not required.

The B rating has been stratified into B0, B1, and B2, to recognize the spectrum of peripheral blood tumor burden that ranges from minimal blood involvement, which can be seen in both early leukemic MF or SS as well as in patients with benign erythroderma, to significant blood involvement (B2), which qualifies for stage IV disease. Analysis of the peripheral blood for morphologic atypia (with Sézary count), immunophenotypic aberrations (with flow cytometry), and clonal expansion of TCR gene rearrangement (by PCR or Southern blot) are recommended to assess the B status. The TNMB status is then incorporated into a clinical stage (Table 1-8).

It is important to note that staging has prognostic implications and, thus, applies to the workup and ultimate tumor stage at the time of the *initial* diagnosis. This clinical stage is not altered with disease progression or remission. However, reassessment of the TNMB status is often performed in order to tailor the therapy to progression or regression of disease. Recommended workup for patients with MF/SS is listed in Table 1-9.

TABLE 1-8   International Society for Cutaneous Lymphoma/European Organization for Research and Treatment of Cancer Revision to the Staging of Mycosis Fungoides and Sézary Syndrome

Clinical Stage	T	N	M	B
IA	1	0	0	0,1
IB	2	0	0	0,1
II	1,2	1,2	0	0,1
IIB	3	0-2	0	0,1
III	4	0-2	0	0,1
IIIA	4	0-2	0	0
IIIB	4	0-2	0	1
IVA1	1-4	0-2	0	2
IVA2	1-4	3	0	0-2
IVB	1-4	0-3	1	0-2

B, blood; M, metastasis; N, node; T, tumor.
Adapted from Olsen E, Vonderheid E, Pimpinelli N, Willemze R, Kim Y, Knobler R, et al. Revisions to the staging and classification of mycosis fungoides and Sézary syndrome: a proposal of the International Society for Cutaneous Lymphomas (ISCL) and the cutaneous lymphoma task force of the European Organization of Research and Treatment of Cancer (EORTC). *Blood*. 2007;110:1713–1722.

TABLE 1-9   Suggested Recommended Evaluation of the Patient with Mycosis Fungoides/Sézary Syndrome*

Physical Examination (Skin, Mucous Membranes, Genitalia)
Document morphology of skin lesions: patch, plaque, tumor, erythroderma
  Note hypopigmentation, poikiloderma, erosions, ulceration, alopecia
Estimate percentage of body surface area involved (patch/plaque/erythroderma)
  Note if restricted to palms/soles
  Note mucous membrane involvement
Assess number, maximum size, aggregate volume, and region of tumors

Extracutaneous Evaluation
Comment on presence or absence of adenopathy and distribution (cervical, axillary, epitrochlear, inguinal)
  Any palpable lymph node, especially those ≥1.5 cm in largest diameter or firm, irregular, clustered, or fixed
Document presence or absence of organomegaly

Skin Biopsy
Sample the most indurated area if only one biopsy: best to biopsy more than 1 if different morphologies
  Procedure: punch, excision, shave, depending on morphology of lesion
Immunophenotyping to include at least the following markers: CD2, CD3, CD4, CD5, CD7, CD8, and a B-cell marker such as CD20. CD30 may also be indicated in cases in which lymphomatoid papulosis, anaplastic large cell lymphoma, or large-cell transformation are considered. If CD4–/CD8– or CD4–/CD8+, consider βF1, TIA-1
Evaluation for clonality of TCR gene rearrangement (PCR preferred over Southern blot): consider two samples or skin + blood for dual PCR

Blood Tests
CBC with manual differential, liver function tests, LDH, comprehensive chemistry panel
  Consider HIV or HTLV-1 testing
TCR gene rearrangement and relatedness to any clone in skin (dual PCR)
  Isolated PCR of blood should be assessed with caution because clonality may be seen in healthy elderly persons
Analysis for abnormal lymphocytes by Sézary cell count and/or flow cytometry (including assessment of CD4+/CD7– and CD4+/CD26– levels)

Radiologic Tests
Limited studies (chest x-ray or ultrasound of the peripheral nodes):
  In healthy patients with T1N0B0 stage disease or in selected patients with T2N0B0 disease with limited skin involvement, without signs or symptoms of visceral disease
CT scans of chest, abdomen, and pelvis alone ± FDG-PET scan (MRI if cannot undergo CT:
  In patients with more than stage IA disease, or selected patients with limited T2 disease and no adenopathy or blood involvement)

Lymph Node Biopsy
Excisional biopsy: if a node either is 1.5 cm or larger in diameter and/or is firm, irregular, clustered, or fixed
Site of biopsy:
Preference is largest lymph node draining an involved area of the skin or if FDG-PET scan data are available, the node with highest SUV

(Continued)

TABLE 1-9   Suggested Recommended Evaluation of the Patient with Mycosis Fungoides/Sézary Syndrome* (Continued)

If no imaging information and multiple similar-appearing enlarged nodes, the order of preference is cervical, axillary, and inguinal regions.
Analysis: pathologic assessment by light microscopy, flow cytometry, and TCR gene rearrangement.

CBC, complete blood count; CT, computed tomography; FDG, fluorodeoxyglucose; HIV, human immunodeficiency virus; HTLV-1, human T-cell lymphotropic virus-1; LDH, lactate dehydrogenase; MRI, magnetic resonance imaging; PCR, polymerase chain reaction; PET, positron emission tomography; SUV, standardized uptake value; TCR, T-cell receptor.
Adapted from Olsen E, Vonderheid E, Pimpinelli N, Willemze R, Kim Y, Knobler R, et al. Revisions to the staging and classification of mycosis fungoides and Sézary syndrome: a proposal of the International Society for Cutaneous Lymphomas (ISCL) and the cutaneous lymphoma task force of the European Organization of Research and Treatment of Cancer (EORTC). *Blood.* 2007;110:1713–1722.

Staging of Non–Mycosis Fungoides/Sézary Syndrome Cutaneous Lymphoma

Non-MF and non-SS cutaneous lymphomas do not fit well into the standard TNMB staging classification. Thus, prognostication for these tumors is determined by the WHO/EORTC classification because it best incorporates the clinical, histopathologic, and immunophenotypic features that distinguish the indolent, intermediate, and aggressive subtypes. Nonetheless, in hopes of capturing longitudinal data that might allow better distinction within these subtypes, the ISCL/EORTC has proposed a TNM classification system for primary cutaneous lymphomas other than MF and SS. These include the T, NK, B, and precursor neoplasms from Table 1-1, excluding, MF, MF variants, LyP, SS, and ATLL. It also applies to lymphomas designated as "primary cutaneous peripheral T-cell lymphoma, unspecified, other." Because these tumors are too heterogeneous to extract prognostic information, this system offers only anatomic documentation of disease extent, with the intention to supplement the TNM designations with additional prognostically relevant data in future revisions (Table 1-10).

TABLE 1-10   Tumor-Node-Metastasis Classification of Cutaneous Lymphoma other than Mycosis Fungoides/Sézary Syndrome, Proposed by the International Society for Cutaneous Lymphoma/European Organization for Research and Treatment of Cancer

T		Definition of Body Regions
T1	Solitary skin involvement	Head and neck
T1a	A solitary lesion less than 5 cm diameter	Inferior border: superior border of clavicles and T1 spinous process
T1b	A solitary greater than 5 cm diameter	Chest
T2	Regional skin involvement: multiple lesions limited to one body region or two contiguous body regions	Superior border: superior border of clavicles Inferior border: inferior margin of rib cage Lateral borders: midaxillary lines, glenohumeral joints (including axillae)
T2a	All-disease-encompassing in a less than 15-cm-diameter circular area	Abdomen/genital
T2b	All-disease-encompassing in a greater than 15- and less than 30-cm-diameter circular area	Superior border: inferior margin of rib cage Inferior border: inguinal folds, anterior perineum Lateral borders: midaxillary lines

(Continued)

T

T2c	All-disease-encompassing in a greater than 30-cm-diameter circular area
T3	Generalized skin involvement
T3a	Multiple lesions involving two noncontiguous body regions
T3b	Multiple lesions involving three or more body regions

Definition of Body Regions

Upper back
  Superior border: T1 spinous process
  Inferior border: inferior margin of rib cage
  Lateral borders: midaxillary lines
Lower back/buttocks
  Superior border: inferior margin of rib cage
  Inferior border: inferior gluteal fold, anterior perineum (include perineum)
  Lateral borders: midaxillary lines
Each upper arm
  Superior borders: glenohumeral joints (excluding axillae)
  Inferior borders: ulnar/radial-humeral (elbow) joint
Each lower arm/hand
  Superior borders: ulnar/radial-humeral (elbow) joint
Each upper leg (thigh)
  Superior borders: inguinal folds, inferior gluteal folds
  Inferior borders: mid-patellae, midpopliteal fossae
Each lower leg/foot
  Superior borders: midpatellae, midpopliteal fossae.

N

N0	No clinical or pathologic lymph node involvement
N1	Involvement of one peripheral lymph node region that drains an area of current or prior skin involvement
N2	Involvement of two or more peripheral lymph node regions or involvement of any lymph node region that does not drain an area of current or prior skin involvement
N3	Involvement of central lymph nodes

Definition of Lymph Node Regions

Peripheral node regions
  Antecubital, cervical, supraclavicular, axillary, inguinal-femoral, and popliteal.
Central node regions
  Mediastinal, pulmonary hilar, para-aortic, iliac

M

M0	No evidence of extracutaneous non–lymph node disease
M1	Extracutaneous non–lymph node disease present

M, metastasis; N, node; T, tumor.

The staging workup includes

1. Thorough review of systems and physical examination.
2. Imaging studies (CT of chest, abdomen, pelvis; consider integration of CT with whole body FDG-PET scanning; consider ultrasound of neck; consider central nervous system imaging, especially for tumors such as aggressive epidermotropic CD8+ TCL or IVBCL). If imaging reveals lymph nodes larger than 1.0 cm in short axis or if there is significantly increased PET activity, excisional biopsy should be performed.
3. Bone marrow aspirate and biopsy for cutaneous lymphomas with intermediate to aggressive behavior. There is no consensus regarding incorporation of bone marrow evaluation for indolent lymphomas, so regional standard of care guidelines should be considered. Results of staging workup may also provide data requiring marrow evaluation.

SUMMARY

Primary cutaneous lymphomas are a heterogeneous group of neoplasms with variable prognoses, ranging from indolent to aggressive, as determined by clinical, microscopic, and immunophenotypic features. It is important to remember that primary cutaneous lymphomas are distinct from systemic lymphomas, despite the fact that selected subtypes have similar histology and immunophenotype. Some of the indolent T- and B-cell lymphomas may be difficult to differentiate from benign inflammatory dermatoses and from CLH (pseudolymphoma), requiring correlation of clinical morphology, distribution, and course of disease with histopathologic and immunohistochemical features. Documentation of monoclonality may be helpful, but it is not the absolute diagnostic indication of malignancy. Treatment will be dictated by the subtype and stage of the lymphoma. Details of diagnosis and treatment of cutaneous lymphomas are provided in Chapter 19.

SUGGESTED READINGS

Beltraminelli H, Leinweber B, Kerl H, Cerroni L. Primary cutaneous CD4+ small-/medium-sized pleomorphic T-cell lymphoma: a cutaneous nodular proliferation of pleomorphic T lymphocytes of undetermined significance? A study of 136 cases. *Am J Dermatopathol.* 2009;31:317–322.

Berti E, Tomasini D, Vermeer MH, Meijer CJ, Alessi E, Willemze R Primary cutaneous CD8-positive epidermotropic cytotoxic T cell lymphomas. A distinct clinicopathological entity with an aggressive clinical behavior. *Am J Pathol.* 1999;155:483–492.

Campbell JJ, Clark RA, Watanabe R, Kupper TS. Sézary syndrome and mycosis fungoides arise from distinct subsets: a biologic rational for their distinct clinical behaviors. *Blood.* 2010;116:676–671.

Choi YL, Park JH, Namkung JH, Lee JH, Yang JM, Lee ES, et al. Extranodal NK/T-cell lymphoma with cutaneous involvement: "nasal" vs. "nasal-type" subgroups—a retrospective study of 18 patients. *Br J Dermatol.* 2009;160:333–337.

El Shabrawi-Caelen L, Kerl H, Cerroni L. Lymphomatoid papulosis: reappraisal of clinicopathologic presentation and classification into subtypes A, B, and C. *Arch Dermatol.* 2004;140:441–447.

Garcia-Herrera A, Colomo L, Camós M, et al. Primary cutaneous small/medium CD4+T-cell lymphomas: a heterogeneous group of tumors with different clinicopathologic features and outcome. *J Clin Oncol.* 2008; 26:3364–3371.

Garnache-Ottou F, Feuillard J, Saas P. Plasmacytoid dendritic cell leukaemia/lymphoma: towards a well defined entity? *Br J Haematol.* 2007;136:539–548.

Gerami P, Rosen S, Kuzel T, Boone SL, Guitart J. Folliculotropic mycosis fungoides. an aggressive variant of cutaneous T-cell lymphoma. *Arch Dermatol.* 2008;144:738–746.

Golling P, Cozzio A, Dummer R, French L, Kempf W. Primary cutaneous B-cell lymphomas—clinicopathological, prognostic and therapeutic characterisation of 54 cases according to the WHO-EORTC classification and the ISCL/EORTC TNM classification system for primary cutaneous lymphomas other than mycosis fungoides and Sézary syndrome. *Leuk Lymphoma.* 2008;49:1094–1103.

Grogg KL, Jung S, Erickson LA, McClure RF, Dogan A. Primary cutaneous CD4-positive small/medium-sized pleomorphic T-cell lymphoma: a clonal T-cell lymphoproliferative disorder with indolent behavior. *Mod Pathol.* 2008;21:708–715.

Haghighi B, Smoller BR, LeBoit PE, Warnke RA. Sander CA, Kohler S. Pagetoid reticulosis (Woringer-Kolopp disease): an immunophenotypic, molecular, and clinicopathologic study. *Mod Pathol.* 2000;13:502–510.

Jambusaria A, Shafer D, Wu H, Al-Saleem T, Perlis C. Cutaneous plasmablastic lymphoma. *J Am Acad Dermatol.* 2008;58:676–678.

Kempf W, Sander CA. Classification of cutaneous lymphomas—an update. *Histopathology.* 2010;56: 57–70.

Kim Y, Willemze R, Pimpinelli N, Whittaker S, Olsen EA, Ranki A, et al. TNM classification system for primary cutaneous lymphomas other than mycosis fungoides and Sézary syndrome: a proposal of the International Society for Cutaneous Lymphomas (ISCL) and the Cutaneous Lymphoma Task Force of the European Organization of Research and Treatment of Cancer (EORTC). *Blood.* 2007;110:479–484.

Kodama K, Massone C, Chott A, Metze D, Kerl H, Cerroni L. Primary cutaneous large B-cell lymphomas: clinicopathologic features, classification, and prognostic factors in a large series of patients. *Blood.* 2005;106:2491–2497.

Koens L, Vermeer MH, Willemze R, Jansen PM. IgM expression on paraffin sections distinguishes primary cutaneous large B-cell lymphoma, leg type from primary cutaneous follicle center lymphoma. *Am J Surg Pathol.* 2010;34:1043–1048.

Massone C, Chott A, Metze D, Kerl K, Citarella L, Vale E, et al. Subcutaneous, blastic natural killer (NK), NK/T, and other cytotoxic lymphomas of the skin: a morphologic, immunophenotypic, and molecular study of 50 patients. *Am J Surg Pathol.* 2004;28: 719–735.

Massone C, El-Shabrawi-Caelen L, Kerl H, Cerroni L. The morphologic spectrum of primary cutaneous anaplastic large T-cell lymphoma: a histopathologic study on 66 biopsy specimens from 47 patients with report of rare variants. *J Cutan Pathol.* 2008;35:46–53.

Moreno-Giménez JC, Jiménez-Puya R, Galán-Gutiérrez M, Pérez-Seoane C, Camacho FM. Granulomatous slack skin disease in a child: the outcome. *Pediatr Dermatol.* 2007;24:640–645.

Olsen E, Vonderheid E, Pimpinelli N, Willemze R, Kim Y, Knobler R, et al. Revisions to the staging and classification of mycosis fungoides and Sézary syndrome: a proposal of the International Society for Cutaneous Lymphomas (ISCL) and the cutaneous lymphoma task force of the European Organization of Research and Treatment of Cancer (EORTC). *Blood.* 2007;110:1713–1722.

Pimpinelli N, Olsen EA, Santucci M, et al. Defining early mycosis fungoides. *J Am Acad Dermatol.* 2005; 53:1053–1063.

Rodríguez Pinilla SM, Roncador G, Rodríguez-Peralto JL, Mollejo M, García JF, Montes-Moreno S, et al. Primary cutaneous CD4+ small/medium-sized pleomorphic T-cell lymphoma expresses follicular T-cell markers. *Am J Surg Pathol.* 2009;33:81–90.

Shimoyama M. Diagnostic criteria and classification of clinical subtypes of adult T-cell leukemia-lymphoma: a report from the Lymphoma Study Group (1984–87). *Br J Haematol.* 1991;79:428–437.

Thurber SE, Zhang B, Kim YH, et al. T-cell clonality analysis in biopsy specimens from two different skin sites shows high specificity in the diagnosis of patients with suggested mycosis fungoides. *J Am Acad Dermatol.* 2007;57:782–790.

Vergier B, de Muret A, Beylot-Barry M, Vaillant L, Ekouevi D. Transformation of mycosis fungoides: clinicopathological and prognostic features of 45 cases. *Blood.* 2000;95:2212–2218.

Willemze R, Jaffe ES, Burg G, et al. WHO-EORTC classification for cutaneous lymphomas. *Blood.* 2005; 105:3768–3785.

Willemze R, Jansen PM, Cerroni L, Berti E, Santucci M, Assaf C, et al. Subcutaneous panniculitis-like T-cell lymphoma: definition, classification, and prognostic factors: an EORTC Cutaneous Lymphoma Group Study of 83 cases. *Blood.* 2008;111:838–845.

CUTANEOUS LYMPHOMA: EPIDEMIOLOGY

Maria M. Morales Suárez-Varela, MD, PhD,
Maria Teresa Morales-Suárez-Varela, PhD,
and Agustin Llopis-Gonzalez, PhD

EPIDEMIOLOGY

Primary cutaneous lymphomas represent a heterogeneous group of T- and B-cell lymphomas that show considerable variation in histology, phenotype, and prognosis. Recently, the European Organization for Research and Treatment of Cancer (EORTC) Cutaneous Lymphoma Project Group has reached consensus on a new classification for this group of diseases. The EORTC classification for primary cutaneous lymphomas is based on a combination of clinical, histologic, and immunophenotypic criteria, and thus, contains well-defined disease entities rather than histologic subgroups. In addition, this new classification contains a number of provisional entities, which may display characteristic histologic features but are not yet well defined clinically. These provisional entities account for less than 5% of all primary cutaneous lymphomas.

Primary cutaneous lymphomas are, after the group of primary gastrointestinal lymphomas, the second most common group of extranodal non-Hodgkin's lymphomas. The annual incidence is estimated at 0.5 to 1 per 100,000, and until recently, distinction between primary and secondary cutaneous lymphomas was generally not made. Both groups of lymphomas were classified according to histologic classification schemes used by hematopathologists for nodal non-Hodgkin's lymphomas, such as the (updated) Kiel classification and the Working Formulation. However, recent studies demonstrated that patients with primary cutaneous lymphomas, defined as those without concurrent extracutaneous disease at the time of diagnosis, often have highly characteristic clinical and histologic features, and a clinical behavior and prognosis, that are different from primary nodal lymphomas of the same histologic subtype, involving the skin secondarily. In addition, differences in the presence of specific translocations and in the expression of oncogenes, viral

sequences, and adhesion receptors were found, suggesting that primary cutaneous lymphomas should be considered as a distinctive group, both clinically and biologically. New insights into the mechanisms underlying lymphocyte recirculation and organ-specific homing provided an explanation for these differences and led to the present view that morphologically identical lymphomas arising at different sites are clonal proliferations of distinct, organ-related, lymphocyte subpopulations, which have retained many characteristics of their benign counterparts.

These studies on well-defined groups of primary cutaneous lymphomas resulted not only in the delineation of several new disease entities but also in the awareness that the classification schemes used for nodal lymphomas are inadequate to categorize primary cutaneous lymphomas in a clinically meaningful way. First, several types of primary cutaneous large cell lymphomas classified as high-grade malignant lymphomas according to the updated Kiel classification and Working Formulation were found to have an indolent clinical behavior. Second, studies on (cutaneous) T-cell lymphomas revealed that the reproducibility of the Kiel classification for this group of lymphomas was poor. Third, there is mounting evidence that primary cutaneous lymphomas cannot be defined properly by histologic criteria alone. For instance, it has been well-established that primary cutaneous large T-cell lymphomas expressing the CD30 antigen, irrespective of the histologic subtype (anaplastic or nonanaplastic), have a significantly better prognosis than primary cutaneous CD30– large T-cell lymphomas. The difficulty, or sometimes the impossibility, of differentiating between primary cutaneous CD30+ (anaplastic) large cell lymphomas and lymphomatoid papulosis (LyP) is well recognized. Epidermotropic lymphoid infiltrates containing atypical T cells with cerebriform nuclei are the hallmark of plaque stage mycosis fungoides (MF), but can also be found in LyP type

B and some pseudo–T-cell lymphomas. A definite diagnosis in these cases depends on knowledge about the clinical presentation and the results of additional immunologic and genetic investigations. These and other examples clearly illustrate that cutaneous lymphomas can be defined only by a combination of clinical, histologic, and immunologic data.

Cutaneous T-cell lymphoma (CTCL), therefore, is a term that represents a variety of lymphomas with differing clinical presentations, histologic features, and therapeutic considerations. MF and Sézary's syndrome were the first recognized forms of CTCL, but we now recognize additional disease categories characterized by expansions of malignant T cells within the skin and unique combinations of clinical, histologic, and immunophenotypical criteria.

MF makes up the great majority of cases of primary CTCL (80-85%). CTCL is a lymphoproliferative disorder of epidermotropic, neoplastic T cells with a wide range of clinical manifestations. A number of other cutaneous disorders may present as different clinical manifestations of MF. The MF was first described by Alibert and coworkers in 1806. In 1876, Bazin defined the three stages of the disease (patches, plaques and tumors). The term CTCL was introduced by Lutzner and colleagues in 1975 to describe a group of malignant lymphomas with primary manifestations in the skin.

All forms of CTCL are neoplasms of T lymphocytes, which home to the skin and to the T-cell zones of lymphoid structures, but generally not to the bone marrow. General lymphoma pathologists had different classifications of lymphoma, only one of which includes cutaneous lymphoma, as was first introduced by the Kiel classification in 1980, and was updated in 1988. Unfortunately, this classification is of limited value for those involved with cutaneous lymphoma because it is based on a detailed pathologic assessment with no clinical correlation.

The two main classification systems used for cutaneous lymphomas are the Revised European-American Lymphoma (REAL) classification and the system created by the EORTC. Both schema refine and extend older systems such as the Working Formulation because they are based on a combination of clinicopathologic,

immunophenotypical, and molecular biologic characteristics.

INCIDENCE

Ambiguities in *International Classification of Diseases for Oncology (ICD-O)* codes may have caused coding errors that have probably caused an underestimation of the true incidence of CTCL. These ambiguities in *ICD-O-2* morphologic definitions may have resulted in the erroneous classification of several cases of cutaneous B-cell lymphoma as CTCL NOS (not otherwise specified). The *ICD-O-2* (1992-2000) contained the disease classification "cutaneous lymphoma NOS (code 9709)" under the broader disease category "specified cutaneous and peripheral T-cell lymphomas (code 970).

The reported standardized incidence rates for CTCL—of which MF is a subgroup—vary considerably. CTCL is an uncommon neoplasm, and the Surveillance, Epidemiology, and End Results (SEER) program reports that the incidence had increased 3.2-fold between 1973 and 1984, from 0.19 cases to 0.42 cases per 100,000 (Table 2-1). The overall incidence rate is approximately 4 to 5 per 1,000,000, according to data from that particular program in which this tendency is seen in all the age, race, and sex groups (Tables 2-2 to 2-5). In this time period, 721 new cases were diagnosed, and a mean incidence was seen of 0.29 per 100,000 per year in the United States (probably due to an improvement in the diagnosis), which represented 2.2% of all lymphomas.

A similar tendency was seen in different European studies. In Denmark, the MF incidence rate in 1987 was 0.2 per 100,000 in men, whereas only 1 case in 2.6 million was diagnosed in women.

In a North American study, the association that existed between the incidence of the disease and the concentration of doctors in each studied area suggests that the detection of cases could be explained by differences in the geographic distribution because those areas with a greater number of physicians showed a greater incidence level, possibly more consistent with earlier diagnosis. A 3.2-fold increase was described in the incidence of MF during the course of the study, and the proportion of MF cases among lymphomas

TABLE 2-1   Incidence of Mycosis Fungoides and the Total Number of Lymphomas*

Year	Mycosis Fungoides Cases/100,000 Inhabitants/Yr	Total No. of Cases	Total Lymphomas Cases/100,000 Inhabitants/Yr	Total No. of Cases
1973	0.19	30	11.69	1898
1974	0.17	32	11.93	2255
1975	0.23	47	12.18	2505
1976	0.19	39	11.97	2485
1977	0.30	63	12.05	2562
1978	0.25	52	12.51	2700
1979	0.28	60	13.01	2846
1980	0.23	53	12.87	2878
1981	0.34	77	13.66	3097
1982	0.36	83	13.71	3151
1983	0.38	88	14.07	3283
1984	0.42	97	14.79	3498

*Data from the Surveillance, Epidemiology, and End Results Program.

From Weinstock MA, Horm JW. Mycosis fungoides in the United States. *JAMA*. 1988;60:42–46.

TABLE 2-2   Age When the Diagnosis Was Made in a Case Series According to Race and Sex

Age (Yr)	Number (%) of Mycosis Fungoides Cases				
	White Men	White Women	Nonwhite Men	Nonwhite Women	Total
25-29	4 (3.4)	2 (3.2)	0	1 (7.1)	7 (3.3)
30-34	2 (1.7)	0	2 (11.8)	1 (7.1)	5 (2.4)
35-39	3 (2.5)	4 (6.5)	1 (5.9)	1 (7.1)	9 (4.3)
40-44	9 (7.6)	7 (11.3)	0	2 (14.3)	18 (8.5)
45-49	24 (20.3)	8 (12.9)	2 (11.8)	0	34 (16.1)
50-54	15 (12.7)	10 (16.1)	5 (29.4)	2 (14.3)	32 (15.2)
55-59	10 (8.5)	6 (9.7)	1 (5.9)	4 (28.6)	21 (10.0)
60-64	13 (11.0)	9 (14.5)	2 (11.8)	1 (7.1)	25 (11.8)
65-69	14 (11.9)	4 (6.5)	4 (23.5)	1 (7.1)	23 (10.9)
70-74	11 (9.3)	6 (9.7)	0	0	18 (8.5)
75-79	5 (4.2)	4 (6.5)	0	0	9 (4.3)
80-84	4 (3.4)	0	0	0	4 (1.9)
85-89	1 (0.8)	1 (1.6)	0	0	2 (1.0)
Unknown	3 (2.5)	1 (1.6)	0	0	4 (1.9)
Total	118	62	17	14	211

From Greene MH, Dalager NA, Lamberg SI, Arguropoulos CE, Fraumeni JF Jr. Mycosis fungoides: epidemiologic observations. *Cancer Treat Rep*. 1979;63,597–606.

TABLE 2-3　Incidence of Mycosis Fungoides and the Total Number of Lymphomas According to Age, Race, and Sex*

	Mycosis Fungoides		Total Lymphoma	
	Cases/100,000 Inhabitants/Yr	Total No. of Cases	Cases/100,000 Inhabitants/Yr	Total No. of Cases
Age (Yr)				
<40	0.05	90	4.08	7312
40-49	0.34	88	10.94	2830
50-59	0.56	143	21.05	5378
60-69	0.98	190	37.55	7264
70-79	1.28	144	59.72	6744
≥80	1.26	66	67.80	3627
Race				
Whites	0.26	568	13.46	29.977
Men	0.37	367	15.77	15.711
Women	0.17	201	11.56	14.266
Blacks	0.52	98	8.73	1742
Men	0.75	61	11.15	1016
Women	0.33	37	6.71	726
All races	0.29	721	12.95	33.155
Men	0.41	466	15.25	17.559
Women	0.19	255	11.03	15.596

*Data corresponding to the years 1973-1984 from the Surveillance, Epidemiology, and End Results Program.
From Weinstock MA, Horm JW. Mycosis fungoides in the United States. *JAMA.* 1988;60:42–46.

increased from 1.6% to 2.8% over the course of the study.

The present-day incidence rate may be of an order of a higher magnitude, given the possible underreporting and both the difficulty and the confusion in making the diagnosis. The incidence of CTCL rises with age and is approximately twice (2.2 times) as common in men as in women, whereas blacks have twice the incidence of whites (see Table 2-2).

TABLE 2-4　Incidence of Mycosis Fungoides, Specifically by Age, Race, and Sex in Selected Areas*

	White Men No. of Cases/10^5/Yr		White Women No. of Cases/10^5/Yr		Black Men No. of Cases/10^5/Yr		Black Women No. of Cases/10^5/Yr	
Age (Yr)	Population/Yr	Cases	Population/Yr	Cases	Population/Yr	Cases	Population/Yr	Cases
<50	0.10	79	0.05	42	0.23	17	0.20	20
50-59	0.69	74	0.32	36	1.61	15	0.47	5
60-69	1.35	106	0.57	52	2.82	18	0.64	5
≥70	1.92	108	0.77	71	2.97	11	1.28	7

*Data from the Surveillance, Epidemiology, and End Results Program.
From Weinstock MA, Horm JW. Mycosis fungoides in the United States. *JAMA.* 1988;60:42–46.

TABLE 2-5   Incidence of Mycosis Fungoides Adjusted to Age, According to the Year of Diagnosis, Race, Sex, Age, and Registration Date in Selected Areas of the United States*

	1973-1976 Cases/100,000		1977-1980 Cases/100,000		1981-1984 Cases/100,000	
	Population/Yr	Cases	Population/Yr	Cases	Population/Yr	Cases
Total	0.20	148	0.27	228	0.38	345
Race and Sex						
White men	0.28	83	0.34	116	0.47	168
White women	0.11	42	0.15	63	0.23	96
Black men	0.49	12	0.78	22	0.91	27
Black women	0.17	6	0.24	8	0.54	23
Age (Yr)						
<50	0.06	36	0.07	44	0.14	98
50-59	0.27	22	0.69	61	0.69	60
60-69	0.81	46	0.89	58	1.21	86
≥70	0.92	44	1.15	65	1.66	101
Register						
Whites						
San Francisco	0.32	37	0.27	32	0.45	53
Detroit	0.18	23	0.26	35	0.48	62
Connecticut	0.17	21	0.21	27	0.42	55
Blacks						
San Francisco	0.57	7	0.83	11	0.79	11
Detroit	0.24	7	0.36	10	0.90	28
Connecticut	0.63	3	0.69	4	0.81	7

*Data from the Surveillance, Epidemiology, and End Results Program.
From Weinstock MA, Horm JW. Mycosis fungoides in the United States. *JAMA*. 1988;60:42–46.

Although CTCL cases in general, and MF cases in particular, are rarely seen before the age of 30, they have been identified in children and teenagers. However, the mean age at onset is 50 years. Greene and associates observed that the illness predominates in men (85%), generally middle-aged men (64% of patients were found to be between 45 and 69 years of age).

Table 2-2 shows the distribution of 211 MF cases with regard to age, race, and sex according to an American study carried out between 1950 and 1975 (excluding 1972).

According to the data obtained in the county of Los Angeles between 1972 and 1985, a greater incidence continues to be seen among the black race, where the ratio between the sexes is nearly 1:1 (similar to the ratio in the white race).

The data belonging to Third World countries are particularly scarce. In fact, most of the incidence data are limited to developed countries, especially the United States and Europe. MF, however, appears to represent a lesser ratio of non-Hodgkin's lymphoma in China (0.4%) than in the United States (2.2% of all the lymphomas determined between 1973 and 1984).

The gradual increase of incidence with age is presented in all the race and sex strata (see Table 2-3).

During the period 1979 to 1992, Weinstock and coworkers described an incidence rate in the United States of 0.36 per 10 person-years. There was no evidence of increasing incidence rates during the period 1983 through 1992 but the disorder varies greatly among demographic and geographic subgroups (see Tables 2-4 and 2-5).

The incidence of CTCL has risen dramatically and consistently since 1973. Changes in classification schemes may have contributed to the rise in incidence, as have improvements in detection or an increase in the underlying etiologic agent(s). U.S. demographic correlates show that incidence is strongly correlated with the density of physicians. Hence, the rise in incidence may be due, at least in part, to increased efficiency of detection resulting from improvements in medical care since the 1980s. Because of reporting delay, the actual rise in incidence may be greater than the rise found in our data. Reporting delay and reporting error occur when new cases are discovered or erroneous cases are detected in the existing SEER data. Clegg and colleagues found that initial incidence case counts accounted for only 88% to 97% of the estimated final counts in the SEER program and that it would take 4 to 17 years for 99% or more of cancer cases to be reported. The overall annual age-adjusted incidence of CTCL was 6.4 per million persons in United States. Annual incidence increased by 2.9 x 10^{-6} per decade over the study period. Incidence was higher among blacks (9.0×10^{-6}) than among whites (6.1×10^{-6}) and higher among men (8.7×10^{-6}) than among women (4.6×10^{-6}). The racial differences in incidence decreased with age, whereas the sex differences increased with age and decreased over time. Substantial geographic variation in incidence was found. Incidence was correlated with high physician density, high family income, high percentage of population with a bachelor's degree or higher, and high home values. Changes in *ICD-O* morphologic definitions have resulted in the redistribution of the cases of CTCL among specific subclassifications .

ETIOLOGY

Although the etiology of MF is unknown, Rowden and Lewis posed the hypothesis that the start of MF development could be due to a primary alteration in the cellular immune response, mediated by Langerhans cells. The suspicion that a persistent antigenic stimulation could play an important role in MF development was suggested for the first time by Tan and associates in 1974, based on the findings of high immunoglobulin E (IgE) levels in patients affected by MF. Several causative factors have been proposed and subsequently investigated. These include chronic antigenic stimulation as a result of different exposures to bacterial infections, smoking, medications, chronic sun exposure, viral infections, and chemical exposition.

Family History

The marked variation of MF incidence through time and the absence of a documented family association suggest that MF is not a primary genetic disorder, although that does not imply that it does not present a certain grade of genetic predisposition. In addition, the association of MF with a family history of Hodgkin's disease has been documented, although the presence of certain potential factors (environmental or hereditary) has not been determined.

In a study carried out in the United States on 211 patients affected by MF, 56 (26%) were noted to have a close family member who also presented some type of skin disease. Thirty percent (63 patients) had a close family member with a history of cancer. Twenty percent (42 MF patients) had some close family member who was affected by cancer.

Between December 1976 and February 1977, Cohen and coworkers studied family cancer medical histories by means of an interview in which the following data were included: job name, production, activity, the usual work one was assigned to, and a description of its activity. A family medical history was considered as positive if any member who was genetically related to the family was diagnosed with cancer, no matter which type. The finding of a family cancer medical history in both the cases studied and the control subjects had a similar frequency. The probability of finding a positive family medical history of cancer among the study patients was similar to 1 (relative risk [RR] = 1.1).

In the California/Washington study by Cohen and associates, a significant association was noted between MF and a history of other malignant diseases different from non-Hodgkin lymphoma or skin cancer (RR = 3.3, *P* <. 001), probably due to the Berkson bias (this bias deals with the possible existence of spurious associations between different diseases or between a disease and a risk factor). A more extensive and subsequent study performed with data from the Cancer Register in the United States showed the absence of an association between MF and previous malignant diseases and suggested that certain aspects of the California/Washington study could have led to artifactual associations.

Only a strong family history of atopic dermatitis in MF patients has been described. Familial cases of CTCL have rarely been reported. Recently, a case of monozygotic twins with CTCL was reported. This study reported that human leukocyte antigens (HLAs) have shown that the histocompatibility antigens HLA-B8, AW3, and AW31 are more frequent in patients with MF.

Analysis of structural chromosome abnormalities in patients with MF reveals that many chromosomes can have clonal abnormalities. Chromosome 1 seems to be the most frequently affected. The region between 1p22 and 1p36 is thought to contain a gene important in either the malignant transformation or the progression of MF.

Also described are different oncogenes, either the *NFKB-2/lyt-10* gene or the *tal-1* gene, that were mutated in 5 of 38 cases of CTCL. The *tal-1* gene codes for a transcription factor that is not expressed in normal T lymphocytes. Most likely when this is an abnormal deletion of *tal-1*, it becomes activated and may play a role in malignant transformation. In general, more studies are necessary with more cases that clarify the role of family history in development of MF because some of these results are contradictory.

RISK FACTORS

Occupational Factors

The idea that different occupational factors might be involved in the origin of MF fits in quite well with the observation that dermatitis, or more specifically contact dermatitis, may precede the appearance of MF. For example, the operators of different types of machinery are exposed to a wide range of agents such as metals and plastics. They are also exposed to oils used in cutting procedures and to solvents used in grinding operations. Furthermore, some of these agents, which are irritating and sensitizing, have also been recognized as cancer-producing. There are extremely high levels of carcinogenic N-nitrosamine in some makes of fluids used in cutting processes. An appearance of MF has been also described after being exposed to chemical agents (toxic) caused by industrial accidents.

In a case-control study performed by Cohen and coworkers, 40 working periods were detected in industry or in the construction industry and were related to 29 out of the 59 patients affected by MF (49%). Conversely, 19 out of the 54 controls (35%) were employed in industrial jobs, which were comparable with those of the cases (the average duration of the job, both for industrial jobs and for nonindustrial jobs, was similar in the cases and the control subjects). There were only 3 occasions in which the control subjects had industrial jobs and the cases subjects did not (odds ratio [OR] = 4.3; 95% confidence interval [CI]). Consequently, the RR of finding an industrial occupation among the patients affected by MF was 4.3 times greater than among the control subjects. The association between industrial occupation and MF was statistically significant ($P = .020$). The main differences between the industrial occupation of the MF patients and the control subjects were found to be among machinists, construction workers, foundry operators, and industrial electricians. These findings indicate that the MF patients were more greatly involved than the heavy-industry control subjects. However, when reviewing this study, some methodologic defects were observed because many of the occupational medical histories were obtained from the people close to the patients rather than from the patients themselves. This could account for the biases and errors when classifying the medical histories. The patients affected by MF in this study were employed as machinists, machine operators, textile workers, construction workers, foundry operators, wood industry workers, workers in wood cutting processes, and industrial cleaning service workers (with a greater or lesser frequency). But there were also some nonindustrial occupations, such as sales staff managers, clergy, secretaries, social workers, housewives, artists, nursing staff, with a greater or lesser frequency. Such occupations as mechanics, machinery operators, textile workers, construction workers, and overseers were also found among the control subjects, although less frequently.

Employment in the manufacturing industry, especially petrochemicals, textiles, metals, and machinery, was observed in a descriptive study in 29% of a series of patients ($n = 211$) diagnosed with MF. Sixty-three patients (30%) showed exposure to toxic substances, especially petrochemical substances (11%), metals (7%), and solvents (6%), although there were no data regarding the frequency and the duration of such exposure. No correlation was found between MF and the previous exposure to these toxic substances described.

Between 1961 and 1969 in Sweden, 28 cases were diagnosed among working women (1960 census). The risk significantly increased among women employed in hotel business jobs (hotels and restaurants) (6 cases, standardized incidence ratio [SIR] = 3.6 [adjusted by age and region], $P < .05$), and a high risk was observed in the clothing industry (4 cases, SIR = 2.1).

Additional case-control studies carried out in Scotland, California, and Washington state do not confirm the existence of some type of association between industrial occupation and the risk of MF, but others found association in Europe (Table 2-6). Recent results from the European study are in line with what other studies have found: that the working activities in the paper and wood industries were carried out in California/Washington. Furthermore, the same studies identify that those cases with a slightly lower socioeconomic level than the control subjects perform certain occupations, which implies greater exposure to conditions that favor the development of MF, therefore, supporting the hypothesis that workers of a lower socioeconomic level are indeed at greater risk of developing MF.

Radiation

Exposure to solar radiation defined by episodes of severe sunburn does not reveal any association with MF, although farm workers, fishermen, and other groups who work out in the open appear to be at greater risk. From a study carried out among 211 patients, there were 90 who, on being exposed to the sun, burned easily. The data that describe the variations with regard to North-South did not reveal a greater or lesser gradient as far as other skin diseases are concerned, such as cutaneous carcinomas and melanomas.

One case of MF and several of parapsoriasis were detected among the workers at the Thule Air Base when a military airplane crashed and released plutonium, americium, and tritium in 1968. No relation has been found between an exposure to x-rays and the appearance of MF. However, more studies and data are needed.

Given the inherent immunologic nature of the neoplastic cells responsible for this disorder, it has been proposed that chronic exposure to occupational chemicals, pesticides, or tobacco may predispose to the development of CTCL. However, none of these potential associations has survived scrutiny. The observations that the disease is more common in African Americans than in whites and that it often presents first in areas normally shielded from the sun (i.e., "bathing trunk" distribution) collectively suggest that actinic exposure may actually inhibit the evolution of the malignant clone from normal "cutaneous T cells." It is noteworthy that the epidermotropic collections of CTCL cells, referred to as *Pautrier microabscesses,* may represent a congregation of malignant T cells around Langerhans cells (LCs), the dendritic antigen-presenting cells (DCs) of the epidermis, and that LCs are fairly sensitive to ultraviolet (UV) damage. This observation has suggested that the epidermotropic CTCL cells may receive growth signals from their contact with LCs. Therefore, it is possible that UV damage of LCs, more significant in whites than in African Americans (whose darker pigment shields the LC), may interrupt this growth signal and inhibit the replication of CTCL cells in UV-exposed skin sites. It is also intriguing that the often profound response of patch/plaque CTCL to UV treatment may reflect this phenomenon as well. The observation that individuals infected with the human T-cell leukemia virus type 1 (HTLV-1) often develop T-cell leukemias with skin involvement indistinguishable from those of CTCL has led some to hypothesize that CTCL may be a consequence of infection with HTLV-1, or with another unknown retrovirus, a possibility that remains the subject of active investigation.

Lifestyle: Alcohol and Tobacco Consumption

In the European Rare Cancer Study, wine had no protective effect and yet, quite to the contrary,

TABLE 2-6 Odds Ratios for Mycosis Fungoides in Participants Who Have Always Worked in Industries (NACE)* Represented with at Least Two Exposed Cases

SEX	Male				
NACE Code	Description	Cases	Controls	OR[†]	95% CI[‡]
26	Manufacture of other nonmetallic mineral products	4	21	5.3	1.7-16.2
51	Wholesale trade and commission trade	3	46	3.6	1.2-10.5
63	Transport activities	2	17	3.4	0.8-15.3
65	Financial intermediation, except insurance and pension funding	3	31	3.0	0.9-10.5
80	Primary school	2	46	2.1	0.5-9.1
75	Public administration	3	102	1.7	0.6-4.7
36	Manufacture of furniture, manufacturing	2	44	1.6	0.4-6.8
29	Manufacture of machinery and equipment	3	85	1.3	0.4-4.2
52	Retail trade, except of motor vehicles and motorcycles	2	160	1.2	0.5-3.0
1	Agriculture, hunting, and forestry	8	304	0.9	0.4-1.7
SEX	Female				
NACE Code	Description	Cases	Controls	OR[†]	95% CI[‡]
21	Manufacture of pulp, paper and paper products	2	33	14.4	2.17-95.1
74	Other managerial activities	2	26	4.1	1.3-12.7
18	Manufacture of wearing apparel; dressing and dyeing of fur	4	43	2.4	0.9-6.5
95	Private households with employed persons	4	112	1.8	0.7-4.4
15	Manufacture of food products and beverages	2	33	1.3	0.3-5.5
1	Agriculture, hunting and forestry	5	76	1.1	0.4-2.9
52	Retail trade, except of motor vehicles and motorcycles	4	134	0.9	0.4-2.3

*Industries classified by the Nomenclature of Activities of the European Community (NACE) Rev.1, 1993.
†ORs adjusted by age, country, and number of jobs.
‡95% confidence interval.
CI, confidence interval; OR, odds ratio.
From Morales-Suárez-Varela M, Olsen J, Johansen P, Karelev L, Guénel P, Arveux P, et al. Occupational risk factors for mycosis fungoides: a European multicenter case-control study. *J Occup Environ Med.* 2004;46:205–211.

the daily consumption of more than 24 g of alcohol was associated with a high risk of MF. There was a dose-dependent increase in the risk of MF with increased smoking habits, albeit the observed trend was not statistically significant. A combined exposure to high tobacco and alcohol use yielded a significantly increased risk for MF (Table 2-7).

TABLE 2-7 Odds Ratio* for Mycosis Fungoides According to the Combined Use of Wine and Tobacco†

Wine Intake (G Alcohol/Day)	Tobacco Use (Pack-Yr) 0			1-24 (≤2 Units/Day)			>24 (≥2 Units/Day)			Tobacco Use Adjusted for Wine Intake
	Cases	Controls	OR (95% CI)	Cases	Controls	OR (95% CI)	Cases	Controls	OR (95% CI)	OR (95% CI)
0	11	348	1.0	26	797	1.93 (0.90-4.10)	1	90	0.42 (0.05-3.47)	1.0
1-25	1	193	0.41 (0.05-3.33)	14	617	1.71 (0.70-4.14)	3	81	1.75 (0.43-7.08)	0.92 (0.50-1.70)
>25	1	191	0.45 (0.06-3.69)	15	441	2.47 (1.0-6.10)	4	140	1.25 (0.35-4.45)	1.19 (0.64-2.23)
Wine Intake Adjusted for Tobacco Use			1.0			2.41 (1.26-4.63)			1.29 (0.49-3.40)	76 cases/2899 controls

*Adjusted for country, age, sex, and education. Logistic regression.
†The table for definite and possible cases combined.
CI, confidence interval; OR, odds ratio.
From Morales-Suárez-Varela M, Olsen J, Kaerlev L, Guénel P, Arveux P, Wingtren G, et al. Are alcohol intake and smoking associated with mycosis fungoides? A European multicentre case-control study. *Eur J Cancer.* 2001;37:392–397.

Marital Status and Level of Education

In the Green and colleagues study on 211 MF patients, 75% were married, 14% were widowed, 7% were single, and 4% were divorced. With regard to the patients' educational level, the average number of complete school years was 12 (60% had graduated high schools, including 34% whose education went beyond high schools).

Cutaneous Evolution

In the same study, when medical histories were considered in allergic conditions or cutaneous infections, a history of cancer in the family, exposures to toxic substances, occupation in manufacturing industries, and sensitivity to the sun, all possible risk factors, out of 211 patients, 18 (8%) were seen to not present any factor. From the remaining 92%, 168 (80%) presented two or more and 108 (51%) presented three or more risk factors. Generally speaking, if there was any type of allergy demonstrated by cutaneous tests, no differences were found between cases and controls. By means of the medical histories, Cohen and coworkers' study was able to verify that many patients affected by MF had histories of rashes prior to diagnosis, mainly nonspecific rashes or dermatitis, and also contact dermatitis. Some patients had atopic or nummular eczema, psoriasis and contact dermatitis including a general exfoliative dermatitis, with a greater or lesser frequency. Personal histories of contact dermatitis, asthma, rhinitis, or atopic dermatitis have not been related to an increase in the risk of MF; although significant differences were seen in the association with family medical histories of atopic dermatitis. Family medical histories of benign inflammatory dermatosis appear to be a risk factor for MF, but its study proves complicated.

Others

Some MF cases have been described in immunosuppressed patients caused by organ transplants or by human immunodeficiency virus (HIV) infection, although it appears to be infrequent.

Occasionally, lesions similar to those produced by CTCL have been observed in acquired immunodeficiency syndrome (AIDS) patients. Patients infected with HIV concomitantly with CTCL, even in the absence of severe immunosuppression, develop an atypical course of the disease, and its progress is more rapid.

Although there are different hypotheses regarding the etiology of MF (viral agents or an alteration in the cellular immunity), if other benign diseases are compared with similar clinical characteristics (e.g., dermatosis, parapsoriasis, eczema), the main hypothesis continues to be that of an alteration in cellular immunity.

In the European multicenter case-control study, information on infections, skin pathology, and the clinical history 5 years before the diagnosis of MF was used to estimate the risk. The highest risk of MF was found in patients who reported a history of psoriasis 5 years before the diagnosis. Infections and atopic diseases were not closely associated. Whether this can be a causal background or simply reflects early diagnostic uncertainty is not known (Table 2-8).

In a study carried out by Fischmann and colleagues on 43 patients affected by MF or by Sézary syndrome, 86% were regular smokers, 20% habitually used painkillers, 18% used tranquillizers, and 14% used thiazides.

There appears to be no evidence that marital status, smoking habits, mobility (taking journeys), the use of drugs, being exposed to UV light, or consuming alcohol are related to MF. Nevertheless, according to the Fischmann and colleagues study, those patients with chronic cutaneous pathologies and those who have been exposed to a combination of chemical, physical, and biologic agents for a long time, those who smoke a lot, and those who have had recurrent herpes simplex appear to be the first candidates to develop MF.

MORTALITY AND SURVIVAL

In the United States, fewer than 100 deaths per year are attributed on average to this neoplasm. In the period between 1950 and 1975 (excluding 1972), 1948 deaths were attributed to MF (see Table 2-6). The annual average rates of mortality, specified by age, revealed a greater rate in men than in women, and likewise the same happened between the nonwhite and the white race. The annual average rate of mortality, adjusted by age and according

TABLE 2-8   Odds Ratios for Definitive and Possible Cases of Mycosis Fungoides According to Infection or Atopic Dermatitis Reported Present 5 Years before Mycosis Fungoides Was Diagnosed

	Cases Pos	Controls	Definitive Cases			Possible Cases		
			ORc	ORa	95% CI	ORc	ORa	95% CI
Infection								
No	18	8	733	1	1	Ref.	1	1	Ref.
All*	36	14	1367	1.1	1.5	0.8–2.7	1.0	1.3	0.6–3.2
Dermatitis								
No	53	19	2276	1	1	Ref.	1	1	Ref.
Yes	13	7	417	1.4	1.6	0.8–3.0	2.0	2.3	0.9–5.5

* Missing data on infection or dermatitis were excluded.

All, mumps or herpes or hepatitis; CI, confidence interval; OR, odds ratio; ORa, odds ratio adjusted by sex, age, and country; ORc, crude odds ratio.

From Morales-Suarez-Varela M, Olsen J, Johansen P, Kaerlev L, Guenel P, Arveux. P, et al. Viral infection, atopy and mycosis fungoides: a European multicentre case-control study. *Eur J Cancer.* 2003;39:511.

to race during this 25-year period, was men from the white race, 0.53×10^6; women from the white race, 0.28×10^6; men from the nonwhite race, 0.84×10^6; and women from the nonwhite race, 0.54×10^6. The mortality rate increases with age, with a mortality peak found between 65 and 69 years of age for men from the nonwhite race and between 75 and 84 years of age for men from the white race.

By means of data in the United States between 1950 and 1975, greater mortality rates were observed among men from the white race and in northeastern urban areas. No consistent difference was noted as far as the socioeconomic level is concerned. Mortality was greater in the counties having the following industries: oil, rubber, metal, machinery, and printing, although no consistent difference was noted as far as the socioeconomic level is concerned.

In summary, the survival of patients with MF and other forms of CTCL depend on the diagnosis and treatment but the data remain challenging. There is a multitude of clinical and histopathologic presentations (>20 forms have been described) as well as a variety of therapeutic options with a lack of randomized trials to establish efficacy with adequate epidemiologic surveillance.

ACKNOWLEDGMENT

I am indebted to Prof. J. Olsen from Aarhus University, Denmark.

SUGGESTED READINGS

Alibert JLM. *Description des Maladies de la Peau Observées a l'Hôpital St. Louis.* Paris: Barrois L'aire et Fils; 1806:413.

Bazin PAE. *Maladies de la Peau Observées a l'Hôpital St. Louis.* Paris, 1876.

Beljaards RC, Meijer CJLM, Scheffer E, Toonstra J, Van Vloten W, Avan der Putte SCJ, et al. Prognostic significance of CD30 (Ki-1/Ber-H2) expression of primary cutaneous large-cell lymphomas of T-cell origin. A clinicopathologic and immunohistochemical study in 20 patients. *Am J Pathol.* 1989;135:1169–1178.

Berger CL, Eisenberg A, Soper L, Chow J, Simone J, Gapas Y, et al. Dual genotype in cutaneous T cell lymphoma: immunoglobulin gene rearrangement in clonal T cell. *J Invest Dermatol.* 1988;90:73–77.

Berkson J. Limitations of the application of fourfold table analysis to hospital data. *Biometrics.* 1946;2:47.

Bernstein L, Deapen D, Ross RK. Mycosis fungoides. *JAMA.* 1989;261:1882.

Burke JS, Hoppe RT, Cibull ML, Dorfman RF. Cutaneous malignant lymphoma. A pathologic study of 50 cases with clinical analysis of 37. *Cancer*. 1981;47:300–310.

Clegg LX, Feuer EJ, Midthune DN, Fay MP, Hankey BF. Impact of reporting delay and reporting error on cancer incidence rates and trends. *J Natl Cancer*. 2002;94(20):1537-1545.

Cohen SR, Stenn KS, Braverman IM, Beck GJ. Clinicopathologic, relationships, survival, and therapy in 59 patients with observations on occupation as a new prognostic factor. *Cancer*. 1980;46:2654–2666.

Evans H, Winkelmann R, Banks P. Differential diagnosis of malignant and benign cutaneous infiltrates. *Cancer*. 1979;44:699–717.

Fischmann AB, Bunn PA Jr, Guccion JG, Matthews MJ, Minna JD. Exposure to chemicals, physical agents, and biologic agents in mycosis fungoides and the Sézary syndrome. *Cancer Treat Rep*. 1979;63:591–596.

Greene MH, Dalager NA, Lamberg SI, Arguropoulos CE, Fraumeni JF Jr. Mycosis fungoides: epidemiologic observations. *Cancer Treat Rep*. 1979;63,597–606.

Kaudewitz P, Stein H, Dallenbach F. Primary and secondary Ki-1+ (CD30+) anaplastic large cell lymphomas. *Am J Pathol*. 1989;135:1169.

Koch SE, Zackheimer HS, Williams ML, Fletcher V, Boit PE. Mycosis fungoides beginning in childhood and adolescence. *J Am Acad Dermatol*. 1987;17:563–568.

Lutzner MA, Edelson R, Schein R, Green I, Kirkpatrick C, Ahmed A. Cutaneous T-cell lymphomas: the Sézary syndrome, mycosis fungoides, and related disorders. *Ann Intern Med*. 1975;83:534–552.

McFadden N, Nyfors A, Tanum G, Granholt A, Helme P, Kavli G. Mycosis fungoides in Norway 1960-80. *Acta Derm Venereol Suppl (Stockh)*. 1983;109:1–13.

Non-Hodgkin's lymphoma pathologic classification project. National Cancer Institute sponsored study of classification of non-Hodgkin's lymphomas: summary and description of a Working Formulation for clinical usage. *Cancer*. 1982;49:2112–2135.

Noorduyn L, Avan der Valk P, van Heerde P, Vroom TM, Blok P, Willemze R, et al. Stage is a better prognostical indicator than morphological subtype in primary non-cutaneous T-cell lymphomas. *Am J Clin Pathol*. 1990;93:49–57.

Olivan Ballabriga A, Reparaz Prados J, Sala Bonita J. Micosis fungoide asociada a infección por VIH. *Anal Med Intern*. 1990;7:83.

Rowden G, Lewis MG. Langerhans cells: involvement in the pathogenesis of mycosis fungoides. *Br J Dermatol*. 1976;95:665.

Stansfeld AG, Diebold J, Kapanci Y, Kelenyi Gleaner K, Mioduszewska O, Noel H, et al. Updated Kiel classification for lymphomas. *Lancet*. 1989;9:7–9.

Tan RA, Butterworth CM, McLaughlin H, Malka S, Samman PD. Mycosis fungoides—a disease of antigen persistence. *Br J Dermatol*. 1974;91:607–616.

The Non-Hodgkin's Lymphoma Pathologic Classification Project. National Cancer Institute–sponsored study of classifications of non-Hodgkin's lymphomas: summary and description of working formulation for clinical usage. *Cancer*. 1982;49:2112.

Tuyp E, Burgoyne A, Aitchison T, MacKie R. A case-control study of possible causative factors in mycosis fungoides. *Arch Dermatol*. 1987;123:196–200.

Weinstock MA, Horm JW. Mycosis fungoides in the United States. *JAMA*. 1988;60:42–46.

Weinstock MA, Horn JW. Mycosis fungoides in the United States: increasing incidence and descriptive epidemiology. *JAMA*. 1988;260:42–46.

Weiss LM, Hu E, Wood GS, Moulds C, Cleary ML, Warnke R, et al. Clonal rearrangements of T-cell receptor genes in mycosis fungoides and dermatopathic lymphadenopathy. *N Engl J Med*. 1985;313,539.

Whittemore AS, Holly EA. Mycosis fungoides in relation to environmental exposures and immune response: a case-control study. *J Natl Cancer Inst*. 1989;81:1560.

Willemze R, Meijer CJ, Scheffer E, Kluin PM, Van Vloten WA, Toonstra J, et al. Diffuse large cell lymphomas of follicular center cell origin presenting in the skin. A clinicopathologic and immunologic study of 16 patients. *Am J Pathol*. 1987;126:325–333.

Willemze R, Meijer CJLM, Van Vloten WA, Scheffer E. The clinical and histological spectrum of lymphomatoid papulosis. *Br J Dermatol*. 1982;107:131–144.

Yang K, Li YW, Li JY, Zhang YH. T-cell lymphoma. Natl Cancer Inst Monogr. 1989;69:35–37.

APPROACH AND ASSESSMENT FOR A PATIENT WITH SUSPECTED CUTANEOUS LYMPHOMA

John C. Hall, MD

There is no more difficult task as a clinician than to decide whether a skin lesion has the potential for malignancy. Nowhere is this task more daunting that with lymphoma of the skin. This is in part due to the protean manifestations of cutaneous lymphoma and in part due to the confusing nomenclature used to define this condition.

If it is considered a possibility, a workup is mandatory. A skin biopsy is the essential first step, but other parts of the workup may involve repeat biopsy of the skin or other organs, evaluation of other organs by laboratory testing or imaging, and often most important of all, persistent and adequate follow-up.

To begin this discussion, it is necessary to review the circumstances in which cutaneous lymphoma should be suspected. The early markers need to be emphasized because early diagnosis may improve outcome and this is when the disease is often missed. Cutaneous T-cell lymphoma (CTCL) is the most common skin lymphoma and

will be emphasized (Figure 3-1). Sun-protected skin is the most common location for CTCL to begin and can be an early clue that a lymphoma may be present.

The following conditions indicate where lymphoma should be most highly suspected as a skin disease:

Pruritus is often the first sign of cutaneous lymphoma. It can even be the only sign in patients with in cognito CTCL. These patients can only be diagnosed with a high degree of suspicion for a localized area of recalcitrant, and often severe, pruritus by a skin biopsy.

Dry skin in a localized area that does not respond to moisturizers or corticosteroid ointments. This dryness often is accompanied by redness and/or scaling (Figure 3-2).

Asymmetrical areas of hypopigmentation, especially if there is accompanying dryness, scaling, pruritus, or induration (Figure 3-3).

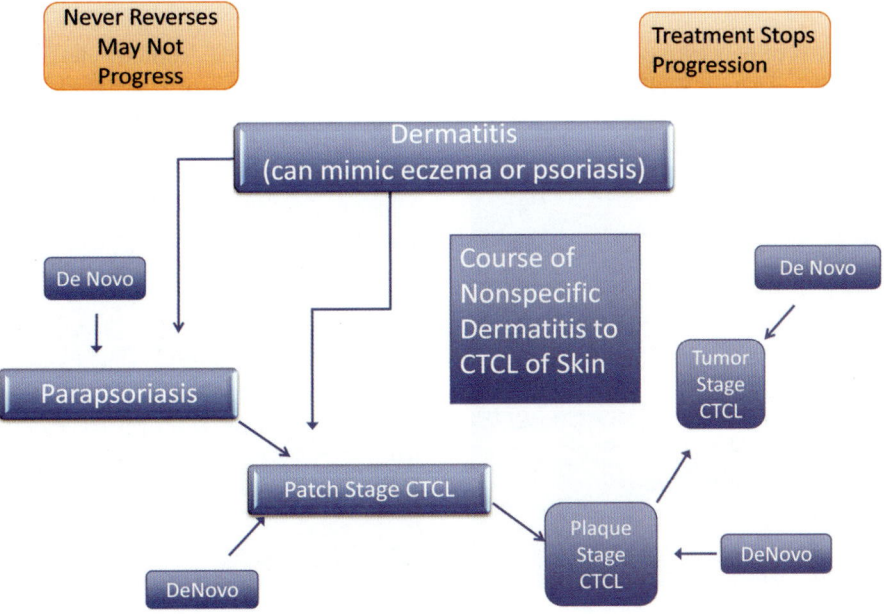

Figure 3-1 Progression of cutaneous T-cell lymphoma (CTCL).

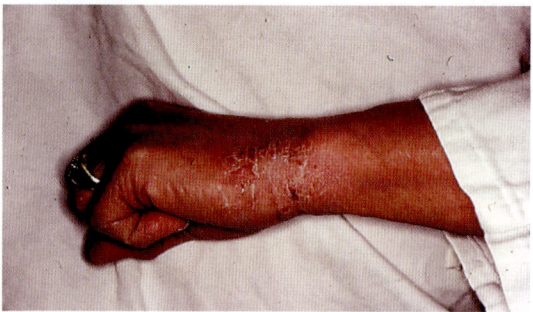

Figure 3-2 Dry, scaling skin with excoriations indicative of pruritus in CTCL.

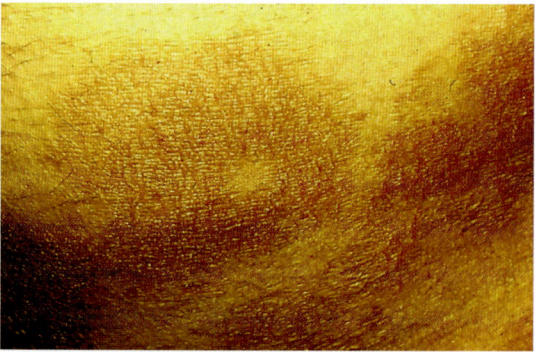

Figure 3-5 Reticulate hyperpigmentation on the abdomen of a patient with CTCL.

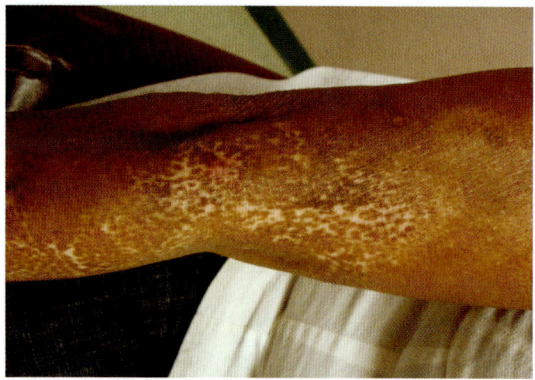

Figure 3-3 Hypogmentation on the extensor forearm with lichenification indicating the patient has been scratching this area of CTCL.

Asymmetrical areas of hair loss, especially if there is accompanying dryness, scaling, pruritus, or induration (Figure 3-4).

Hyperpigmentation, especially in a reticulate or lacy configuration. Alternating bands of hyper- and hypopigmentation may appear (Figure 3-5).

Livedo reticularis in which a reticulate or lacy configuration of purplish bands appears.

Cigarette paper wrinkling atrophy is subtle but helpful. The fine wrinkling can be brought out by squeezing the skin to emphasize the crinkled skin (Figure 3-6).

Induration with a firm woodiness of the skin is important not only as an initial marker but also as a sign that early patch stage disease is progressing.

General signs that should alert the clinician include recalcitrance of a dermatitis to therapy that would normally respond to treatment, longevity

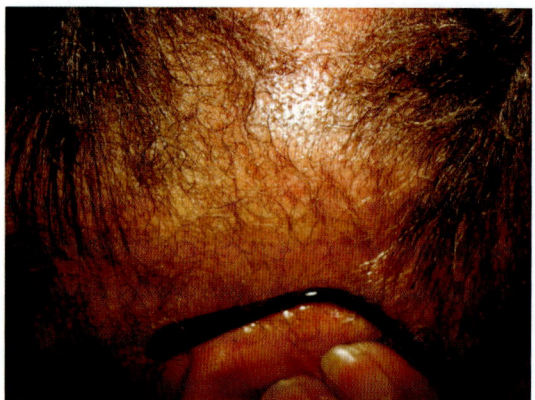

Figure 3-4 Asymmetrical temporal alopecia in a patient with CTCL.

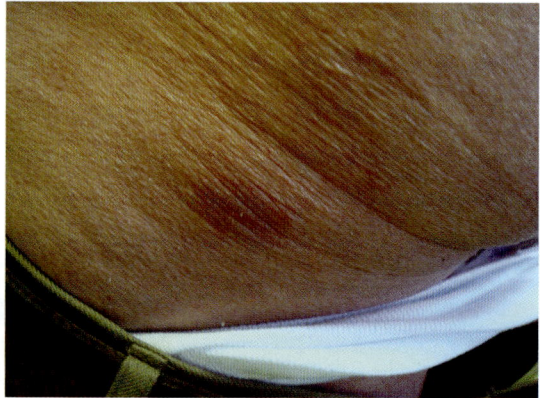

Figure 3-6 Cigarette paper wrinkling atrophy on the waist of a patient with CTCL.

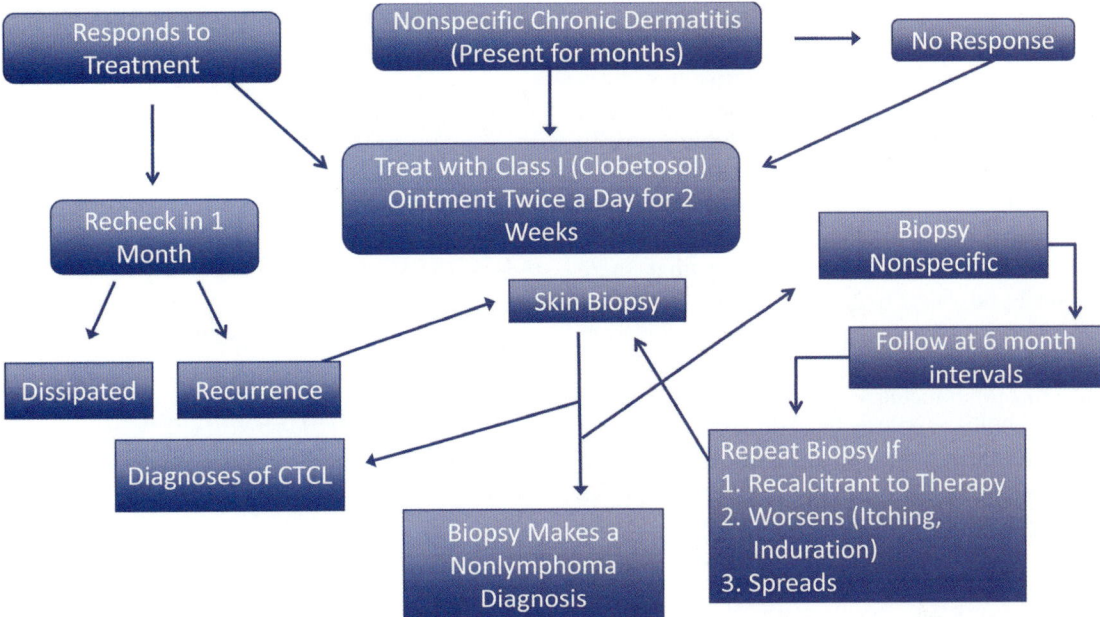

Figure 3-7 Evaluation of nonspecific skin inflammation for CTCL (a suggestion).

of a dermatitis (months to years instead of days to weeks), unusual location (only away from sun-exposed sites), asymmetrical (vs. symmetrical drug eruption, viral exanthema, or autoimmune disease), and severity of symptoms (more pruritic, redder, indurated, or desquamative than expected).

Remember that skin a biopsy is easily done with minimal pain and inconvenience and lawsuits are rarely done for failure to restrain from doing a biopsy.

Late markers of disease are less easily confused with nonspecific skin irritation. They can arise de novo in stages II or III (Figure 3-7). Although more suspicious, these signs are much less common.

Plaques, which are often pink to red or hyperpigmented, are asymmetrical in location and configuration.

Papules (Figure 3-8) and tumors (Figure 3-9) can be of any size and may be seen singly or more often in a cluster or asymmetrical clusters. The color tends to pink, red, or purplish (plum-colored). The surface may be ulcerated.

Parapsoriasis is a curious nonspecific dermatitis that may or may not be a precursor to CTCL. In spite of the name, it is not related to psoriasis.

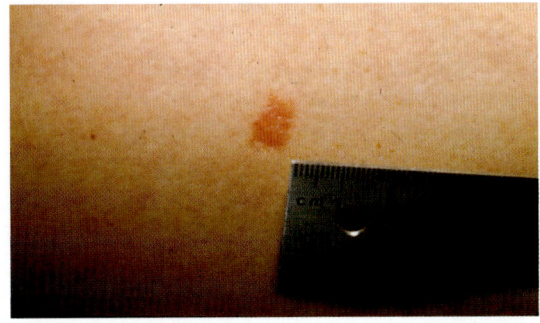

Figure 3-8 Nonspecific pink papule on the lower back that, on biopsy, was CTCL.

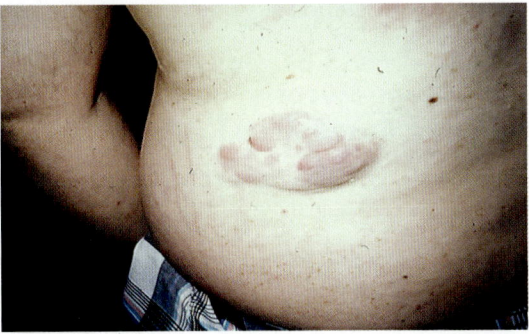

Figure 3-9 Large purple-pink tumor that was the presenting sign of cutaneous B-cell lymphoma. The diagnosis was confirmed only on the third biopsy, that was deeper than the first two.

Generalized pruritus is more a sign of systemic lymphoma, especially Hodgkin's disease. Generalized exfoliative erythroderma may be a sign of CTCL up to 50% of the time especially in patients older than 50 years. It is ominous if no other reason for the skin findings are evident such as a previously existing skin disease or a pertinent medication.

The rule of skin presentation is that there are really no rules. Expect the unexpected. Rare clinical variants are not rare and are discussed in Chapter 6. These rare presentations include vasculitis, thrombophlebitis, panniculitis, nonhealing ulcer, cellulitis, carbuncle, and epidermal cyst. These diagnoses may be seen on biopsy along with the cutaneous lymphoma or may simply be a mimic of the lymphoma; on biopsy, all that is seen is the lymphoma. If the skin condition does not react to therapy as expected, consider a significantly deep biopsy. Superficial biopsies can be misleading and show only a surrounding area of inflammation. Repeat biopsies should be done if suspicion is high because sampling error is always a possibility. Not sending a tissue specimen for histologic examination, even if suspicion is low, is not recommended.

The single most important principle is to err on the side of overdiagnosis instead of underdiagnosis.

CTCL can mimic psoriasis and eczema so biopsy if the course is atypical.

SUGGESTED READINGS

Ann Diagn Pathol. 2010;14:369–385.

Early Stage Mycosis Fungoides Variants: Case-based Review

Cho-Vega JH, Tschen JA, Duvic M, Vega F.
St. Joseph Dermatopathology, Houston, TX 77030, USA. Available at: vegaelena@ymail.com
Oncology (Williston Park). 2010;24:491–501.

Diagnosis and Management of Mycosis Fungoides

Galper SL, Smith BD, Wilson LD.
Department of Therapeutic Radiology, Yale University School of Medicine, New Haven, CT 06520.
Semin Oncol Nurs. 2006;22:90–96.

Cutaneous T-cell Lymphoma

Gemmill R.
Acta Derm Venereol. 2010;90:12–17.

Pruritus in Cutaneous T-cell Lymphomas: Frequent, Often Severe, and Difficult to Treat

Meyer N, Paul C, Misery L.
Cancer Treat Res. 2009;146:343–351.

Cutaneous Lymphomas

Seçkin D, Hofbauer GF.
Department of Dermatology, Faculty of Medicine, Başkent University, 06490, 5. sokak No. 48, Bahçelievler, Ankara, Turkey.
Curr Probl Cancer. 2008;32:43–87.

Cutaneous Lymphoma

Smith BD, Wilson LD.
USAF Medical Corps, Wilford Hall Medical Center, Lackland AFB, TX.
PMID: 18325433 [PubMed - indexed for MEDLINE]
Ann Oncol. 2009;20(Suppl 4):115–118.

Primary Cutaneous Lymphoma: European Society for Medical Oncology (ESMO) Clinical Recommendations for Diagnosis, Treatment, and Follow-up

Willemze R, Dreyling M; ESMO Guidelines Working Group.
Department of Dermatology, Leiden University Medical Center, Leiden, The Netherlands.

APPROACH AND ASSESSMENT OF SKIN BIOPSY FOR A PATIENT WITH SUSPECTED CUTANEOUS LYMPHOMA

Wang L. Cheung, MD, PhD, and Jennifer R. Kaley, MD

INTRODUCTION

Cutaneous lymphomas, comprised of clonal proliferations of T or B lymphocytes, historically represent a diagnostic challenge to both pathologists and clinicians. When a biopsy is performed under clinical suspicion, the pathologist needs to determine whether a neoplasm is present and, if so, to classify the lesion to the appropriate diagnostic category. Accurate diagnosis is critical in determining the treatment plan, surveillance, and prognosis of the disease. Several tools are available to the pathologist to aid in diagnosis, including histology, immunohistochemistry (IHC), and molecular studies. Whereas none of these are diagnostic when analyzed alone, they should be interpreted in context of one another in order to arrive at a complete diagnostic picture.

The latest WHO (World Health Organization)/EORTC (European Organization for Research and Treatment of Cancer) classification scheme takes into account the unique morphologic, immunohistochemical, and genetic properties of primary cutaneous lymphomas, which are considered entities separate from their nodal counterparts because primary cutaneous lymphomas behave different clinically, have a different prognosis, and require different treatment than systemic lymphomas with cutaneous manifestation.

Other systemic conditions may initially present in the skin, such as natural killer (NK) cell lymphoma, adult T-cell lymphoma, or less commonly, precursor B-lymphoblastic leukemia/lymphomas and acute myeloid leukemia. These should be considered but are not discussed.

HISTOPATHOLOGY

Any biopsy suspected of cutaneous lymphoma will be examined routinely with a hematoxylin-and-eosin (H&E) stain. We typically decide quickly where the inflammatory cells are located. Normally, determining whether the inflammatory cells are located only at the superficial dermis and epidermis or at the dermis as a nodular infiltrate is very helpful. Cells in the superficial dermis and epidermis could represent mycosis fungoides (MF), whereas cells in the dermis could represent other cutaneous T-cell lymphoma or B-cell lymphoma. The next step is to determine what types of inflammatory cells are in these infiltrate (e.g., lymphocytes, histiocytes, eosinophils, neutrophils, or enlarged atypical cells). In general, a mixture of different inflammatory cells favors a reactive process; however, there are cases of cutaneous T-cell lymphoma that can contain many eosinophils.

When the infiltrate is predominantly superficial and involving the epidermis (epidermotropic), the main histologic differential diagnosis is cutaneous T-cell lymphoma such as MF. There are some histopathologic features that one can use to determine whether further histology workups (i.e., immunohistochemical stains or gene rearrangement) are needed. Some of these features are shown in Figure 4-1 and listed here:

1. Pautrier microabscesses.
2. Hyperchromatic and irregular nuclear contour of the lymphocytes.
3. "Tagging" of the dermoepidermal junction by the lymphocytes.
4. Enlarged lymphocytes.
5. Thickened collagen bundles within the papillary dermis.
6. Halo lymphocytes.

In the dermis, we always look for enlarged cells and determine whether these are histiocytes or enlarged (activated) lymphocytes. Histiocytes usually have enlarged nuclei with vesicular chromatin and irregular nuclear contours. In contrast, CD30+ cells have more euchromatic nuclei with prominent irregular shaped nucleoli. Again, immunostains can be used to help differentiate these cell types.

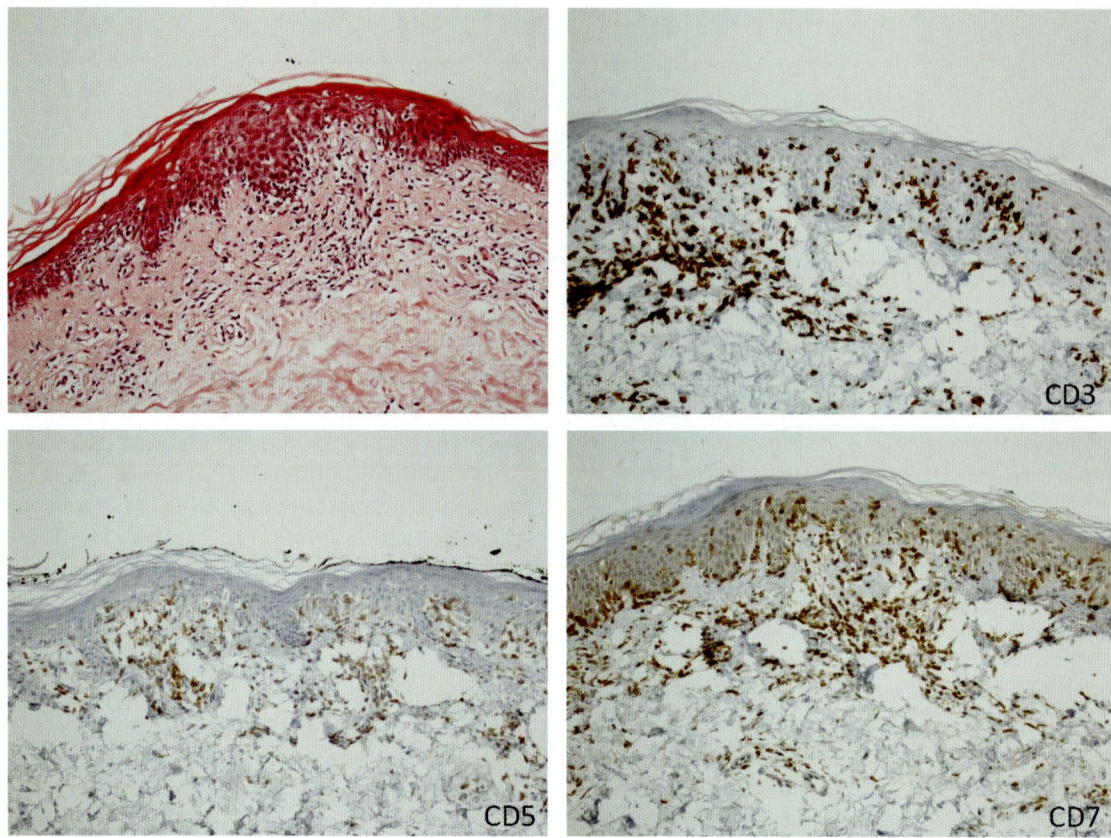

Figure 4-1 Mycosis fungoides and immunophenotypes. Routine hematoxylin and eosin stain and immunostains for CD3, CD5, and CD7 demonstrate epidermotropic lymphocytes with some loss of expression of T-cell antigen CD5.

When the infiltrate is predominantly in the dermis, one needs to determine whether the lymphocytes are involving the follicular epithelium to rule out the possibility of a folliculotropic mycosis fungoides (FMF). If the infiltrate is dermal-based and if the cells are predominantly lymphocytes, it is critical to determine whether the cells are T cells or B cells. Because most infiltrates in the skin are T cells, any clusters of B cells are unusual unless they are forming a reactive germinal center. Even then, a follicular lymphoma or a marginal zone lymphoma (MZL) needs to be ruled out with further immunohistochemical studies.

Because it is impossible to tell the phenotypes of lymphocytes from histopathology, pathologists do rely heavily on IHC (see the next section) for making the diagnosis of cutaneous lymphoma.

IMMUNOHISTOCHEMISTRY

As an adjunct to histolopathology, IHC is a tool used by pathologists in assessing the neoplastic nature of the lymphoid population in question, and if it is neoplastic, IHC is used to classify the infiltrate into a specific type of lymphoma. Immunohistochemical staining is performed by the laboratory on formalin-fixed, paraffin-embedded tissue specimens and basically consists of a primary antibody that binds to the antigen in question. Then, using a secondary antibody linked to an enzyme will create a specific color of choice in cells that are interpreted as positive.

When the pathologist is presented with an atypical lymphocytic infiltrate, it is helpful to determine whether the infiltrate is composed of T lymphocytes (CD3+) or B lymphocytes (CD20+).

In consideration of morphologic clues, a panel of immunohistochemical stains can then be strategically chosen in order to arrive at the best diagnosis. Characteristic immunophenotypical features have been established for many cutaneous lymphomas. However, aberrant expressions and inconsistencies are not uncommon, and therefore, IHC results must always be interpreted in concert with histology rather than independently. We first discuss the T-cell lymphomas and then the B-cell lymphomas. Some of the common cutaneous lymphomas and their IHC pattern are discussed in the following sections.

Cutaneous T-cell Lymphomas

Mycosis Fungoides

Immunohistochemistry
Diagnostic Highlights

- Classic immunophenotype: CD2+, CD3+, CD4+, CD5+. CD45RO+, CD8−, T-cell receptor-beta–positive (TCR-β+), and CD30−.
- Full or partial deletion of multiple T-cell antigens.
- Increased CD4/CD8 ratio.

MF is the most common cutaneous lymphoma accounting for nearly 50% of all primary cutaneous lymphomas. Routine morphologic features (discussed previously) are the gold standard for diagnosing MF (see Figure 4-1), although ancillary studies can be helpful in providing additional evidence in suspicious cases. This disease evolves in a stepwise fashion, from patches to plaques and eventually dissemination of tumor to lymph nodes, blood, bone marrow, and other organs. The term MF should be used only for the classic "Alibert-Bazin" type, characterized by this clinical evolution.

The classic phenotype of MF is CD2+, CD3+, CD4+, CD5+, CD45RO+, CD8−, TCR-β+, and CD30−. A panel including CD2, CD3, CD5, CD7, CD8, and CD79a is reasonable in evaluating loss of T-cell markers in a possible MF (see Figure 4-1). Loss of expression of pan–T-cell antigens such as CD7 (most common), CD5, and CD2, especially in the epidermotropic cerebriform cells, has been previously reported to be of diagnostic value in MF, especially in later disease. However, CD7 deletion

may be considered nonspecific because this may also occur in the benign lymphocytic infiltrates or atypical MF. A diagnosis of MF was also more likely when multiple epidermal T-cell antigens were deleted. Figure 4-1 shows focal loss of CD5 expression in the epidermotropic lymphocytes. Deletions in T-cell antigens of the dermal component were not significant predictors of MF.

Elevation of CD4/CD8 due to clonal expansion of CD4+ cells can also be diagnostically useful. Harvell and coworkers performed a detailed study of lymphocyte subsets in MF and other dermatoses, evaluating intraepidermal lymphocytes (where most of the neoplastic lymphocytes reside, especially in early disease) and found that, for spongiotic dermatoses, the CD4/CD8 ratio was 2, lichen planus 2.1, lichen sclerosis and psoriasis 0.1, and MF 6.2. A cutoff of value of at least 2.4:1 in the epidermal compartment maximizes sensitivity (69%) and specificity (93%) for a diagnosis of MF. Figure 4-2 illustrates a plaque stage MF, which shows a CD4/CD8 ratio of greater than 100:1. In early MF, there may be a brisk infiltrate of CD8+ cells in response to the neoplastic cells, thus altering the CD4/CD8 ratio. Other cutaneous conditions may contain lymphocytes that express CD8, which can alter the CD4/CD8 ratio. Actinic reticuloid usually has a predominant CD8+ phenotype, and so does human immunodeficiency virus (HIV)–associated dermatitis, pityriasis lichenoides et varioliformis acuta, lichen sclerosis, and psoriasis. In addition, Langerhans cells that populate the dermis and epidermis can falsely elevate the CD4/CD8 ratio.

When the disease progresses and large cell transformation occurs, CD4+ epidermotropic cells can express a cytotoxic phenotype (TIA-1 and granzyme B) and CD30. CD30 positivity in the majority of the neoplastic population is most frequently observed in the later stages of disease (plaque or tumor); however, care must be taken not to mistake nodules of histiocytes for transformed MF (CD3 and CD68 will help confirm the nature of the population). As the disease progresses, there is greater likelihood of T-cell antigen loss and Ki-67 activity. Rare cases of otherwise classic MF can have a CD4−, CD8+ mature T-cell phenotype; these cases have the same clinical behavior and should not be considered as separate entities.

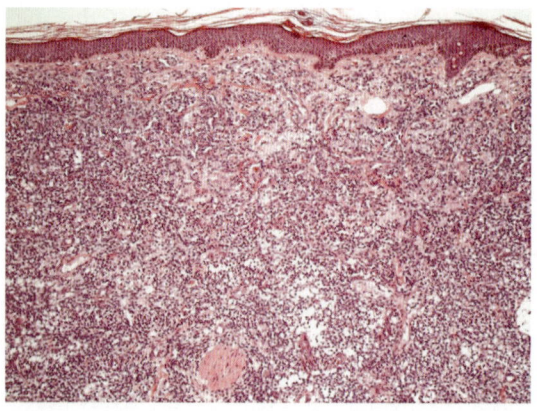

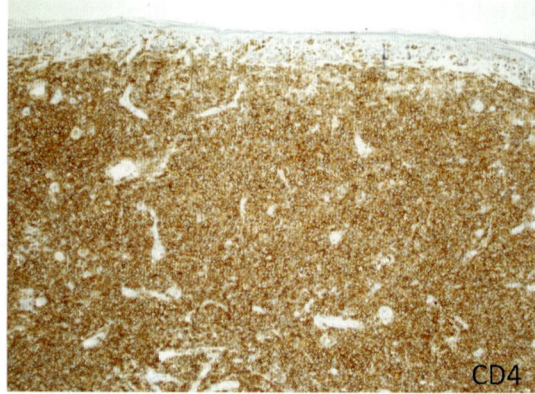

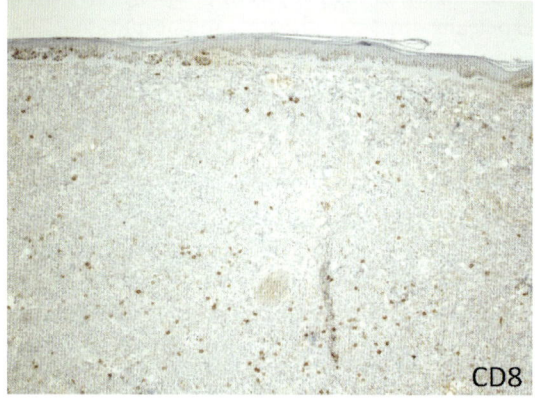

Figure 4-2 Mycosis fungoides, plaque stage. Hematoxylin and eosin stain, CD4 and CD8 immunostains. The H&E shows a dense dermal nodular proliferation of atypical lymphocytes. The immunostains demonstrate a lymphoid population with a CD4/CD8 ratio of greater than 100:1.

Variants of Mycosis Fungoides

Folliculotropic Mycosis Fungoides

FMF is a variant of MF that is classified as its own entity. Compared with conventional MF, this variant has a more aggressive course and poorer prognosis, with poorer response to treatment. The characteristic finding in FMF is small to medium atypical CD3+ CD4+ CD8– T lymphocytes around and within the epithelium of the hair follicles. The neoplastic infiltrates are deep, making them less accessible to skin-targeted therapies. In FMF, the CD4/CD8 ratio is frequently 10:1 and the follicles show abundant CD1a+ cells. The CD4+ cells are seen mainly in the infundibular and isthmic epithelium.

Immunophenotype is useful when attempting to distinguish between primary follicular mucinosis and lymphoma-associated follicular mucinosis, an important diagnostic challenge among pathologists. Primary follicular mucinosis (PFM) is a spontaneously remitting process that

occurs in children and young adults. Lymphoma-associated follicular mucinosis occurs in elderly patients. Follicular mucinosis is positive when stained with colloidal iron and negative for periodic acid–Schiff (PAS). A stain for Alcian blue will frequently be positive. Rongioletti and colleagues found that in four of five cases of lymphoma-associated follicular mucinosis, CD4+ cells were more numerous than CD8+ cells with a 3:1 ratio, whereas in seven of the eight PFM cases, they were almost as numerous as CD8+ cells. Clinical information such as the location, size, and number of lesions and the age and medical history should be considered in these cases.

Pagetoid Reticulosis

Pagetoid reticulosis is characterized by a solitary patch or plaque, localized to the extremities, with an intraepidermal proliferation of neoplastic T cells. The neoplastic T cells may have either a CD3–, CD4+, CD8– or a CD3+, CD4–, CD8+ phenotype. CD30 is commonly expressed.

Granulomatous Slack Skin

Granulomatous slack skin is an extremely rare variant of MF. The tumor cells display a T-helper immunophenotype (CD3+, CD4+, CD8–, CD45RO+) with possible loss of T-cell markers (CD 3, CD5, and CD7). Giant cells of histiocytic origin are present and are positive for CD68 and Mac 387+. In rare cases, the tumor cells express CD30. Scattered S-100+ cells may also be detected in the infiltrate.

Sézary's Syndrome

Immunohistochemistry Diagnostic Highlights

- Mature T-helper cells with a memory cell phenotype with the following immunohistochemical profile: CD2+, CD3+, CD4+, CD5+, CD45RO+, CD8–, and CD30–.
- The majority of Sézary cells are also CLA+ and CD7–.

Sézary's syndrome (SS) is a leukemic form of cutaneous lymphoma characterized by erythroderma, lymphadenopathy, and presence of neoplastic T cells (Sézary cells) in skin, lymph nodes, and peripheral blood with an absolute Sézary cell count of at least 1000 cells/mm^3. Some studies confirmed the importance of identifying circulating clonal T cells in making the diagnosis. Other useful criteria include a CD4/CD8 ratio of more than 10 and loss of any or all T-cell antigens including CD2,

CD3, CD4, and CD5. Sézary cells also frequently lose expression of CD26and CD7.

CD30+ Lymphoproliferative Disorders

Primary cutaneous CD30+ lymphoproliferations represent the second most common group of cutaneous T-cell lymphomas and comprise a spectrum of diseases including lymphomatoid papulosis (LyP), primary cutaneous anaplastic large-cell lymphoma (C-ALCL), and so-called borderline cases. Borderline cases include those that cannot be specifically classified as either C-ALCL or LyP. So classified, these entities share expression of CD30, and thus, the final diagnosis must include careful histologic and clinical correlation. In addition, many benign reactive conditions can contain large CD30+ cells. Figure 4-3 shows the histopathologic picture of a CD30+ lymphoproliferative disorder and immunostain indicating CD30 positivity.

Lymphomatoid Papulosis

IMMUNOHISTOCHEMISTRY DIAGNOSTIC HIGHLIGHTS

- Tumor cells express the markers of mature T cells (CD3+, CD4+, CD8–, CD30+, and CD56+) and of activated T cells (human leukocyte antigen [HLA]–DR and CD25+).
- CD30+ in LyP types A and C.
- CD30– in LyP type B.

LyP is a chronic, recurrent, self-healing papulonodular eruption with histologic features suggestive

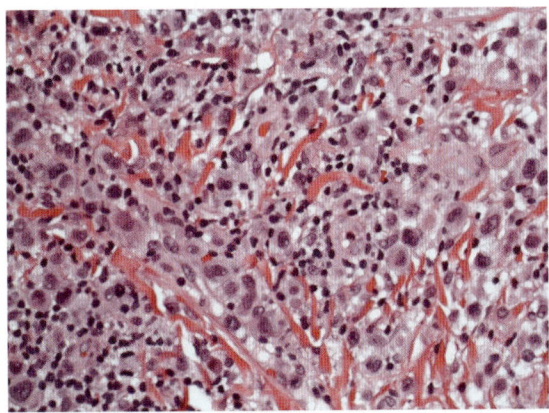
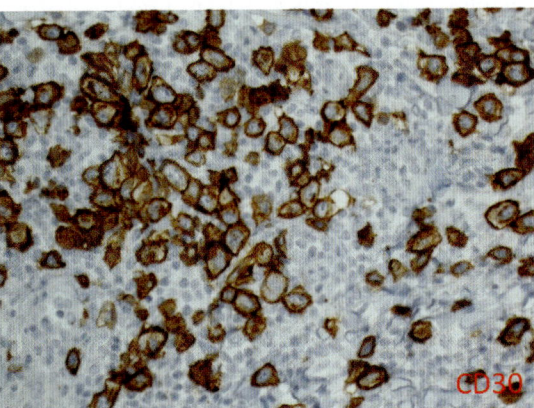

Figure 4-3 CD30+ lymphoproliferative disorder. Hematoxylin and eosin stain and CD30 immunostain highlight a dermal lymphoid population of enlarged lymphocytes with CD30 positivity.

of a malignant lymphoma but with a benign clinical course. These lesions are found in various stages of healing on the trunk and limbs, most commonly in adults. Three subtypes have been described (A, B, and C) that represent a spectrum of overlapping features. In type A lesions, multinucleate Reed-Sternberg–like CD30+ cells are intermingled with inflammatory cells. Type C lesions contain a monotonous population of CD30+ cells with little to no admixed inflammatory cells. Type B is uncommon (10%) and is characterized by an epidermotropic infiltrate of atypical lymphocytes with cerebriform nuclei, as seen in MF. In all types, T antigens such as CD2 and CD5 are often expressed, and CD7 is often absent. CD15 (characteristic marker for Reed-Sternberg cells in Hodgkin's lymphoma) is not expressed by tumor cells in LyP A. Small tumor cells with the classic cerebriform nuclei (LyP B) are usually negative for CD30.

Primary Cutaneous Anaplastic Large-cell Lymphoma

IMMUNOHISTOCHEMISTRY DIAGNOSTIC HIGHLIGHTS

■ Tumor cells with activated T-cell phenotype with expression of T-cell antigens CD2, CD3, CD4, CD45RO and activation markers CD25, CD30, CD71, and HLA-DR.
■ Variable loss of expression (CD2, CD3, CD5).
■ Anaplastic lymphoma-related tyrosine kinase (ALK) negative.

Primary cutaneous anaplastic large-cell lymphoma (ALCL) presents as a single nodule or group of nodules, often ulcerated, which are confined to one area of the body. It is characterized by CD30 expression of at least 75% of the large pleomorphic or anaplastic cells seen within the nonepidermotropic infiltrate. As in LyP, an activated T-cell phenotype along with variable loss of T-cell antigens is seen. When compared with nodal ALCL, C-ALCL does not express EMA but instead may express cutaneous lymphocyte antigens (CLA and HECA-452) and homeobox gene HOXC5.

Another differential diagnosis in the CD30+ lymphoproliferative disorder is blast transformation of MF. In these cases, there is usually some evidence of MF in the biopsy or in a biopsy from another location. In addition, many benign reactive conditions exist in which CD30+ cells can be found; however, in these conditions the CD30+ population does not usually form a majority of the infiltrate or gather in dense cohesive clusters. Clinical and histologic correlation is essential.

Subcutaneous Panniculitis-like T-cell Lymphoma

Immunohistochemistry Diagnostic Highlights

■ Tumor cells originate from α/β T cells with a cytotoxic profile.
■ T-cell–associated antigens CD2+, CD3+, CD4–, CD5+, CD8+, CD43+.
■ Cytotoxic proteins TIA-1+, granzyme B+, perforin+.

Subcutaneous panniculitis-like T-cell lymphoma (SPTCL) originates and presents primarily in the subcutaneous fat, often involving the legs, and includes neoplastic T cells of the α/β receptor class; others with γ/δ phenotypes are included in the group of peripheral T-cell lymphomas, not otherwise specified (NOS). A common diagnostic conundrum is the distinction between SPTCL and a lobular panniculitis, for example, lupus profundus. Lupus profundus may be confined to the subcutis and display atypical lymphocytes; however, the monomorphic immunoprofile of SPTCL contrasts the polymorphic infiltrate in lupus profundus.

Other T-cell Lymphomas

Adult T-cell Leukemia/Lymphoma

Adult T-cell leukemia/lymphoma is a T-cell neoplasm associated with infection of human T-cell leukemia virus 1 (HTLV-1). The neoplastic T cells express a CD3+, CD4+, CD8– phenotype. CD25 is highly expressed.

Cutaneous γ/δ T-cell Lymphoma

Cutaneous γ/δ T-cell lymphoma is a clonal proliferation of mature, activated, γ/δ T cells expressing a cytotoxic phenotype. These cells can involve the epidermis, dermis, and subcutis. The clinical course is quite aggressive when compared with the α/β type, which reaffirms the need to separate the entities into two groups.

Primary Cutaneous Aggressive Epidermotropic CD8+ Cytotoxic T-cell Lymphoma

Also known as "Berti's lymphoma," primary cutaneous aggressive epidermotropic CD8+ cytotoxic T-cell lymphoma presents with erosive plaques and exhibits a rapid, aggressive course.

Primary Cutaneous CD4+ Small/Medium-sized Pleomorphic T-cell Lymphoma

Primary cutaneous CD4+ small/medium-sized pleomorphic T-cell lymphoma is a noncytotoxic cutaneous T-cell lymphoma characterized by a predominance of small to medium-sized CD4+ pleomorphic T cells. Clinical features in this entity are incompatible with MF.

Extranodal Natural Killer/T-cell Lymphoma, Nasal Type

Extranodal NK/T-cell lymphoma, nasal type, is nearly always an Ebstein-Barr virus–positive (EBV+) lymphoma of small, medium, or large cells with an NK-cell or possibly a cytotoxic T-cell phenotype. Skin involvement may be a primary or secondary manifestation of the disease; however, each has an aggressive clinical course and the treatment is the same, and so distinction between primary and secondary is not required.

Cutaneous B-cell Lymphomas

In contrast to T cells, a substantial infiltrate of B lymphocytes is a rare feature of a reactive process. Therefore, the presence of a heavy B-cell population even with little or insignificant atypia is sufficient grounds for suspecting a B-cell lymphoma. The architecture of the infiltrate and the histologic features of the cells should help guide the interpretation of the IHC when diagnosing B-cell lymphomas. Evaluation of the presence or absence markers of germinal centers (CD10 and bcl-6), postgerminal center cells (MUM-1), and follicular dendritic networks (CD21 and CD23) are useful when evaluating B-cell lymphomas.

Primary Cutaneous Follicle Center Lymphoma

Immunohistochemistry Diagnostic Highlights

- CD19+, CD20+, CD79a+, bcl-6+, bcl-2–.
- CD23 and CD10 variable.
- MUM-1 may highlight a minority of cells scattered among the infiltrate.
- Absence of detectable surface immunoglobulin.

Primary cutaneous follicle center cell lymphoma (PCFCCL) occurs commonly on the scalp, forehead, and trunk. The most important differential diagnosis includes follicular pseudolymphoma, MZL, and diffuse large B-cell lymphoma. The identification of the neoplastic B cells as of germinal center origin is crucial in making the diagnosis. There is usually a vague follicle center with CD79+ and bcl-6+ (Figure 4-4). In contrast to their nodal counterparts, PCFCCLs generally do not express bcl-2 and are not associated with t(14;18). These lymphomas rarely disseminate to extracutaneous sites and have an excellent prognosis.

Cutaneous Marginal Zone Lymphoma

Immunohistochemistry Diagnostic Highlights

- CD19+, CD20+, CD22+, CD79a+, CD5–, CD10–, CD23–, bcl-6–, bcl-2+, and monotypic light chain expression in the majority of cases.
- Aberrant expression of CD43 is helpful.
- CD21 reveals regular and irregular networks of follicular dendritic cells corresponding to sites of involved follicles.

The interfollicular infiltrate represents the neoplastic portion of cutaneous MZL. Distinguishing this entity from cutaneous lymphoid hyperplasia (CLH) is a diagnostic challenge, and histology, architecture, clinical history, and IHC must be considered. IHC or in situ hybridization (ISH) for kappa and lambda light chain can be helpful

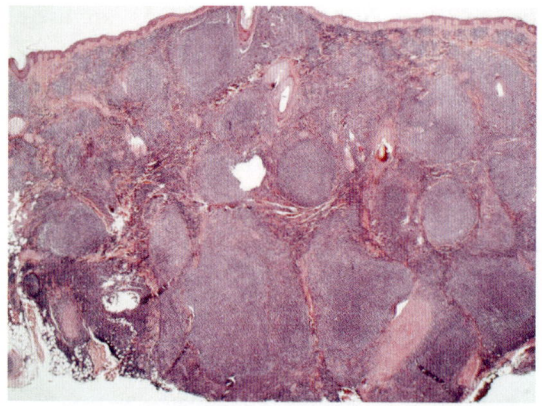

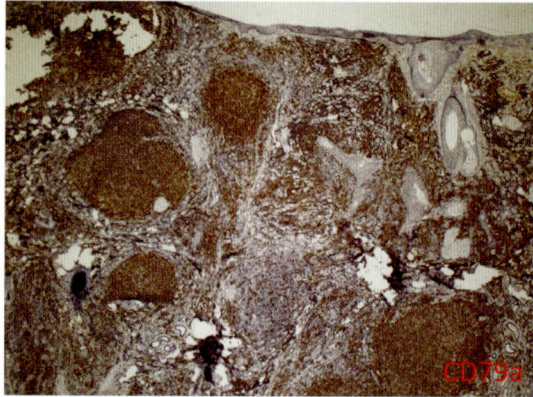

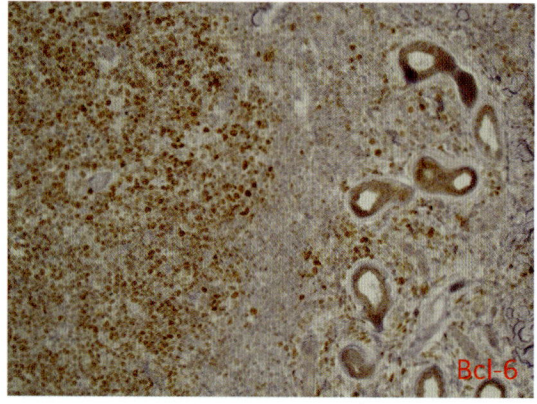

Figure 4-4 Primary cutaneous follicle center cell lymphoma. Hematoxylin and eosin stain and immunostains for CD79a and bcl-6. The H&E shows a proliferation of lymphocytes in follicle centers pattern. Both CD79a and Bcl-6 highlight the follicle center cells.

to show the presence of a light chain restriction. ISH uses deoxyribonucleotide probes to detect kappa or lambda mRNAs in paraffin-fixed tissues. Figure 4-5 shows a case of cutaneous MZL with plasma cells and lymphoplasmacytoid cells with ISH showing lambda light chain restriction. Dissemination to extracutaneous sites has not been reported in primary cutaneous MZL.

Cutaneous Diffuse Large B-cell Lymphoma

Primary cutaneous diffuse large B-cell lymphomas (DLBCL) include two forms: DLBCL, leg-type (DLCBL,LT), and DLBCL, other. The most common is the leg type, and as named, it occurs most frequently on the leg. In fact, location on the leg is the most significant factor in predicting adverse prognosis. The other variants comprise T-cell–/histiocyte-rich DLBCL, intravascular large B-cell lymphoma, plasmablastic lymphoma, and others, which do not fit into the leg type.

Diffuse Large B-cell Lymphoma, Leg Type

IMMUNOHISTOCHEMISTRY DIAGNOSTIC HIGHLIGHTS

- CD19+, CD20+, CD22+, CD79a+, CD5–, CD10–, CD138–, cyclin D1–.
- Bcl-2 and MUM-1/IRF4+.
- Bcl-6 is mostly positive.

DLBCL,LT, affects primarily the elderly and shows a higher relapse rate and a more unfavorable prognosis than those forms arising on the head and trunk. Multiple skin lesions correlate with a more unfavorable prognosis. As the name implies, these cells are enlarged and atypical with high proliferative index as shown by Ki-67 immunostain (Figure 4-6). There is a significantly higher incidence of bcl-2 expression in DLBCL,LT, than in those arising in the upper body. Some cases may co-express bcl-6 and CD10, indicating that a proportion of these lymphomas are of follicle center origin.

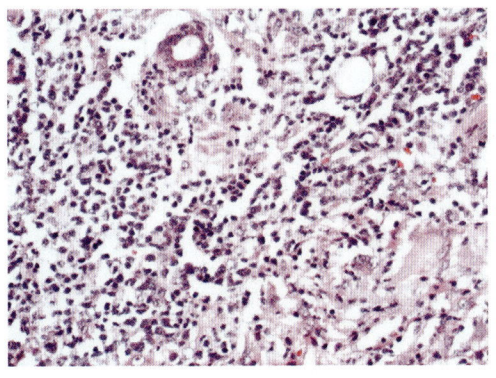

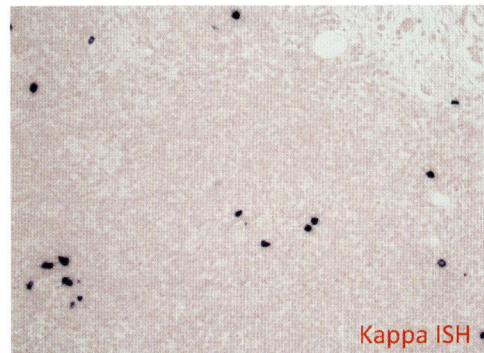

Kappa ISH

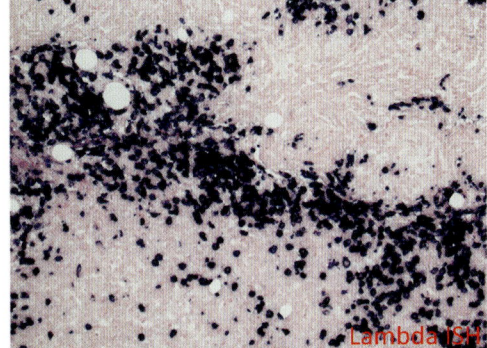

Lambda ISH

Figure 4-5 Cutaneous marginal zone lymphoma. Hematoxylin and eosin stain shows plasma cells and lymphoplasmacytoid cells in the dermis. The in situ hybridization for both kappa and lambda reveals a lambda light chain restriction which supports a clonal proliferation.

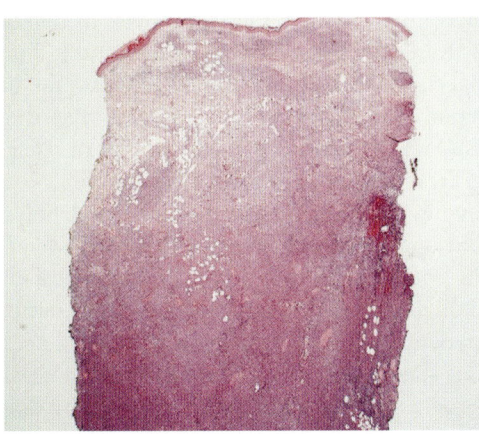

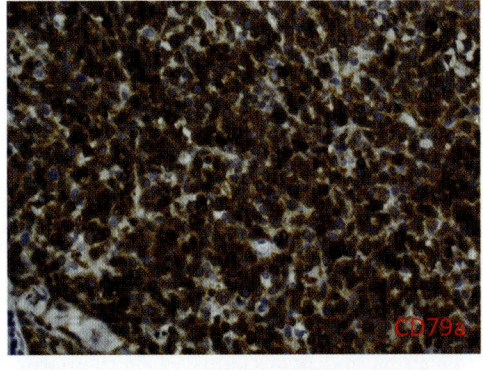

CD79a

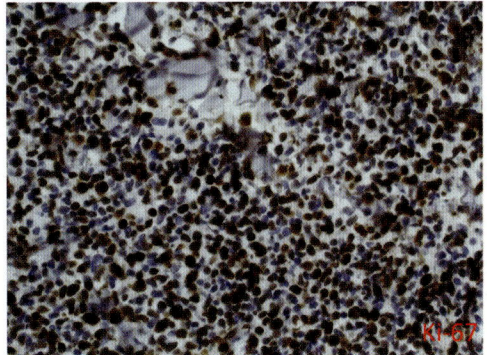

Ki-67

Figure 4-6 Diffuse large B-cell lymphoma, leg type. Hematoxylin and eosin stain shows a dense dermal lymphoid infiltrate containing large and atypical cells. These cells are CD79a positive. Immunostain for Ki-67 demonstrates a very high proliferative index.

Diffuse Large B-cell Lymphoma, Other

DLCBL, other, comprises large B-cell neoplasms that lack the typical features of DLBCL,LT, and do not fit into the follicular category. These cases include anaplastic or plasmablastic variants of DLBLC, T-cell–/histiocyte-rich large B-cell lymphomas and intravascular large B-cell lymphoma. Plasmablastic lymphomas are seen almost exclusively in the setting of immune deficiency (e.g., HIV infection). These lymphomas will have immunophenotypic characteristics similar to the other B-cell lymphomas and are rather categorized according to clinical features and histology.

GENE REARRANGEMENT

Cutaneous lymphoproliferative disorders are usually diagnosed based on morphologic and immunophenotypic characteristics; however, in 5% to 15% of cases, the differential diagnosis between a malignant lymphoma and a reactive lymphoproliferation is difficult. In these cases, molecular clonality studies of immunoglobulin or T-cell receptor (TCR) rearrangements can be employed to assist the pathologist in distinguishing these lesions. Molecular results must be interpreted in the context of clinical, histologic, and immunohistochemical findings because some clinically benign cutaneous entities may demonstrate clonal expansion of lymphocytes.

T and B cells each express unique surface antigen receptors that serve as a specific marker for that cell and all of its clonal progeny. For T cells, this is the TCR, and for B cells, the immunoglobulin (Ig) molecule. Ig molecules are composed of heavy chains and light chains. TCRs are composed of either alpha and beta chains (95% of mature T cells) or gamma and delta chains. Each of these contain unique rearrangements of several variable (V), diversity (D), and joining (J) regions, a process that occurs sequentially in the earliest stages of lymphoid differentiation. These unique rearrangements are present in almost all immature and mature lymphoid cells. Because a neoplasm arises from the clonal expansion of a malignantly transformed cell, virtually all cells composing the neoplasm will contain one or several clonal Ig and/or TCR gene rearrangements. In a reactive process, several different T cells are present and a polyclonal or oligoclonal pattern would be expected; therefore, monoclonality is a key feature of malignant lymphoid cell populations.

Gene amplification techniques involving the polymerase chain reaction (PCR) has essentially replaced Southern blotting in detecting clone-specific rearrangements. In a European collaborative study known as BIOMED-2, standardized techniques in TCR gene rearrangement analysis were developed and are now widely used by clinical molecular laboratories today. Advantages of PCR over Southern blotting include suitability for smaller tissue samples, enhanced sensitivity, more rapid results, avoidance of radioactive labeling, and decreased cost. Analysis can be performed on formalin-fixed tissue; however, it is preferable to submit fresh tissue in order to ensure intact DNA. Gene rearrangement analysis of the TCR-gamma gene is most commonly used for studying T-cell clonality; the gamma gene is targeted because its relatively simple structure requires fewer sets of PCR primers and because the gamma gene is rearranged early in T-cell development. For B-cell clonality, Ig heavy chain (IgH) gene rearrangement analysis is often preferred.

In interpreting gene rearrangement studies, it is important for the pathologist to be familiar with the specific assay being used and to know its special features and limitations. Several limitations exist that must be considered. Based on the BIOMED-2 study of PCR analysis of TCR gene rearrangements, the sensitivity is limited (~10%), owing to the presence of the normal polyclonal background and to the low tumor burden found in cutaneous lymphomas. For instance, monoclonality in skin and peripheral blood samples of patients with MF is more likely to be detected in late stages of the disease or in patients with disease progression. In addition, monoclonality does not necessarily equate to malignancy. Several clinically benign conditions have a clonal origin, for example, CD8+ and CD4+ T-cell lymphocytosis, LyP, initial phase of EBV+ lymphoproliferations, pityriasis lichenoides, and lupus panniculitis. This further emphasizes the importance of interpreting molecular results in the context of clinical, histologic, and immunophenotypic findings. An integrated, multidisciplinary approach to diagnosis of cutaneous lymphomas should be utilized to ensure the arrival at the correct diagnosis.

CONCLUSION

Accurate classification of cutaneous lymphomas represents a unique diagnostic challenge to pathologists. Characteristic histologic features and immunophenotyping are essential tools when attempting to classify a lesion, and gene rearrangement studies are available in more difficult cases that require additional testing. Each of these aspects of pathologic diagnosis must be interpreted in context of one another and in consideration of the clinical picture. As in all realms of pathology, aberrancies and exceptions are not uncommon; thus, in establishing a diagnosis, a good pathologist will consider the entire picture rather than one piece of the puzzle. Finally, effective communication with the patient's clinician, other pathologists, molecular biologists, and laboratory technicians is an invaluable tool in making the correct diagnosis and providing exceptional patient care.

SUGGESTED READINGS

Boon DL, Guitart J, Gerami P. Follicular mycosis fungoides: a histopathologic, immunohistochemical, and genotypic review. *G Ital Dermatol Venereol.* 2008;143:409–414.

Burg G, Kempf W, Cozzio A, Feit J, Willemze R, Jaffe A, et al. WHO/EORTC classification of cutaneous lymphomas 2005: histologic and molecular aspects. *J Cutan Pathol.* 2005;32:647–674.

Florell S, Cessna M, Lundell RB, Boucher KM, Bowen GM, Harris RM, et al. Usefulness (or lack thereof) of immunophenotyping in atypical cutaneous T-cell infiltrates. *Am J Clin Pathol.* 2006;125:727–736.

Gallardo F, García-Muret MP, Servitje O, Estract T, Bielsa I, Salar A, et al. Cutaneous lymphomas showing prominent granulomatous component: clinicopathologic features in a series of 16 cases. *J Eur Acad Dermatol Venereol.* 2009;23:639–647.

Gerami P, Guitart J. The spectrum of histopathologic and immunohistochemical findings in folliculotropic mycosis fungoides. *Am J Surg Pathol.* 2007; 31:1430–1438.

Goodlad J, Krajewski A, Batstone PJ, McKay P, White JM, Benton EC, et al. Primary cutaneous diffuse large B-cell lymphoma—prognostic significance of clinicopathologic subtypes. *Am J Surg Pathol.* 2003;27:1538–1545.

Groenen PJ, Langerak AW, van Dongen JJ, van Krieken JH. Pitfalls in TCR gene clonality testing: teaching cases. *J Hematop.* 2008;1:97–109.

Harvell JD, Nowfar-Rad M, Sundram U. An immunohistochemical study of CD4, CD8, TIA-1, and CD56 subsets in inflammatory skin disease. *J Cutan Pathol.* 2003;30:108–113.

Ismail SA, Han R, Sanborn SL, Stevens SR, Cooper KD, Wood GS, et al. Immunohistochemical staining for CD45R isoforms in paraffin sections to diagnose mycosis fungoides-type cutaneous T-cell lymphoma. *J Am Acad Dermatol.* 2007;56:635–642.

Kandolf Sekulovic L, Cikota B, Stojadinovic O, Basanovic J, Skiljevic D, Medenica LJ, et al. TCRgamma gene rearrangement analysis in skin samples and peripheral blood of mycosis fungoides patients. *Acta Dermatovenerol Alp Panonica Adriat.* 2007;16:149–155.

Langerak AW, Molina TJ, Lavender FL, Pearson D, Flohr T, Sambade C, Schuuring E, et al. Polymerase chain reaction–based clonality testing in tissue samples with reactive lymphoproliferations: usefulness and pitfalls. A report of the BIOMED-2 Concerted Action BMH4-CT98-3936. *Leukemia.* 2007;21:222–229.

Robson A. Immunocytochemistry and the diagnosis of cutaneous lymphoma. *Histopathology.* 2010; 56:71–90.

Ronglioletti F, De Lucchi S, Meyes D, Mora M, Rebora A, Zapo S, et al. Follicular mucinosis: a clinicopathologic, histochemical, immunohistochemical and molecular study comparing the primary benign form and the mycosis fungoides–associated follicular mucinosis. *J Cutan Pathol.* 2010;37:15–19.

van Dongen JJM, Langerak AW, Brüggemann M, Evans PAS, Hummel M, Lavender FL, et al. Design and standardization of PCR primers and protocols for detection of clonal immunoglobulin and T-cell receptor gene recombinations in suspect lymphoproliferations: report of the BIOMED-2 Concerted Action BMH4-CT98-3936. *Leukemia.* 2003;17:2257–2317.

Willemze R, Jaffe ES, Burg G, Cerroni L, Berti E, Swerdlow SH, et al. WHO-EORTC classification for cutaneous lymphomas. *Blood.* 2005;105:3768–3785.

Willemze R. Primary cutaneous lymphomas. *Curr Opin Oncol.* 2000;12:419–425.

Wood GS. T-cell receptor and immunoglobulin gene rearrangements in diagnosing skin disease. *Arch Dermatol.* 2001;137:1503–1506.

MYCOSIS FUNGOIDES (CUTANEOUS T-CELL LYMPHOMA)

Amy Musiek, MD, and Ellen J. Kim, MD

SETTING THE STAGE AND HISTORY

Over the past 200 years, our understanding of mycosis fungoides (MF) and Sézary syndrome (SS) has grown from a clinical description in 1806 by Alibert, a French physician, who described a patient with skin tumor resembling mushrooms, to a complex field of diagnosis, tumor staging, treatment algorithms, and pathophysiologic mechanisms.

Alibert provided the first clinical description of MF in 1806 by describing a 56-year-old man with skin tumors. In 1870, Bazin described the natural progression of the disease from the premycotic stage to the infiltrative plaque stage and, finally, the tumor stage. These classic stages have transcended time and remain integrated into even the current staging system. Today, MF that follows this classic progression is described as the *Alibert-Bazin variant.* The concept of mycosis d'emblee (eruptive tumors in the absence of patch or plaque disease) was introduced in 1885 by Vidal and Brocq, although they may have been describing what we know today as the recently more clearly characterized group of aggressive cutaneous cytotoxic T-cell or natural killer (NK)/T-cell lymphomas (such as aggressive epidermotropic CD8+ cutaneous T-cell lymphoma [CTCL], γ/δ CTCL, NK/T-cell lymphomas). The erythrodermic stage of the disease was described in 1892 by Besnier and Hallopeau, but it was not until 1938 that Sézary and Bouvrain reported a patient with erythroderma, adenopathy, pruritus, hair loss, and circulating mononuclear cells that had convoluted nuclei. Louis Winer referred to the intraepidermal abscess of Pautrier in 1946, but these lesions had originally been described by Darier in 1889. SS appeared in the U.S. literature in 1961 when Taswell and Winkelmann described seven cases observed at the Mayo Clinic from 1946 to 1960. Finally, in 1975, the term *cutaneous T cell lymphoma (CTCL)* was coined when the cell of origin of MF and SS was determined to be skin-homing T cells.

Reflecting on the current treatment of MF and SS, many organizations have contributed to propose diagnostic, staging, and clinical practice guidelines to ensure that patients receive the highest quality care. In 1992, the International Society of Cutaneous Lymphoma (ISCL) was founded to increase knowledge of lymphoproliferative diseases and related skin disorders. Then, in 2005, a joint classification of cutaneous lymphomas was published by the World Health Organization (WHO) and European Organization for Research and the Treatment of Cancer (EORTC) reclassifying the diseases that, only 30 years earlier, had been combined under the term *CTCL.* In 2007, the ISCL and EORTC announced an updated staging system for MF and SS that incorporated further classification of blood involvement as well T-cell receptor clonality status, and the U.S. National Comprehensive Cancer Network (NCCN) added MF and SS to their online Non-Hodgkins Lymphoma Clinical Practice of Oncology Treatment Guidelines in 2008. Finally, in 2009, the U.S. Cutaneous Lymphoma Consortium (USCLC) was formed with the goal of providing a collaborative platform for research, clinical trials, and treatment guidelines on this disease (similar to the EORTC CTCL platform in Europe).

PATHOGENESIS

Defining the pathogenesis of MF is complicated by its many variants and relationship with other CTCL variants. Particularly complex is the relationship between MF and SS. At its simplest, MF is characterized by malignant skin-homing mature T cells. This discussion includes a characterization of these T cells and discussion of the malignant transformation of these cells with the hope that an understanding of these mechanisms will lead to more targeted and effective treatments.

GENETICS

MF and SS are not strictly genetically determined cancers and no discrete genetic abnormality has been uniformly detected in early patch/plaque disease. In early disease, defects in apoptosis caused by decreased Fas signaling and increased STAT activation likely contribute to slow tumor cell "accumulation" rather than rapid proliferation. In more advanced tumor and erythrodermic disease, numerous genetic abnormalities have been detected including chromosomal deletions (1p, 10q, 17p) and gains (4q, 18, 7q). In addition, defects in tumor suppressor genes such as p53, p14, p15, p16, and PTEN, defects in JunB and human leukocyte antigen (HLA)–G signaling, as well as hypermethylation of mismatch repair genes have been reported in advanced stages as well.

THE MALIGNANT T-CELL/ SKIN-HOMING T-CELLS

As the field of immunology continues to grow, so does our understanding of the malignant T cell in MF. In 1971, the cell of origin in SS was confirmed to be a lymphocyte. We now know that the origin of the malignant T cell in MF is a skin resident effector memory T cell. These effector memory T cells are long-term residents in the skin produced during the normal physiologic immune response. Studies demonstrate that greater than 95% of the T cells in normal skin are memory T cells. These cells proliferate after keratinocyte damage from infection or environmental exposures and stimulate antigen-presenting cells. Dendritic cells (DCs) and macrophages are activated after the phagocytosis of antigen or after ligation of various receptors including those in the Toll-like receptor family. After activation, the antigen-presenting cells migrate to the skin-draining lymph nodes where they interact with naïve T cells. Subsequent to this interaction, CD4+ skin resident effector memory T cells and central memory T cells are produced. The skin resident effector memory T cells will be redistributed to the skin, particularly at the site of antigen exposure. The central memory T cells express the lymph node–homing

cell surface markers L-selectin and CCR7 and remain in the lymph nodes and blood awaiting activation via antigenic rechallenge. In contrast to MF, it appears that the central memory T cells are the cells of origin of the malignant T cells in SS.

The skin-homing mechanism for effector memory T cells begin with the up-regulation of E-selectin on postcapillary venules. Binding of the effector memory T- cell to E-selectin occurs via common lymphocyte antigen (CLA) and causes lymphocyte rolling. The CLA+ cells also express CC chemokine receptor 4 (CCR4), which binds CC chemokine ligand 17 and CC chemokine ligand 22 on endothelial cells/basal keratinocytes and Langerhans cells, respectively. These cells also co-express CCR10, whose ligand CC chemokine ligand 27 is expressed on basal keratinocytes. Studies have shown that greater than 90% of CLA+ T cells are in the skin under normal conditions. The chemokine receptors discussed previously are expressed on the skin-homing malignant T cell of MF. Other chemokine receptors expressed in MF include CXCR3 and CXCR4, and other cell surface molecules include integrin $\alpha E/\beta 7$ and LFA-1. Basal keratinocytes, Langerhans cells, and endothelial cells all express ligands for these receptors.

In more advanced stages of MF when epidermotropism is lost, the cell surface molecule expression profile changes. Tumor stage lesions demonstrate decreased CCR4 and CXCR3 expression but an increase in CCR7 expression. In addition, studies have shown lower intercellular adhesion molecule-1 (ICAM-1) expression in tumor stage disease and SS. Finally, as alluded to previously, the cell of origin of MF and SS appear to be different, thus, explaining some variability between the cell surface molecule expression profiles in these two diseases.

Aberrant activation of malignant T cells is believed to play a crucial role in disease pathogenesis. Several T-cell activation markers are overexpressed in CTCL, including CD45ρ, CD25/ interleukin-2 (IL-2) receptor, proliferating cell nuclear antigen (PCNA), and phosphorylated STAT3. As mentioned earlier, anti-apoptotic strategies are also employed by malignant T cells in CTCL including decreased Fas/Fas ligand expression and down-regulation of p53. As our understanding of the molecular events involved in T-cell transformation in CTCL evolves, new diagnostic and therapeutic targets are rapidly being identified.

Several lines of evidence suggest the importance of a host immune deficit in MF patients. There is decreased complexity of the T-cell repertoire in MF patients, which has been described even in early patch disease patients and is most pronounced in tumor and erythrodermic MF patients. The contracted normal T-cell repertoire is similar to that observed in human immunodeficiency virus (HIV) infection. This may explain the susceptibility of late stage MF and SS patients to a variety of infections. It has been suggested that this relative immunosuppression is due to the elaboration of a soluble factor by malignant T cells that impairs normal host T-cell maturation, although the identity of this factor remains elusive.

The activated malignant T-cell clone causes significant immune dysregulation in MF. The malignant skin effector memory T cells are typically CD4+ T-helper cells with a Th2 phenotype. They express increased levels of cytokines IL-4, IL-5, and IL-10. Expression of these cytokines increases as the density of the malignant clone increases (with highest levels seen in erythrodermic MF and SS). This increase in Th2 cytokines leads to increased immunoglobulin E (IgE) production and drives eosinophilia, explaining the atopy-like symptoms associated with the disease.

It has also been hypothesized that this increased expression of Th2 cytokines allows malignant T cells to suppress the host Th1 response and, thus, evade destruction by the host immune system. In early limited patch stage disease, there is a vigorous CD8+/TIA1+ T-cell host response evident in skin biopsies that is diminished in late stage (extensive patch/plaque, tumor, and erythrodermic) disease. In keeping with this, levels of the Th1 cytokines IL-12 and interferon-alpha (IFN-α) in peripheral blood from SS patients decline as the percentage of malignant T cells increases. This decrease in host Th1 response leads to diminished dendritic cell production, which further cripples the host Th1 response and impairs host IFN-γ production. Thus, preserving the host immune response is critical for controlling disease progression.

More recently, Samimi et al. reported Sezary Syndrome patients have upregulation of programmed death-1 (PD-1) on their malignant T-cells in contrast to MF patients or normal controls which may further contribute attenuated immune responses in this group.

EPIDEMIOLOGY

CTCL represents a subgroup of extranodal non-Hodgkin's lymphomas. The 2005 WHO/EORTC joint classification of cutaneous lymphoma classified MF in the CTCL and/or NK-cell lymphoma category. MF is the most common subtype of CTCL and represents greater than 50% of all CTCLs. CTCL has an incidence rate of 7.7 per 1 million person-years, with MF incidence rate accounting for 4.1 per 1 million person-years, based on Surveillance, Epidemiology, and End Results (SEER) program data. Overall, the incidence rates of cutaneous lymphoma and CTCL have risen since 1980, and although the trend also exists for MF, it is less robust. The incidence of MF and SS is similar to Merkel cell carcinoma. Underreporting likely remains an issue for MF and SS.

Whereas incidence rates vary from country to country, risk factors for MF remain consistent. Incidence increases with age before peaking around 80 years. The mean age of onset is approximately 65 years. MF is less common in children. Overall, the incidence is higher in men than in women and in blacks than in non-Hispanic whites. An increased risk of CTCL has been associated with HLA-DR5 and HLA-DQB1*03 alleles, suggesting a genetic predisposition. Cases of familial MF have been reported (particularly from Israel), but the vast majority of MF cases are sporadic (including a few cases of married spouses both having MF, suggesting an environmental trigger).

Despite numerous studies no specific infectious or environmental exposures are known to conclusively trigger MF or SS. Infections studied have included human T-cell lymphotropic virus-1 (HTLV-1), *Borrelia* spp., human herpesvirus-8 (HHV-8), cytomegalovirus, Epstein-Barr virus (EBV), *Chlamydia* spp., and *Staphylococcus aureus*. Chemical exposures studied have included halogenated hydrocarbons. Incidence rates may be higher in metropolitan areas; however, the specific regional incidence rates for MF are not known. As classifications of CTCL are further refined through increased recognition and improved diagnostic techniques, the accuracy of incidence rates and risk factors will continue to improve.

CLINICAL FINDINGS

Clinically, classic MF still follows the Alibert-Bazin progression from patch to plaque to tumor stage disease and favor sun-protected or "double-covered" areas in a bathing trunk distribution. However, there are numerous clinical variants of MF (see Chapter 6) and some variants have a distinct anatomic distribution (e.g., folliculo-tropic MF presents frequently on the scalp, face, and hair-bearing areas and pigmented purpura-like MF presents on the lower extremities). All skin stages may present with pruritus ranging from asymptomatic to debilitating itch generally reflecting the burden of malignant T cells. It is now known that the vast majority of MF patients with early patch disease will not progress (to either more aggressive tumor stage or extracuta-neous involvement).

In patch disease, patients may present with anything from a single lesion to extensive body surface area (BSA) involvement. Patches tend to appear first in sun-protected or "double-covered" regions including the upper inner arms, periax-illary, breasts, waist, hips, buttocks, and upper proximal thighs (Figure 5-1A). The patches tend to be ill-defined erythematous or pink patches with a fine, slightly atrophic "cigarette paper" scale (in contrast to the thicker white scale seen in psoriasis). They are often several centimeters in size. Patches may have a poikilodermatous appearance (atrophic patches with reticulated hypo and hyperpigmentation). Some patches will have a finger-like or "digitate" shape. In patients with skin of color, in addition to the classic pink or red color, hypopigmented or hyperpigmented patches are extremely common. It is not unusual to see a patient with skin of color having patches of varying colors. In such patients, hyperpig-mentation can become even more pronounced when patients undergo treatment (due to postin-flammatory hyperpigmentation); this can take months to years to fully resolve. Patients with thin patches often report a waxing and waning course with spontaneous improvement in summer

months and more pronounced lesions in colder winter months (likely due to seasonal variations in ultraviolet exposure and humidity). Heat can exacerbate lesions (hot showers, exercise or exer-tion, and for some patients, hot weather). Limited patch disease (<10% BSA, T1a classification—see "Staging" section) is frequently asymptomatic and may remain indolent for years. More extensive patch or plaque disease will often be itchy.

The average time to diagnosis of patch MF/CTCL is often years and after multiple biopsies. The reasons for this are multifactorial: early MF lesions when biopsied are often nondiagnostic owing to a brisk host immune response that obscures the tumor cells on histopathology. Furthermore, there are precursor inflammatory disorders character-ized by chronic skin T-cell inflammation without overt phenotypic atypia (sometimes referred to as *T-cell dyscrasias*) that, over time, may in a small subset of patients evolve into MF. Such condi-tions include small plaque parapsoriasis, pityriasis lichenoides, chronic dermatitis, chronic idiopathic erythroderma, alopecia mucinosa, and benign follicular mucinosis. The percentage of patients who evolve from these benign but chronic condi-tions into MF are unknown.

Plaque disease often mirrors patch disease in location and shape, but the lesions become more indurated and well-defined (see Figure 5-1B). Subtle erythema gives way to a red-brown appear-ance. Patients who develop tumor MF (see Figure 5-1C) always give a history of concurrent patches, plaques, or erythroderma. The concept of "tumor d'emblee" disease, presenting initially as tumor nodules only, is outdated and likely represents recently more precisely classified separate aggres-sive cytotoxic CTCL entities. Tumors can appear on mucosal surfaces (oropharyngeal mucosa, vulvovaginal mucosa), face, and scalp and can become ulcerated. MF lesions that are treatment-resistant or undergo an abrupt increase in growth or symptomatology should be biopsied to deter-mine whether there is histologic evidence of large cell transformation (>25% of infiltrate with large cell morphology, frequently but not always CD30+; see Figure 5-1D).

In patients with exfoliative erythroderma, it is difficult clinically to distinguish erythrodermic MF from SS, although classically, SS has a more abrupt and rapid onset whereas erythrodermic MF often arises out of preceding patches/plaques. Patients with exfoliative erythroderma can be a diagnostic challenge and the diagnosis of erythrodermic MF and SS often requires molecular genetic studies and peripheral blood and/or lymph node flow cytometry for accurate diagnosis. The eruption often initially appears eczematous and can progress to a more infiltrative erythroderma with fine white scale (see Figure 5-1E Severe erythroderma due to MF or SS will present with extensive exfoliation or, at times, generalized edema (particularly pedal and lower extremity edema seen in older patients with underlying venous stasis), maceration of body folds, skin fissures, and frequent bacterial impetiginization with yellow crusting or oozing. The vast majority of these patients are severely pruritic and some will have a burning or tingling quality to their itch symptoms or frank peripheral neuropathy. Hyperkeratosis or keratoderma with or without fissuring of the palms and soles

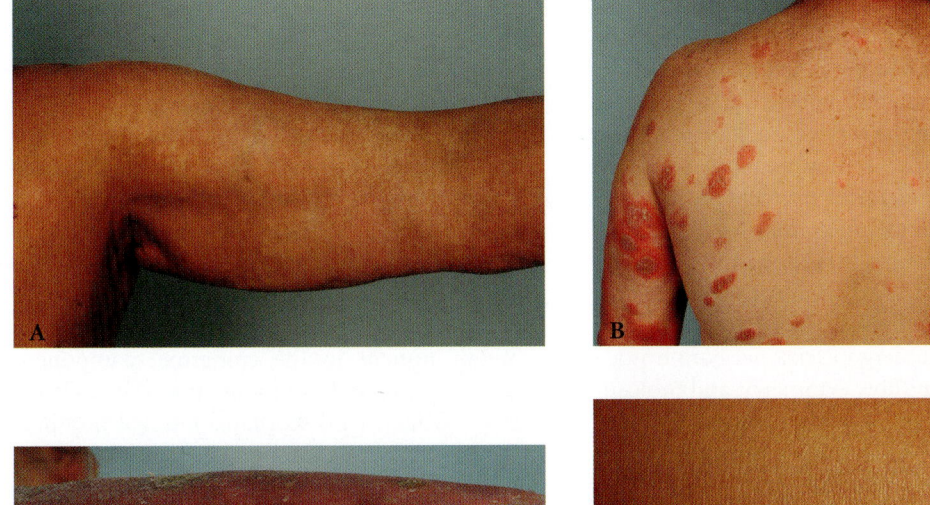

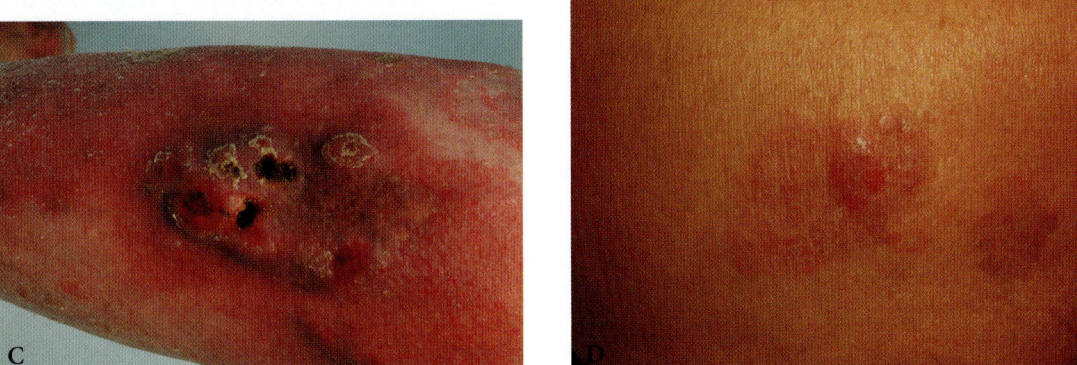

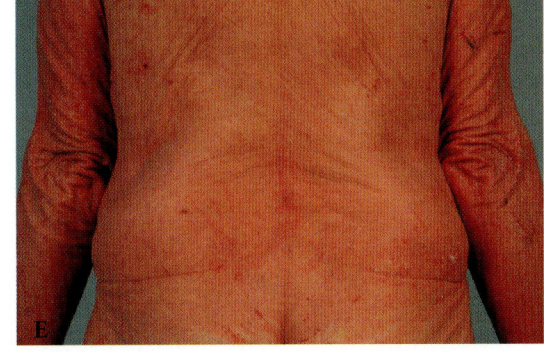

Figure 5-1 a, Patch MF. b, Patch/plaque MF. c, Tumor MF. d, Plaque MF with new nodule emerging (large cell transformation). e, Erythrodermic MF. f, Erythrodermic MF

is common. Alopecia (scalp and body hair areas), ectropion (eversion of the eyelids exposing the eye conjunctiva), and nail dystrophy can occur. Some patients report alterations in sweat gland function. Exfoliative erythrodermic patients may experience low-grade fevers, chills, night sweats, and unintentional weight loss.

Extracutaneous involvement can occur at any site, although the lymph nodes (most common), lungs, spleen, liver, oro-/nasopharynx, and central nervous system (CNS) are the most frequent locations. The risk of extracutaneous involvement is generally related to the degree and severity of skin activity; it is rare for MF to progress systemically if skin activity is in remission. Exfoliative erythrodermic MF or SS patients frequently have palpable peripheral nodes in the cervical, axillary, inguinal, femoral, and rarely, inframammary areas on physical examination. It is difficult to clinically differentiate dermatopathic nodes (N1 classification) from nodes with lymphomatous involvement (N2 and N3 classification), and patients with peripheral lymph nodes larger than 1.5 cm in long axis should undergo excisional lymph node biopsy for histology, flow cytometry, and molecular studies (see "Staging" section). Recent studies indicate that even patients with dermatopathic nodes have a poorer survival than patients with no lymph node involvement. Patients with bulky lymphadenopathy (>3 cm in long axis) may have either nodal large cell transformation due to MF or a separate concomitant lymphoma (such as Hodgkin's disease).

HISTOLOGY

Similarly to the clinical description, the histopathology of MF can be divided into patch, plaque, tumor, and erythrodermic disease. The clinicopathologic correlation is generally present, but in cases in which a disconnect occurs, vigilance is required to ensure the disease does not behave in an unpredictable manner. Punch biopsy specimens for routine histology and immunohistochemistry should be taken from untreated skin. Prior treatment with steroids or phototherapy can make a histopathologic diagnosis difficult. It is often helpful to obtain two biopsies from different sites to aid in the interpretation of clonality

assessments (two skin sites: one skin and one extracutaneous site). T-cell receptor (TCR) gene rearrangement studies for clonality can be performed on paraffin tissue blocks or fresh tissue (which has higher sensitivity).

In early patch disease, the histopathologic features are often subtle and can be overlooked (Figure 5-2A). Generally, there is mild hyperkeratosis, a psoriasiform epidermal hyperplasia, and a superficial perivascular lymphocytic infiltrate. The characteristic atypical lymphocytes, with convoluted and hyperchromatic nuclei surrounded by clear halos, are seen in the epidermis. Often, this is subtle, and they only appear in the lower dermis or even as single cells found along the dermal-epidermal junction ("tagging"). The epidermotropism should be prominent compared with the amount of spongiosis in the epidermis (in contrast to eczematous dermatitis). As noted, the lymphocytic infiltrate should be composed of atypical lymphocytes, although the size of the lymphocytes varies (small vs. medium, less commonly large size). The atypia should be more prominent in the epidermal component than in the dermal component of the infiltrate (epidermal/dermal discordance). Small numbers of eosinophils and plasma cells can be present, and in many cases, papillary dermal fibrosis (indicating chronicity) is seen. Given the difficulty of obtaining a histopathologic diagnosis of MF in early patch patients, the ISCL proposed a point-based diagnostic algorithm to aid in the diagnosis of early MF (Table 5-1). When patients have a clinical presentation highly suspicious for patch MF, but the histology remains nonspecific, TCR/polymerase chain reaction (PCR) studies on two skin specimens or skin and blood can be extremely helpful.

When well-developed plaques are present, the classic histopathologic changes are more likely apparent (see Figure 5-2B). Again the epidermis may demonstrate compact hyperkeratosis, a psoriasiform epidermal hyperplasia, and a lymphocytic infiltrate along the dermal-epidermal junction. There is usually significant epidermotropism or atypical lymphocytes. The classic Pautrier's microabscesses (atypical lymphocytes in close proximity to Langerhans cells) are present in approximately 20% of cases. The perinuclear halos are more prominent, and there may

TABLE 5-1   Algorithm for diagnosis of early mycosis fungoides according to the ISCL

Criteria	Scoring system
Clinical -Basic Persistent and/or progressive patches/thin plaques	2 points for basic criteria and 2 additional criteria
-Additional 1) Non-sun exposed location 2) Size/shape variation 3) Poikiloderma	1 point for basic criteria and 1 additional criterion
Histopathologic -Basic Superficial lymphoid infiltrate -Additional 1) Epidermotropism without spongiosis 2) Lymphoid atypia	2 points for basic criteria and 2 additional criteria 1 point for basic criteria and 1 additional criterion
Molecular biological 1) Clonal TCR gene rearrangement Immunopathologic 1) <50% CD2+, CD3+, and/or CD5+ T-cells 2) <10% CD7+ T-cells 3) Epidermal/dermal discordance of CD2, CD3, CD5 or CD7	1 point for clonality 1 point for 1 or more criteria

*A total of 4 points is required for the diagnosis Of MF based on any combination of points from the clinical, histopathologic, molecular biological, and immunopathologic criteria.

be slightly more spongiosis. The lymphocytic infiltrate is more dense in plaque stage disease and occurs in a superficial and bandlike pattern. Dermal fibrosis is also more prominent than in early stage disease. Eosinophils and plasma cells may still be present. Establishing a diagnosis in the plaque stage is often more straightforward than in patch stage disease.

Tumor lesions tend to lose their epidermotropism (see Figure 5-2C). The infiltrate often occupies the entire dermis and extends into the underlying subcutaneous tissue. The atypical lymphocytic infiltrate has atypical cells that are larger and more pleomorphic in nature. They often have large vesicular nuclei with prominent nucleoli. At this stage, it might become harder to differentiate MF from other lymphomas.

In erythrodermic MF and SS, the disease maintains highly convoluted cerebriform lymphocytes,

but the characteristic epidermotropism is often lost (see Figure 5-2D). One third of biopsies are nondiagnostic or show a nonspecific eczematous pattern. Skin biopsies can demonstrate varied histologic patterns including superficial perivascular lymphocytic infiltrate, spongiosis, parakeratosis, and papillary dermal fibrosis. Commonly, there is a papillary dermal lymphocytic infiltrate with fibrosis of the dermal collagen.

As noted previously, large cell transformation occurs in approximately 5% to 20% of patients with MF (represents molecular evolution of the original malignant T-cell clone) and can occur in skin lesions, lymph nodes, or less commonly, the peripheral blood. Large cell transformation is diagnosed based on histopathologic criteria. The T cell must be four or more times the size of a small lymphocyte and the infiltrate must contain 25% or more large cells or a discrete tumor cell

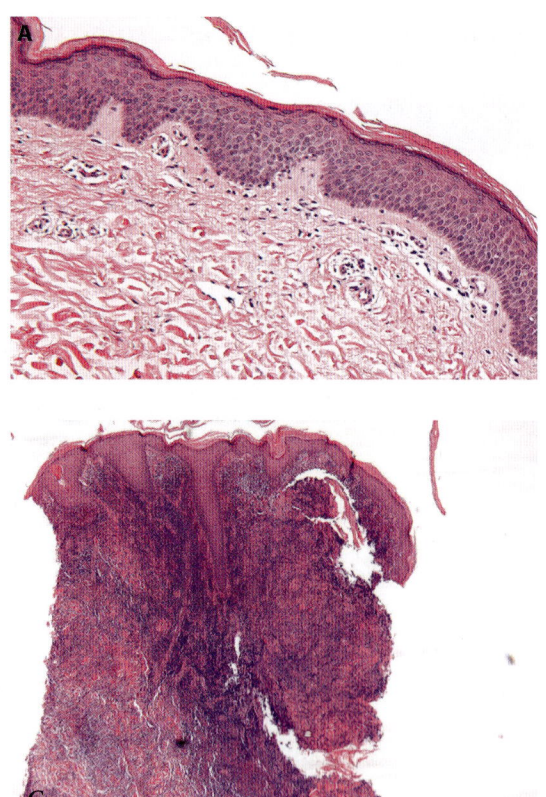

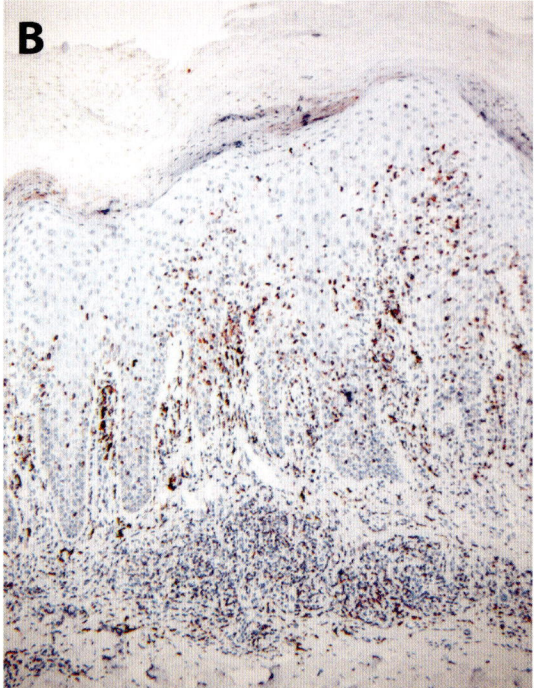

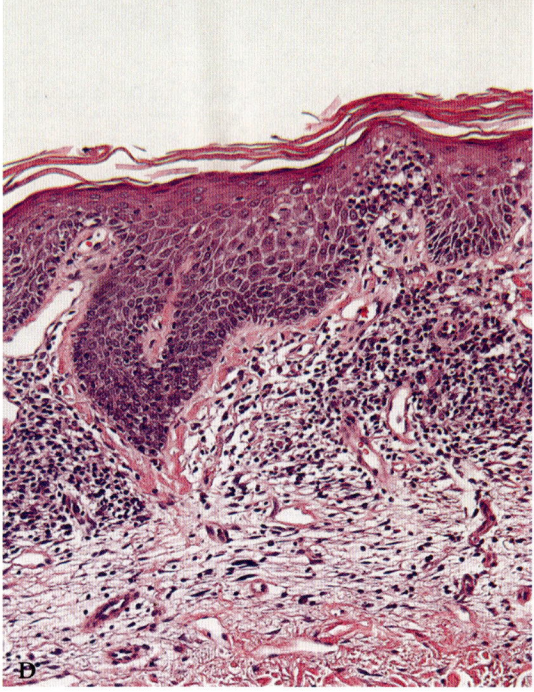

Figure 5-2 a, patch stage mycosis fungoides. A) H&E B) CD3 staining highlighting the subtle "tagging" of atypical lymphocytes at the dermal epidermal junction. **b,** Plaque stage mycosis fungoides demonstrating a skewed CD4:CD8 ratio. A) H&E B) CD3 C) CD4 D) CD8. **c,** Tumor stage mycosis fungoides with the atypical lymphocytic infiltrate extending deep into the dermis. **d,** Sezary syndrome with mild exocytosis and prominent spongiosis. **e,** Large cell transformation A) H&E B) CD30 staining highlighting the large atypical lymphocytes

nodule. The large cells have marked nuclear pleomorphism including prominent vesicular and hyperchromatic nuclei with prominent nucleoli and more abundant cytoplasm than their nontransformed counterparts. CD30 is often (but not always) expressed.

Immunohistochemical studies often aid in making the diagnosis of MF and are listed as useful under certain circumstances in the diagnosis section of the NCCN practice guidelines. Most commonly, MF demonstrates CD4+, CD45RO+ skin effector memory T cells. A CD8+ suppressor phenotype is occasionally observed. This variant does not exhibit different clinical behavior. The malignant clone expresses CD2, CD3, and CD5, but these along with CD7 can be lost in advanced stage disease. An elevated CD3+/CD8+ or CD4+/CD8+ ratio, particularly in the epidermis, can suggest MF.

Molecular pathology techniques detecting a monoclonal TCR gene rearrangement (originally performed with Southern blot analysis, but more recently with PCR-based assays) can provide additional information. Approximately 60% of early stage disease will be positive using the standardized BioMed-2 PCR primer sets. TCR gene rearrangement positivity must be interpreted with caution because many benign inflammatory conditions can also demonstrate clonality, and therefore, clinicopathologic correlation is absolutely essential for correctly interpreting the results of gene rearrangement testing. TCR gene rearrangement results are particularly helpful when the patient has matching clones from multiple biopsy sites or tissues.

STAGING

Cancer *stage* is defined as the extent or severity of a cancer diagnosis based on information about the tumor (traditionally strictly speaking, at the *time of diagnosis*). Staging is important to determine prognosis and to guide proper treatment. Since 1979, MF/CTCL staging has been based on the original National Cancer Institute/Mycosis Fungoides Cooperative Group Tumor-Node-Metastases (TNM) Staging system. To incorporate newer diagnostic techniques such as immunohistochemistry, flow cytometry molecular gene histochemistry, flow cytometry molecular gene

rearrangement assays, and imaging modalities, in 2007, the MF staging system was revised by the ISCL and the EORTC (Table 5-2). In this updated staging system, blood (B) classification now affects staging (whereas in the 1979 system it did not) and newer, potentially prognostic variables were incorporated for subsequent tracking and validation. Of note, the 2007 revision emphasized that the staging system for MF and SS does *not* apply to other non-MF CTCLs (a separate staging system for non-MF CTCLs was also published in 2007 by the ISCL/EORTC).

Staging of a newly diagnosed MF/CTCL patient starts with identifying the primary skin lesion morphology and BSA involved to determine T classification (T1 = patch, papule, or plaque < 10% BSA; T2 = patch/plaque ≥ 10% BSA; T3 = tumor; T4 = erythroderma). The 2007 revised staging system separates T1 and T2 disease into patch alone (T1a, T2a) versus patch/plaque (T1b, T2b).

Physical examination of peripheral lymph nodes (anterior and posterior cervical, supraclavicular, epitrochlear, axillary, inguinal areas) and palpation of liver and spleen for organomegaly should be performed at the initial staging. If examination reveals clinically abnormal peripheral lymph nodes (defined as firm, irregular, clustered fixed, or ≥ 1.5 cm in diameter) or organomegaly, patients should undergo imaging studies to assess extent of nodal involvement and additional extracutaneous disease (ultrasound, computed tomography of neck/chest/abdomen/pelvis with contrast, whole body ^{19}F-fluorodeoxyglucose positron emission tomography [FDG-PET]), or magnetic resonance imaging (in the event of contrast dye allergy). Excisional lymph node biopsy of an abnormal lymph node with histopathologic, immunohistochemistry, flow cytometry, and/or TCR gene rearrangement testing is recommended to precisely determine the N classification (Table 5–2). Patients who have clinically abnormal peripheral nodes but without histologic confirmation are designated N_x. Visceral involvement should be histologically confirmed and is designated as M_1 involvement.

If no lymphadenopathy or organomegaly is detected on physical examination, which patients require additional staging blood and imaging tests? T3 and T4 patients have higher risk of

TABLE 5-2   Revised staging system of mycosis fungoides and Sézary Syndrome (ISCL-EORTC 2007)

Skin
T1   Limited patches (T1a), papules, plaques (T1b) covering <10% of the skin surface.
T2   Patches (T2a), papules, plaques (T2b) covering ≥ 10% of the skin surface
T3   One or more tumors (≥ 1 cm diameter)
T4   Confluence of erythema covering ≥ 80% body surface area

Lymph nodes
N0   No clinically abnormal peripheral lymph nodes, biopsy not required
N1   Clinically abnormal peripheral lymph nodes, histopathology Dutch grade 1 or NCI LN0-2
    N1a   Clone negative
    N1b   Clone positive
N2   Clinically abnormal peripheral lymph nodes, histopathology Dutch grade 2 or NCI LN3
    N2a   Clone negative
    N2b   Clone positive
N3   Clinically abnormal peripheral lymph nodes, histopathology Dutch grades 3-4 or NCI-
    LN4, clone positive or negative
Nx   Clinically abnormal peripheral lymph nodes; no histologic confirmation

Visceral
M0   No visceral organ involvement
M1   Visceral involvement (must have pathology confirmation and organ involved should be
    specified)

Blood
B0   Absence of significant blood involvement: ≤5% of peripheral blood lymphocytes are
    atypical (Sézary) cells.
    B0a   Clone negative
    B0b   Clone positive
B1   Low blood tumor burden >5% of peripheral blood lymphocytes are atypical Sezary cells
    but does not meet the criteria of B2
    B1a   Clone negative
    B1b   Clone positive
B2   High blood tumor burden ≥1000/ul Sezary cells with positive clone
    If Sezary cells cannot be used to determine tumor burden for B2, then one of the
    following modified ISCL criteria along with a positive clonal rearrangement of the
    TCR may be used instead: 1) expanded CD4+ or CD3+ cells with CD4:CD8 ratio of 10
    or more, 2) expanded CD4+ cells with abnormal immunophenotype including loss of
    CD7 or CD26.

Stage
IA   T1N0M0B0-1
IB   T2N0M0B0-1

IIA   T1-2N1-2M0B0-1
IIB   T2N0-2M0B0-1

III   T4N0-2M0B0
IIIB   T4N0-2M0B1

IVA1   T1-4N0-2M0B2
IVA2   T1-4N3M0B0-2
IVB   T1-4N0-3M1B0-2

extracutaneous disease and full staging blood work and imaging are recommended. T1 and T2 patients with either (1) high-risk features clinically (folliculotropic subtype) or histologically (large cell morphology or transformation), (2) systemic symptoms (fever, chills, night sweats, unintentional weight loss, severe fatigue), or (3) concomitant immunosuppression (HIV+, organ transplantation on extensive immunosuppressive medications) should be considered for more extensive staging workup. Patients with limited patch disease in the absence of high-risk or poor prognostic features do not require imaging studies.

Assessment of the peripheral blood compartment includes complete blood count with differential, peripheral blood flow cytometry or $V\beta$ specific analysis using monoclonal antibodies, manual Sézary preparation peripheral smears (less commonly done currently owing to significant interobserver variability and subjectivity and is less quantitative than flow cytometry techniques), and TCR gene rearrangement status. Chromosomal analysis, once commonly done during the 1980s, is not now routinely done in the clinical setting (chromosomal abnormalities are more commonly detected in advanced disease—tumors, erythroderma). Currently, the NCCN guidelines recommend checking the specialized blood tests for staging in patients with higher likelihood of peripheral blood involvement: patients with T2, T3, or T4 skin classification.

Since the original staging system in 1979, several published studies have demonstrated the prognostic importance of "significant" peripheral blood involvement (defined as Sézary count > 20% of total lymphocytes, >1000 cells/mm³). The 2007 revised staging system has clarified the definition of the B (blood) classifications: B_0 5% or fewer Sézary cells; B_1 greater than 5% Sézary cells but fewer than 1000 cells/mm³ or no clonal TCR gene rearrangement detected; B_2 = clonal TCR gene rearrangement detected AND Sézary cells greater than 1000 cells/mm³ or CD4/CD8 ratio 10 or higher or increase in CD4+ T cells with an abnormal phenotype (defined as ≥ 40% CD4+CD7– or ≥ 30% CD4+CD26– lymphocytes of total lymphocyte population). In the 2007 staging revision, erythrodermic patients (without frank nodal involvement) with B_1 involvement are designated as stage IIIB (vs. erythrodermic

patients with B_0 involvement = stage IIIA). B_2 involvement is assigned stage IVA_1, now equivalent to N_3 overt nodal involvement (which now has the designation *stage IVA₂*).

Skin TCR gene rearrangement studies play primarily a diagnostic role, and lymph node and blood TCR gene rearrangement testing is done for both diagnosis and staging purposes. Peripheral blood flow cytometry to detect CD4+ T cells that lose expression of CD7 and/or CD26 does not have 100% specificity for MF/SS because patients with benign inflammatory dermatoses can also occasionally demonstrate such CD4+CD7– or CD26– T cells at low level in the peripheral blood; the presence of a blood clone that matches a skin clone can validate the flow cytometry findings. Furthermore, recently, the presence of a relevant (i.e., matching) peripheral blood TCR clone in the absence of frank phenotypic/morphologic blood involvement ($B0_b$ vs. $B0_a$ status) was found to be a significant poor prognostic marker in a multivariate analysis. It is important to stress that blood TCR gene rearrangement testing should always be done in concert with skin lesion or lymph node tissue testing, with the goal of identifying a matching clone (although admittedly erythrodermic MF and SS patients can at times have more than one clonal population). A subset of normal control patients (particularly > 60 yr) will have a monoclonal TCR gene rearrangement in their peripheral blood of unclear significance.

Additional blood studies for staging include lactate dehydrogenase (LDH) and comprehensive metabolic panel. Elevated serum LDH is a prognostic factor and can be followed over time to monitor disease activity in patients with more advanced disease.

Brain imaging is not routinely done, although patients with large cell transformed disease can develop CNS involvement. If such high-risk patients report neurologic or cognitive signs and symptoms (which may be subtle), neurologic evaluation and imaging is recommended.

Bone marrow biopsy is not routine part of the staging workup (even for erythrodermic MF or SS patients) but can be considered if the patient has B² blood involvement or initial blood testing reveals unexplained cytopenias or other findings.

Clinical stage should always refer to the stage assigned at *initial diagnosis*. Naturally, many patients will experience changes in disease tumor burden/activity but the clinical stage should not change; rather, the current disease activity should be indicated by the TNMB rating (e.g., a patient diagnosed with T2aN0M0B0a = stage IB MF in 2007, developed new tumors and dermatopathic lymphadenopathy in 2011). Current disease status is T3N1M0B0a—do not revise the original clinical numeric "stage."

PROGNOSIS

The prognosis of MF is heterogeneous: early limited patch disease has excellent prognosis with no difference in overall survival versus age-matched controls, whereas tumor MF, erythrodermic MF, and SS have a more aggressive course and poor prognosis. Numerous retrospective studies have been published by large referral centers demonstrating that initial stage at diagnosis and T classification have strong prognostic significance. The most recent study was published in 2010 examining 1502 patients from a single referral center in the United Kingdom over nearly 30 years of follow-up. The mean age at presentation was 54 years old and 74% of the patients had early stage MF (stages IA-IIA). Overall survival of the entire cohort was 74.5% and disease progression was observed in one third of all patients, and one fourth of patients died from MF. This study looked at the significance of some of the newer variables captured by the 2007 ISCL/EORTC revised staging system and validated that plaque disease (T1b, T2b) had worse prognosis than patch disease (T1a, T2a) and the presence of a matching TCR/PCR clone (B0b status) in the peripheral blood even in the absence of frank blood involvement was a poor prognostic marker. In their multivariate analysis, the major prognostic factors associated with decreased overall survival and increased disease progression were advanced T classification, folliculotropic subtype of MF, increased LDH, an B0b status.

Other previously published clinical prognostic factors have included age (older patients have poorer prognosis), race, certain clinical subtypes (hypopigmented and pagetoid reticulosis subtypes of MF seem to have better prognosis, folliculotropic has a worse prognosis), presence of multiple tumors (vs. single tumors), nodal involvement, and degree of peripheral blood malignant T-cell tumor burden. Histologic or laboratory prognostic factors include presence of CD8+ T cells (better prognosis), peripheral eosinophilia (worse prognosis), and presence of large cell transformation (worse prognosis, particularly for nodal or blood transformation).

Specific genotyping and molecular typing of MF patients at diagnosis to help predict prognosis or response to treatment are experimentally available (using cDNA- or PCR-based microarray analysis), but are not yet routinely done as standard clinical care.

TREATMENT

Treatment of MF and SS is primarily stage-based, and it is crucial that treatment goals for each patient be specifically defined. Sixty percent to 70% of patients will have early stage disease (stages IA-IIA) with an overall indolent course, but are unlikely to achieve a durable "cure." In these patients, the risks versus benefits of the various skin-directed and systemic treatments need to be weighed. Itching and cosmetic disfigurement are the primary reasons to treat in these patients; some patients with limited patch disease that is asymptomatic and with a clear history of indolent behavior over years can elect for "watchful observation." For patients with more advanced disease (extensive plaques, tumors, exfoliative erythroderma), particularly those with rapid "momentum" of their disease course, treatment needs to be instituted more quickly and often requires both skin-directed and systemic treatments together at the outset and a multidisciplinary approach. These patients often require maintenance therapy or repeat courses of therapy over the long term.

The paradigm of treatment of MF/CTCL has shifted over the past 50 years—conventional cytotoxic systemic chemotherapy does not result in durable response and cannot be continued indefinitely; in the paper by Bunn and coworkers, it did not result in survival benefit versus more conservative cycled skin therapies. Cycled therapies (returning to the same therapy even after relapse/recurrence) is another concept unique to MF/CTCL in the field of oncology.

The treatment of MF is challenging owing to the inherent heterogeneity among the various stages of the disease and the lack of adequate evidence-based data (owing to the rarity of the disease), randomized, blinded, controlled trials comparing existing treatments have been difficult. However, owing to the efforts of several cutaneous lymphoma organizations, several practice guidelines based on consensus conferences are now available from organizations including the NCCN, EORTC, European Society of Medical Oncology (ESMO), ISCL, and USCLC.

Skin-directed Therapies

Skin-directed therapies are the first-line treatment for newly diagnosed early stage MF (stages IA-IIA MF) and are divided into topical agents, phototherapy, and radiation therapy (see Table 5-3). Radiation therapy has the highest efficacy of all the skin-directed treatments but is generally first line only for either single-lesion MF (such as pagetoid reticulosis) or thicker plaques and tumors. Early patch and thin-plaque patients are treated with topicals or phototherapy initially and moved to radiation therapy if lesions are refractory.

Localized patch or plaque disease can be treated with topical corticosteroids (generally superpotent class I steroids for the scalp and body, class III or V for the face), topical retinoids (e.g., topical bexarotene, topical tazarotene), topical compounded chemotherapy (mechlorethamine/ nitrogen mustard ointment or solution; carmustine/BCNU [bischloroethylnitrosourea] ointment or solution). Efficacy rates are fairly similar (50-80%) and the major distinctions between the subtypes are side effect profiles and availability. Corticosteroids are readily available and well tolerated in the short term, but prolonged use results in skin atrophy, fragility, striae, and easy bruising. Topical retinoids cause retinoid irritant dermatitis requiring either frequent emollients or adjunctive topical steroids. Topical chemotherapy requires compounding at a specialized pharmacy and has a 5% to 20% incidence of allergic or irritant contact dermatitis and, for carmustine, frequent postinflammatory hyperpigmentation and telangiectasias. Topical imiquimod 5% cream is useful for very localized lesions but can cause inflammation in a subset of patients. Topical

TABLE 5-3 Therapies for mycosis fungoides and Sezary Syndrome (based on National Comprehensive Cancer Network 2011 guidelines)

SKIN DIRECTED THERAPIES
Limited skin involvement
Topical corticosteroids
Topical retinoids (bexarotene, tazarotene)
Topical imiquimod
Topical chemotherapy (mechlorethamine/ nitrogen mustard, carmustine)
Phototherapy (UVB, nbUVB, PUVA)
Localized electron beam radiation therapy

Generalized skin involvement
Topical corticosteroids (short term)
Topical chemotherapy (mechlorethamine/ nitrogen mustard, carmustine)
Phototherapy (UVB, nbUVB, PUVA)
Total skin electron beam radiation therapy

SYSTEMIC THERAPIES
CATEGORY A
Interferons (interferon alpha, interferon gamma)
Retinoids (bexarotene, acitretin, all trans retinoic acid)
Extracorporeal photopheresis
Histone deacetylase inhibitors (vorinostat, romidepsin)
Denileukin diftitox
Methotrexate (<100 mg/week)

CATEGORY B
First line
Liposomal doxorubicin
Gemcitabine
Second line
Chlorambucil
Pentostatin
Etoposide
Cyclophosphamide
Temozolamide
Bortezemib
Methotrexate (.>100 mg/week)
Low dose pralatrexate
(Alemtuzumab – Sezary Syndrome)

CATEGORY C
Liposomal doxorubicin
Gemcitabine
Denileukin diftitox
Romidepsin
Low or standard dose pralatrexate

calcineurin inhibitors are not listed in any of the treatment guidelines for MF/SS (likely related to concerns regarding its controversial black box warning and risk of lymphoma), although there are reports of its efficacy, particular on the face or in body folds. Topical photodynamic therapy and excimer laser are novel skin-directed agents that are not formally listed on clinical practice guidelines as yet.

Not all topicals can be used for more generalized skin involvement. Topical steroids, particularly after bathing and under occlusion with a sauna suit ("soak and smear" regimen with triamcinolone ointment 0.025% or 0.1%) can be used neck to feet once or twice daily for a few weeks for rapid-acting and significant symptom relief, but they should not be used in this manner for more than a few weeks owing to the risks of systemic absorption and skin atrophy. Topical retinoids cannot be applied in a generalized way. Topical chemotherapy with nitrogen mustard ointment or solution can be used as a whole body treatment without significant systemic absorption. Patients should be warned that whole body topical nitrogen mustard can cause initial disease flare in the first month of application due to unmasking of subclinical lesions. Topical carmustine may be systemically absorbed if applied to a large BSA.

Phototherapy (currently with either narrowband UVB [NBUVB] or psoralen plus ultraviolet A [PUVA]) is another skin-directed therapy that is effective for both localized and generalized skin disease. Patients receive treatments at a dermatologist's office two to three times a week for several months to years. This treatment is not messy, but it does require travel to the physician's office. Phototherapy is not effective for lesions that are in relatively photoprotected "sanctuary sites" such as the periorbital, pubic/genital, or axillary fold areas. Short-term side effects of phototherapy include phototoxicity and photosensitivity, nausea, or dizziness when taking the oral 8-methoxypsoralen pills; long-term side effects include increased photodamage, lentigines, and risk of skin cancers (both nonmelanoma and melanoma skin cancers).

Similar to topical nitrogen mustard whole body application, phototherapy can initially cause disease flare during the first 1 month. Full clinical responses can take 6 to 12 months of either therapy. Patients should continue skin-directed treatment for at least 1 to 3 months after they are clinically clear and then either stop and observe or taper treatment to a maintenance regimen. Maintenance regimens have not shown in published studies to improve disease-free survival, although many physicians do utilize maintenance treatments for their MF patients. NBUVB is more readily available and does not require administration of any oral photosensitizing agent (unlike PUVA), but PUVA is still recommended for thicker plaque lesions or lesions resistant to NBUVB.

Radiation therapy (generally electron beam) is extremely effective for localized refractory patches, plaques, and first line for tumors (24-36 Gy) and is relatively readily available. For relapsed skin disease, however, even lower-dose radiation therapy (2 Gy × 2) can still be effective palliation for clearing lesions, although the duration of response is likely to be lower than the higher doses. In contrast to localized radiation therapy, total skin electron beam (TSEB) therapy is available only at a few specialized centers and requires particular equipment setup and expertise. It is very effective for generalized refractory patch or plaque or tumor disease—for initial treatment, doses of 30 to 36 Gy have been traditionally recommended. More recently, however, a low-dose TSEB regimen (10-20 Gy, 20-30 Gy) has been reported that is less time-intensive for patients with still satisfactory clinical responses. For erythrodermic MF and SS, opinions on role of TSEB vary from center to center. In our experience, erythrodermic patients can tolerate TSEB, and furthermore, it can result in debulking of peripheral blood malignant T-cell burden in a subset of SS patients who are also on concomitant systemic medications at the time of TSEB.

Systemic Therapy

Early stage disease that is refractory to skin-directed treatments alone or patients with advanced stage disease will require systemic therapies. Since 1999, no less than four systemic agents have been approved for MF/SS (CTCL) in the United States by the Food and Drug Administration (FDA). Systemic agents can be used either as single agents or in combination with skin-directed therapies or other systemic medications. The current NCCN guidelines divide the systemic medications into categories A, B and C (see Table 5-3). Category A agents are the least immunosuppressive and consist of oral retinoids (bexarotene, acitretin), IFNs (α, γ; given as subcutaneous injections), oral low- to mid-dose weekly methotrexate, denileukin diftitox (a fusion protein of diphtheria toxin and IL-2 targeting IL-2R–bearing tumor cells), extra-corporeal photopheresis, and histone deacetylase inhibitors (vorinostat and romidepsin). Several category A agents can be combined with either skin-directed therapies or other systemic category A agents (Table 5-4). Our group often employs an immunomodulatory multimodality combination therapy approach in our erythrodermic MF and SS patients that includes multiple treatments simul-taneously: skin-directed topicals or phototherapy or TSEB therapy + extracorporeal photopheresis + IFN-α and/or -γ + oral bexarotene. The newest group of agents in category A are the histone deacetylase (HDAC) inhibitors oral vorinostat and intravenously administered romidepsin. These agents should be used if patients are refractory to the other category A agents because their side effect profile and effect on host immune responses place them closer to the category B chemothera-peutic agents than the other category A agents.

Category B agents are suggested in patients who are refractory to category A and comprise more traditional chemotherapeutic agents, with

TABLE 5-4 Combination therapies for mycosis fungoides and Sezary Syndrome (based on NCCN 2011 guidelines)

Skin-directed + Systemic
Phototherapy + interferon
Phototherapy + retinoid
Phototherapy + extracorporeal photopheresis
Total skin electron beam radiation therapy + photopheresis
Systemic + systemic
Retinoid + interferon
Bexarotene + denileukin diftitox
Photopheresis + interferon
Photopheresis + retinoid
Photopheresis + interferon + retinoid

initial preference given to single-agent rather than combination chemotherapy (given the overly immunosuppressive effects of CHOP [cyclo-phosphamide, hydroxydaunoimycin, Oncovin, prednisone]–based and other combination chemotherapy regimens that do not have durable efficacy in MF/SS). For stage III or IV SS refrac-tory to category A, alemtuzumab (anti-CD52 mAb) is now listed in the NCCN guidelines as a treatment option, particularly the lower-dose regimen. Category C agents are recommended as initial therapy for patients with non-SS stage IV disease (nodal, visceral involvement).

Systemic agents are selected on an individual case-by-case basis, taking into account side effect profile and patient comorbidities and the speed at which disease control or response needs to be achieved. MF has few randomized studies that directly compare systemic agents to help guide choices based on "best response rate." Because of this and the chronic and recurrent nature of the disease, patients who have disease refractory to standard therapies are encouraged to consider clinical trials if appropriate.

Novel Agents

Agents that are currently under investigation include forodesine, Toll-like receptor agonists (CpG, resiquimod), cytokines, monoclonal anti-bodies (anti-CD4 mAB, anti-CCR4 mAb), and newer-generation histone deacetylase inhibitors including topical formulations.

More recently, there is increasing literature on the role of allogeneic hematopoietic stem cell transplantation in refractory, high-risk MF and SS. Autologous transplantation results in disease relapse as it lacks the "graft-versus-tumor" effect in allogeneic transplantation that results in long-term disease control (or even cure). Nonmyeloablative regimens have been developed to minimize imme-diate transplant-related morbidity. In 2010, two separate publications detailed the largest series of CTCL patients transplanted to date (19 MF/SS patients from M. D. Anderson and 60 MF/SS patients from a European cohort). Transplant-related mortality remains high (20%) and long-term sequelae include a high incidence of graft-versus-host disease of varying severity. The optimal timing and conditioning regimens for transplant also are not well established. However, young patients (<60 yr) with high-risk disease (tumors, folliculotropic plaques, erythrodermic MF or SS) should be counseled about this option. Of note, disease relapse can still occur after transplant, although withdrawal of immunosuppression or donor lymphocyte infusion can result in either complete remission or "downgraded" residual disease that is more manageable than disease before transplant.

Associated Issues

MF and SS patients suffer from skin barrier impairment due to the scaling and exfoliation. Once- or twice-daily tub or shower soaks immediately followed by bland emollients is an important adjunctive regimen. Ulcerated plaques and tumors are susceptible to infection and patients can develop life-threatening sepsis. Exfoliative erythroderma patients in particular are susceptible to bacterial colonization (especially methicillin-resistant *S. aureus*) that clinically presents as yellow crusting, fissures, and oozing. Actively impetiginized areas should be cultured. Dilute bleach baths, chlorhexidine cleansers, or dilute acetic acid soaks/sprays can minimize colonization, and topical antibiotics (mupirocin, silver sulfadiazine) can be used as initial therapy, with oral or systemic antibiotics reserved for more active cases. Some erythrodermic patients will have dramatic improvement with chronic courses of systemic antibiotics, but the benefits must be weighed with the risks of increased antibiotic resistance. Superficial skin infections by *Tinea* or *Candida* are more frequent in MF patients, and viral reactivation of herpes simplex or herpes zoster has a higher chance of dissemination in MF/SS patients owing to barrier compromise and also inherent immunosuppression due to their disease.

Treatment of itch is important, yet it remains an area where improvement is sorely needed and there is scant literature in MF/SS. Only recently has pruritus relief been a major outcome measure in clinical trials and reports. Topical emollients with various anti-itch agents (menthol, topical anesthetics such as pramoxine, topical steroids, topical calcineurin inhibitors, topical antihistamines), and phototherapy (broadband UVB [BBUVB], narrowband UVB [NBUVB], psoralen UVA [PUVA]) can be used.

Systemic anti-itch agents most commonly include oral antihistamines, gabapentin, mirtazapine, and more recently, aprepitant.

ASSOCIATIONS

Patients with MF and SS have a higher risk of developing a second lymphoproliferative disorder than those in the general population. Primary cutaneous CD30+ lymphoproliferative disorders (e.g., lymphomatoid papulosis and cutaneous anaplastic large cell lymphoma) can be seen concomitantly with MF lesions. Hodgkin's disease is also more common in MF patients, as are other non-Hodgkin's lymphomas (both B- and T-cell–derived), and the presentation may be dyssynchronous with the MF activity.

MF patients often receive chronic skin-directed treatments that results in photodamage, increased lentigines (PUVA and NBUVB lentigines), and increased risk of melanoma and nonmelanoma skin cancers. This issue is particularly relevant for younger MF patients who will have their disease longer—their risk of disease progression is not worse than older patients, but they have a higher risk of associated treatment-related skin malignancies. Immunomodulatory systemic therapies rarely can result in unmasking of autoimmune conditions (e.g., thyroiditis, hepatitis, nephritis, psoriasis, vitiligo, colitis).

SUGGESTED READINGS

Bernengo MG, Novelli M, Quaglino P, Lisa F, De Matteis A, Savoia P, et al. The relevance of the CD4+ CD26– subset in the identification of circulating Sézary cells. *Br J Dermatol*. 2001;144:125–135.

Bernengo MG, Quaglino P, Comessatti A, Ortoncelli M, Novelli M, Lisa F, et al. Low-dose intermittent alemtuzumab in the treatment of Sézary syndrome: clinical and immunologic findings in 14 patients. Haematologica. 2007;92:784–794.

Criscione VD, Weinstock MA. Incidence of cutaneous T-cell lymphoma in the United States, 1973–2002. *Arch Dermatol*. 2007;143:854–859.

Dummer R, Assaf C, Bagot M, Gniadecki R, Hauschild A, Knobler R, et al. Maintenance therapy in cutaneous T-cell lymphoma: who, when, what? Eur J Cancer. 2007;43:2321–2329.

Girardi M, Heald PW, Wilson LD. The pathogenesis of mycosis fungoides. *N Engl J Med.* 2004;350: 1978–1988.

Guitart J, Magro C. Cutaneous T-cell lymphoid dyscrasia: a unifying term for idiopathic chronic dermatoses with persistent T-cell clones. *Arch Dermatol.* 2007;143:921–932.

Huang KP, Weinstock MA, Clarke CA, McMillan A, Hoppe RT, Kim YH. Second lymphomas and other malignant neoplasms in patients with mycosis fungoides and Sézary syndrome: evidence from population-based and clinical cohorts. *Arch Dermatol.* 2007;143:45–50.

Jones GW, Kacinski BM, Wilson LD, Willemze R, Spittle M, Hohenberg G, et al. Total skin electron radiation in the management of mycosis fungoides: consensus of the European Organization for Research and Treatment of Cancer (EORTC) Cutaneous Lymphoma Project Group. *J Am Acad Dermatol.* 2002;47:364–370.

Kari L, Loboda A, Nebozhyn M, Rook AH, Vonderheid EC, Nichols C, et al. Classification and prediction of survival in patients with leukemic phase of cutaneous T-cell lymphoma. *J Exp Med.* 2003;197:1477–1488.

Kim EJ, Hess S, Richardson SK, Newton S, Showe LC, Benoit BM, et al. Immunopathogenesis and therapy of cutaneous T cell lymphoma. *J Clin Invest.* 2005;115:798–812.

Kim EJ, Rook AH. How low can you go? Quality effects of an anti-CD4 antibody. *Blood.* 2007;109:4594–4595.

Kim YH, Duvic M, Obitz E, Gniadecki R, Iversen L, Osterborg A, et al. Clinical efficacy of zanolimumab (HuMax-CD4): two phase 2 studies in refractory cutaneous T-cell lymphoma. *Blood.* 2007;109:4655–4662.

Kim YH, Liu HL, Mraz-Gernhard S, Varghese A, Hoppe RT. Long-term outcome of 525 patients with mycosis fungoides and Sézary syndrome: clinical prognostic factors and risk for disease progression. *Arch Dermatol.* 2003;139:857–866.

Kim YH, Martinez G, Varghese A, Hoppe RT. Topical nitrogen mustard in the management of mycosis fungoides: update of the Stanford experience. *Arch Dermatol.* 2003;139:165–173.

Kim YH, Willemze R, Pimpinelli N, Whittaker S, Olsen EA, Ranki A, et al. TNM classification system for primary cutaneous lymphomas other than mycosis fungoides and Sézary syndrome: a proposal of the International Society for Cutaneous Lymphomas (ISCL) and the Cutaneous Lymphoma Task Force of the European Organization of Research and Treatment of Cancer (EORTC). *Blood.* 2007;110:479–484.

McKenna KE, Whittaker S, Rhodes LE, Taylor P, Lloyd J, Ibbotson S, et al. Evidence-based practice of photopheresis 1987–2001: a report of a workshop of the British Photodermatology Group and the U.K. Skin Lymphoma Group. *Br J Dermatol.* 2006;154: 7–20.

Nashan D, Faulhaber D, Stander S, Luger TA, Stadler R. Mycosis fungoides: a dermatological masquerader. *Br J Dermatol.* 2007;156:1–10.

Nebozhyn M, Loboda A, Kari L, Rook AH, Vonderheid EC, Lessin S, et al. Quantitative PCR on 5 genes reliably identifies CTCL patients with 5% to 99% circulating tumor cells with 90% accuracy. *Blood.* 2006;107:3189–3196.

Pimpinelli N, Olsen EA, Santucci M, Vonderheid E, Haeffner AC, Stevens S, et al. Defining early mycosis fungoides. *J Am Acad Dermatol.* 2005;53:1053–1063.

Rook AH, Wood GS, Yoo EK, Elenitsas R, Kao DM, Sherman ML, et al. Interleukin-12 therapy of cutaneous T-cell lymphoma induces lesion regression and cytotoxic T-cell responses. *Blood.* 1999;94:902–908.

Samimi S, Benoit B, Evans K, Wherry EJ, Showe L, Wysocka M, Rook AH. Increased programmed death-1 expression on CD4+ cutaneous T-cell lymphoma: implications for immune suppression. *Arch Dermatol.* 2010;146:1382-1388.

Smoller BR, Santucci M, Wood GS, Whittaker SJ. Histopathology and genetics of cutaneous T-cell lymphoma. *Hematol Oncol Clin North Am.* 2003; 17:1277–1311.

Steffen C. The man behind the eponym: Lucien Marie Pautrier—Pautrier's microabscess. *Am J Dermatopathol.* 2003;25:155–158.

Taswell HF, Winkelmann RK. Sézary syndrome—a malignant reticulemic erythroderma. *JAMA.* 1961; 177:465–472.

Trautinger F, Knobler R, Willemze R, Peris K, Stadler R, Laroche L, et al. EORTC consensus recommendations for the treatment of mycosis fungoides/Sézary syndrome. *Eur J Cancer.* 2006;42:1014–1030.

Tsai EY, Taur A, Espinosa L, Quon A, Johnson D, Dick S, et al. Staging accuracy in mycosis fungoides and Sézary syndrome using integrated positron emission tomography and computed tomography. *Arch Dermatol.* 2006;142:577–584.

Willemze R, Jaffe ES, Burg G, Cerroni L, Berti E, Swerdlow SH, et al. WHO-EORTC classification for cutaneous lymphomas. *Blood.* 2005;105:3768–3785.

Winkelmann RK, Caro WA. Current problems in mycosis fungoides and Sézary syndrome. *Ann Rev Med.* 1977;28:251–269.

Yawalkar N, Ferenczi K, Jones DA, Yamanaka K, Suh KY, Sadat S, et al. Profound loss of T-cell receptor repertoire complexity in cutaneous T-cell lymphoma. *Blood.* 2003;102:4059–4066.

Zaki MH, Shane RB, Geng Y, Showe LC, Everetts SE, Presky DH, et al. Dysregulation of lymphocyte interleukin-12 receptor expression in Sézary syndrome. *J Invest Dermatol.* 2001;117:119–127.

MYCOSIS FUNGOIDES VARIANTS

Jo-Ann Latkowski, MD, and Neelam Vashi, MD

BACKGROUND

Mycosis fungoides (MF) is an uncommon disorder but it represents the most common type of cutaneous T-cell lymphoma (CTCL). Although generally a disease of the skin, aggressive forms and misdiagnosis may lead to internal progression with increased morbidity and mortality. The name *mycosis fungoides,* loosely meaning "mushroom-like fungal disease," can be misleading to both patients and practitioners unfamiliar with the entity. The rarity, different morphologies, and multiple clinicopathologic variants can make diagnosis a daunting task. This chapter outlines variants and treatment options to aid the practitioner in diagnosing and caring for the patient with MF.

ETIOLOGY AND PATHOGENESIS

The etiology and pathogenesis of MF are not clearly defined. Chronic antigenic stimulation has been postulated as the inciting event in the development of MF, causing an initial inflammatory response in the epidermis with T-cell proliferation and subsequent emergence of a malignant clone. Genetic, environmental, and immunologic factors have all been proposed to have a role in this process.

The disease is an unusual expression and clonal expansion of skin-associated T-helper cells, and more rarely, T-suppressor/killer cells. The neoplastic cells usually have a mature CD3+ CD4+ CD8– CD30– CD45RO+ memory T-cell phenotype. However, in rare cases, a CD3+ CD4– CD8+ mature T-cell phenotype may be seen.

EPIDEMIOLOGY

MF has an incidence of approximately 0.3 per 100,000 persons/yr and typically affects older adults (median age of 55-60 yr at diagnosis) but may also occur in children. Men are generally affected more with a male-to-female ratio of 1.6–0:1.

CLASSIC MYCOSIS FUNGOIDES

"Classic" MF can present with patches, plaques, tumors, or erythroderma. Characteristically, patients progress from patch to plaque to tumor stage and have a protracted clinical course over decades. Location and morphology are important considerations when assessing whether a patient has a classic presentation. Patch/plaque MF is the most common presentation, typically developing in covered, non–sun-exposed areas (e.g., buttock, breasts, inner thigh, inner arms, and trunk below the umbilicus). Classic morphology is characterized by polymorphic lesions with variability in size (most > 5 cm), shape (arcuate, semilunar), and color. Poikilodermatous changes including atrophy, dyspigmentation, and telangiectasia are common along with wrinkling (cigarette-paper–like changes), which some specialists consider pathognomonic for MF. Correlation with histopathology is necessary, especially in early stage disease, and a broad shave biopsy is advised for clinicopathologic correlation and diagnosis.

Early disease is not only difficult to diagnose clinically but also histopathologically and multiple serial biopsies may be needed. Early patch lesions show superficial infiltrates composed of lymphocytes. Findings are subtle and atypical lymphocytes with convoluted (cerebriform) and hyperchromatic nuclei may be few and confined to the epidermis (epidermotropism), often colonizing the basal layer as single cells. Advanced disease shows more pronounced findings, and a minority of cases will demonstrate intraepidermal nests of atypical cells (Pautrier's microabscesses).

Apart from the classic type of MF, many clinical and/or histologic variants have been reported (Table 6-1). In the 2005 European Organization for Research and Treatment of Cancer/World Health Organization (EORTC/WHO) classification

TABLE 6-1   Variants of Mycosis Fungoides

Pagetoid reticulosis
Hypopigmented
Folliculotropic
Syringotropic
Poikilodermatous
Palmar-plantar
Pigmented purpuric
Hyperkeratotic/verrucous
Granulomatous
Granulomatous slack skin
Bullous
Ichthyosiform

for cutaneous lymphomas, three clinical variants of MF—follicular MF, pagetoid reticulosis, and granulomatous slack skin (GSS)—were recognized as distinct entities, behaving differently clinically and pathologically. Most variants have the same prognosis and treatment options as classic MF with the exception of follicular MF, which is discussed later in this chapter.

HYPOPIGMENTED MYCOSIS FUNGOIDES

Hypopigmented MF is the most common variant and affects younger, more darkly pigmented patients (Figure 6-1). It presents as large, asymptomatic hypopigmented patches with irregular borders in the bathing suit distribution. Classic MF lesions and/or hyperpigmented patches may or may not be present. It is easily mistaken for early vitiligo, which can be distinguished with Wood's lamp examination, vitiliginous patches appearing bright white under the Wood's light and MF patches not accentuating. Besides vitiligo, included in the differential diagnosis are sarcoid, leprosy, tinea versicolor, postinflammatory hypopigmentation, and pityriasis alba (Table 6-2). Potassium hydroxide (KOH) preparation of a patch is advised to rule out tinea versicolor, which can easily be diagnosed with the appearance of "spaghetti and meatball" hyphae and spores under light microscopy. In addition to the histopathologic findings of classic MF, hypopigmented

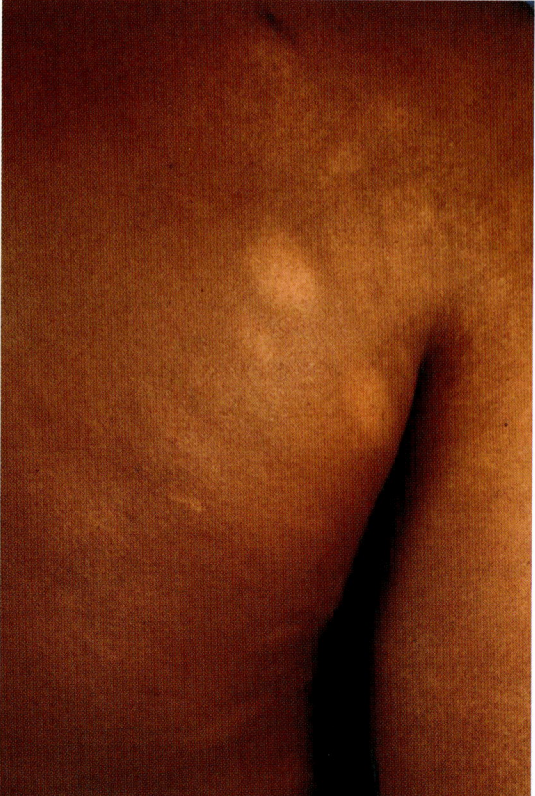

Figure 6-1 Hypopigmented mycosis fungoides (MF).

MF demonstrates pigment incontinence and decreased basal pigmentation. The malignant clone is often of CD8+, rather than CD4+ as seen in classic MF.

Most often, patients with hypopigmented MF present with stage IA (patches or plaques < 10% body surface area [BSA]) or stage IB (patches or plaques >10% BSA) disease, advanced disease being rare in the United States. Given the early stage at presentation, patients with hypopigmented MF have an excellent prognosis and staging workup

TABLE 6-2   Differential Diagnosis of Hypopigmented Mycosis Fungoides

Vitiligo
Tinea versicolor
Postinflammatory hypopigmentation
Pityriasis alba
Leprosy
Sarcoidosis

need not be extensive. Treatment options of hypopigmented MF are similar to those for classic MF. They respond beautifully to narrow-band ultraviolet B (nbUVB) phototherapy or psoralen and ultraviolet A (PUVA) phototherapy with early repigmentation of their lesions. If disease is limited to a few patches, a topical regimen such as potent topical corticosteroids or topical retinoids can be employed. According to literature, recurrence is common in patients with hypopigmented MF. Rather than a true recurrence, this is likely secondary to quicker noncompliance with treatment regimens because lesions can rapidly clear and/or be imperceptible.

PAGETOID RETICULOSIS

Pagetoid reticulosis is a unique variant of MF that does not adhere to the morphology or distribution of classic MF. It presents as a slow-growing, focal patch or plaque with scale on the hands and feet, both locations atypical for MF. It may appear hyperkeratotic or psoriasiform, necessitating a deep punch biopsy for definitive diagnosis. The clinical differential diagnosis includes common dermatoses that occur on the hands and feet such as psoriasis, dermatophytosis, verruca vulgaris, granuloma annulare, and squamous cell carcinoma. Pagetoid reticulosis is referred to as *Woringer-Kolopp disease* when it presents as a focal acral lesion.

The typical histologic picture is distinctive with marked epidermotropism often composed of CD8+ cells rather than CD4+ cells as seen in classic MF. The histologic differential diagnosis for this pattern is Paget's disease, pagetoid melanoma, and Bowen's disease.

Recommended treatment for pagetoid reticulosis includes topical nitrogen mustard, topical corticosteroids, localized radiotherapy, or surgical excision. Phototherapy has also been utilized for this variant of MF.

GRANULOMATOUS SLACK SKIN

GSS is an extraordinarily rare but indolent variant of MF. This condition presents with well-circumscribed, erythematous, and asymptomatic areas of pendulous lax skin with a predilection for the intertriginous areas (e.g., axilla and groin).

Typically, a dense granulomatous infiltrate with atypical T cells is seen on histopathologic sections of GSS. Fully developed lesions show large multinucleated giant cells with a wreath-like appearance. Elastolysis with absence of elastic fibers is also common for GSS. Clinicopathologic correlation is necessary because it is often difficult to distinguish GSS from cases of MF with incidental granulomatous histology.

Although GSS is indolent, patients have an increased risk of acquiring a second lymphoid malignancy, Hodgkin's disease being the most common, and thus, long-term follow-up is necessary. Treatment is difficult but radiotherapy may be effective. Surgical excision is also an option, but disease recurrence has been reported. Despite treatment, changes of lax skin are permanent.

FOLLICULAR MYCOSIS FUNGOIDES

Follicular MF is a distinct variant of MF in which the malignant T cells have a predilection for the hair follicle (Figure 6-2). It has been described as folliculotropic MF, pilotropic MF, folliculocentric MF, and MF-associated follicular mucinosis.

Follicular MF has a significantly higher male-to-female ratio (4-5:1) and presents with acneiform lesions, comedo-like papules, epidermal cysts, erythematous patches, and plaques along with hair loss. Lesions most often appear on the head, neck, and upper chest. It may precede, occur simultaneously with, or occur after classic patch/

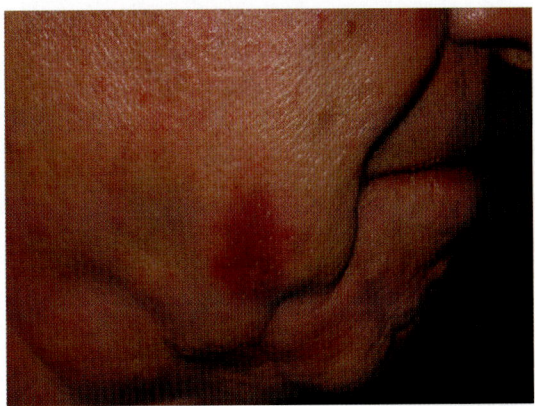

Figure 6-2 Follicular MF.

TABLE 6-3   Differences between Benign and Malignant Follicular Muncinosis

	Benign Follicular Mucinosis	Malignant Follicular Mucinosis
Epidemiology	Younger patients with history of atopy	Older patients, no history of atopy
Clinical presentation	3–15-mm papules on the face, sometimes upper trunk	Polymorphic lesions in location typical of mycosis fungoides
Pathology	No atypia or epidermotropism	Atypia and epidermotropism of lymphocytes may be present

plaque lesions. Clinically, follicular MF must be distinguished from rosacea, acne vulgaris, folliculitis, and benign follicular mucinosis. An elderly man presenting with acne-like lesions on the head and neck with no prior history of rosacea or acne vulgaris raises the suspicion for follicular MF.

The differentiation between benign follicular mucinosis and follicular mucinosis associated with MF is often difficult (Table 6-3). Benign follicular mucinosis presents in younger patients with a history of atopy. Clinically, it appears as small papules on the face or upper trunk, locations atypical of classic MF, or clusters of pink to flesh-colored follicular papules with alopecia, which may form cobblestone or nodular plaques. On histopathologic examination, no atypical cells or epidermotropism is evident. For follicular mucinosis associated with follicular MF, the patient is usually older, has no history of atopy, and has a distribution of lesions typical of classic MF.

Given the deeper infiltrate, a punch biopsy is recommended for definitive diagnosis. In follicular MF, lymphocytes target the hair follicle, often without involvement of the overlying epithelium (folliculotropism rather than epidermotropism). Follicular mucinosis may be seen on histology; however, this does not engender any changes regarding treatment and prognosis. In addition to follicular mucinosis, the pathologic differential includes other forms of CTCL. Of note, in cases of classic MF, follicles are involved over 50% of the time.

The deeper reservoir of malignant cells around hair follicles seen in follicular MF has many implications. First, patients with follicular MF do not respond well to skin-directed therapy such as topical corticosteroids, topical retinoids, or UVB phototherapy. Second, follicular MF has a more aggressive course with a high risk of progression to tumors and/or erythroderma.

It is often equated to tumor stage MF by specialists when workup, treatment, and prognosis are considered.

Given the worse prognosis of follicular MF, a complete staging workup is essential. Basic blood tests including complete blood count with differential, comprehensive metabolic panel, liver function tests, and lactic dehydrogenase should be ordered along with flow cytometry of the peripheral blood to assess for circulating atypical lymphocytes. Lymph node involvement is determined with positron emission tomography/computed tomography (PET/CT). This new technology establishes not only the size of the lymph nodes (via CT) but also the metabolic activity (via PET). Thus, if a lymph node is enlarged and accentuates on PET in the region of cutaneous disease, it might have involvement of atypical cells and should be considered for excision and examination.

Follicular MF is treated much more aggressively than other variants. Oral retinoids, oral antihistone deacetylase inhibitors or interferon-alpha (IFN-α) should be initiated. Often, patients with follicular MF do not respond to the first treatment regimen and combination therapy is necessary (e.g., IFN-α with oral retinoid, UVB with oral retinoid).

SYRINGOTROPIC MYCOSIS FUNGOIDES

Originally reported as syringolymphoid hyperplasia with alopecia, syringotropic MF is a rare variant of MF, similar to follicular MF (Figure 6-3). Whereas in follicular MF, atypical cells have a tropism toward the hair follicle, in syringotropic MF, the atypical cells accumulate around eccrine ducts and glands. Patients present with erythematous to hyperpigmented patches and plaques

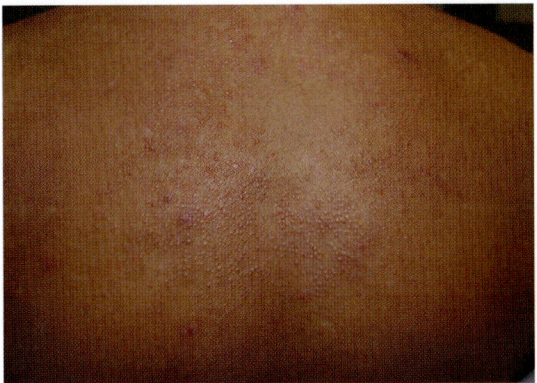

Figure 6-3 Syringotropic MF.

with or without pustules or diffuse tiny papules. Alopecia is common in the areas of involvement.

Histologic findings in syringotropic MF include hyperplastic eccrine glands and eccrine ducts invaded by atypical lymphocytes. Because 30% of classic MF cases show eccrine involvement, a diagnosis of syringotropic MF is made when the predominant pattern is atypical lymphocytic infiltration of the eccrine gland and duct with little epidermotropism.

The workup and treatment for syringotropic MF is similar to that for follicular MF. Given the deep infiltrate, skin-directed therapies may not be efficacious.

POIKILODERMATOUS MYCOSIS FUNGOIDES

Poikilodermatous MF represents a distinct clinicopathologic entity from classic MF (Figure 6-4).

It presents as hypo- and hyperpigmentation with atrophy and telangiectasia. This presentation can be seen in classic MF, but when these changes are the predominant presentation, a diagnosis of poikilodermatous MF can be rendered. In this variant, clinical changes develop slowly and may be permanent despite treatment. Poikilodermatous MF presents at a younger age, with pruritus and burning being common symptoms.

In poikilodermatous MF, histology shows changes of classic MF along with epidermal atrophy and telangiectatic vessels. In addition, the lymphocytic infiltrate is often CD8+ and not CD4+ as in classic MF.

Given the younger demographic of patients who present with this variant, a systemic workup is indicated with stage IB presentation and higher. Treatment is the same as in classic MF and lesions may respond well to phototherapy. In this variant, it is recommended to rebiopsy after treatment because some of the cutaneous changes may be permanent, and it is difficult to assess treatment response on clinical examination alone. It should be noted that poikilodermatous MF is frequently associated with lymphomatoid papulosis (LyP), and thus, long-term follow-up is necessary.

PIGMENTED PURPURIC MYCOSIS FUNGOIDES

Pigmented purpuric mycosis fungoides (PPD MF) is a rare variant of MF that resembles a benign pigmented purpuric dermatosis, presenting with erythematous to brown purpuric macules and patches that may appear atrophic (Figure 6-5).

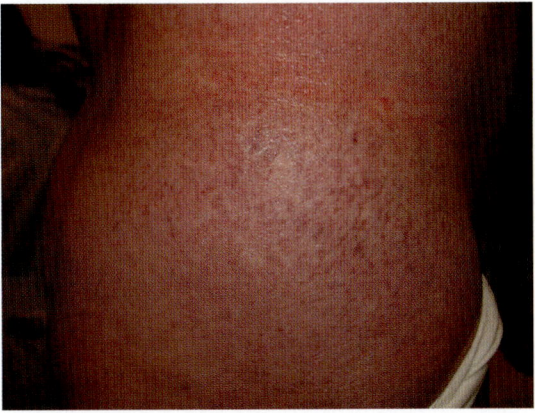

Figure 6-4 Poikilodermatous MF.

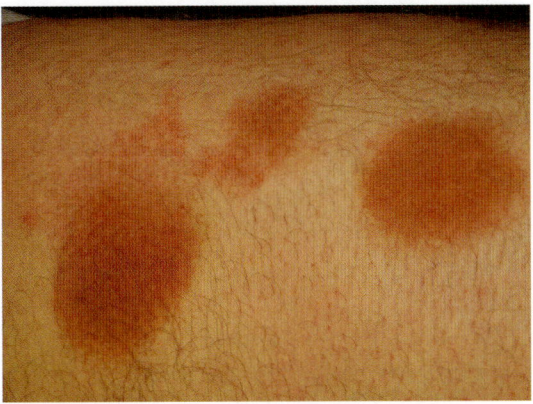

Figure 6-5 Pigmented-purpuric (PPD) MF.

PPD MF usually occurs on the lower trunk and extremities and appears in a younger patient population than classic MF.

The clinical differential diagnosis of PPD MF is benign PPD. One must suspect MF in patients with PPD when the patient is older, the eruption lasts for years and frequently relapses, and involvement is extensive in classic MF locations. Thus, close clinical follow-up is essential in these patients. It should be noted that PPD may simulate MF histologically. The histopathology of PPD MF shows a dense lichenoid infiltrate, similar to classic MF, along with numerous siderphages and extravasated erythrocytes.

Patients respond well to skin-directed therapies of classic MF. Similar to poikilodermatous MF, cutaneous changes may be permanent or slow to resolve, necessitating rebiopsy to evaluate the efficacy of treatment and disease activity.

PALMAR-PLANTAR MYCOSIS FUNGOIDES

Palmar-plantar MF is defined as MF limited to or predominantly affecting the palms and soles (Figure 6-6). Patients with palmar-plantar MF are usually men with a mean age of 50, slightly younger than those presenting with classic MF. Although the definition of this variant correlates to a stage IA presentation, the disease can be quite painful and morbid.

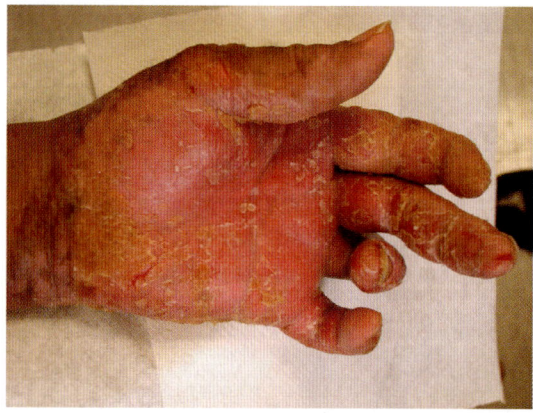

Figure 6-6 Palmar-plantar MF.

Clinically, palmar-plantar MF presents as diffuse erythema with scale, erosions, ulcerations, and fissures that can cause recurrent local infection and subsequent functional difficulties. The clinical differential diagnosis includes psoriasis, tinea manuum/pedis, and eczematous hand/foot dermatitis.

A punch biopsy is necessary for adequate sampling of the thickened squamous layer. Histology findings are similar to those of classic MF.

Treatment of palmar-plantar MF is difficult given the thickness of involved areas. First-line treatment includes high-potency topical corticosteroids, topical retinoids, and topical nitrogen mustard. Phototherapy is another option including topical PUVA and nbUVB to hands and feet only (if no other lesions are present). Although an option, localized radiation is not recommended as first-line treatment because of the high occurrence of side effects including edema and infection. In this difficult-to-treat variant, oral medication, including oral retinoids and methotrexate, may be necessary. Patients are often motivated to start aggressive treatment given the location, discomfort, and limitations of daily activities associated with palmar-plantar MF.

SUMMARY

MF is characterized clinically by an indolent course with evolution of patches, plaques, and tumors and histologically by an epidermal infiltration of atypical T cells. Although the most common type of cutaneous lymphoma, MF is often a very difficult diagnosis to make. Different morphologies, multiple clinicopathologic variants, and similarity to many other disease entities help create this diagnostic conundrum (Table 6-4). Close follow-up and patient education are key to diagnosis and treatment of those with MF.

With the advent of the Internet along with multiple avenues of information, many patients often mistake this usually slow-progressing disease for a fungal infection or a devastating malignancy. If found early and treated appropriately, patients with MF can be expected to have normal lifespans with limited impact on quality of life.

TABLE 6-4   Characteristics of Mycosis Fungoides Variants

Variant	Clinical Presentation	Biopsy Method	Histology	Predominant T-cell Subset
Pagetoid reticulosis	Acral patch with scale	Punch	Marked epidermotropism	CD8+
Granulomatous slack skin	Intertriginous areas with well-circumscribed, erythematous, pendulous lax skin	Shave	Dense granulomatous infiltrate along with elastolysis	CD4+
Follicular	Papules on the face, neck, upper trunk	Punch	Atypical lymphocytes around and within hair follicles	CD4+
Syringotropic	Erythematous to hyperpigmented patches and plaques with or without papules and pustules	Punch	Atypical cells invading hyperplastic eccrine ducts and glands	CD4+
Hypopigmented	Hypopigmented patches with irregular borders in the bathing suit distribution	Shave	Pigment incontinence and decreased basal pigmentation in addition to findings of classic MF	CD8+
Poikilodermatous	Hypo- and hyperpigmentation with atrophy and telangiectasia	Shave	Epidermal atrophy and telangiectatic vessels in addition to findings of classic MF	CD8+
Palmar-plantar	Diffuse erythema with scale, erosions, ulcerations, and fissures on acral locations	Punch	Similar to classic MF	CD4+
Pigmented purpuric	Erythematous to brown purpuric macules and patches	Shave	Siderphages and extravasated erythrocytes in addition to findings of classic MF	CD4+

MF, mycosis fungoides.

SUGGESTED READINGS

Weinstock MA: Epidemiology of mycosis fungoides. Semin Dermatol. 1994;13:154–159.

Willemze R, et al: WHO-EORTC Classification for Cutaneous Lymphoma. Blood. 2005;105:3768–3785.

van Doorn R, et al: Follicular Mycosis Fungoides, a Distinct Disease Entity With or Without Associated Follicular Mucinosis. Arch Dermatol. 2002;138:191–198.

Kazakov DV, et al: Clinicopathological Spectrum of Mycosis Fungoides. JEADV. 2004;18,397–415.

Kempf W, et al: Granulomatous Mycosis Fungoides and Granulomatous Slack Skin. Arch Dermatol. 2008;144(12):1609–1617.

SÉZARY SYNDROME

Agnieszka W. Kubica, MD, Mark D. P. Davis, MD,
and Mark R. Pittelkow, MD

INTRODUCTION

Sézary syndrome (SS), a rare and aggressive type of cutaneous T-cell lymphoma (CTCL), comprises a heterogeneous group of mature T-lymphocyte malignancies. Despite the complexities of this disease, extensive advances in research on SS and CTCL have generated a greater understanding of the immunologic basis and pathogenesis of SS in an effort to better manage affected patients. As the prevalence of CTCL continues to increase, the diagnostic challenges and management of SS prove to be important areas of study. Recently, efforts by the International Society for Cutaneous Lymphomas, the U.S. Cutaneous Lymphoma Consortium, and other national and international collaboratives have provided a greater understanding of this disease and a more uniform consensus on diagnostic, staging, and treatment guidelines. CTCL presents along a disease spectrum defined by the tumor-node-metastasis-blood (TNMB) staging system. SS is, by definition, staged as more advanced disease in which not only cutaneous involvement but also leukemic burden create a potentially more challenging constellation of symptoms and portend poorer outcome.

This chapter outlines the disease pathogenesis of SS, its immunologic basis, and the diagnostic challenges posed by a clinical presentation of erythroderma. Furthermore, molecular advances in our understanding of SS and basic treatment guidelines are reviewed to highlight effective management of this unique malignancy that intertwines dermatologic and hematologic-oncologic manifestations.

EPIDEMIOLOGY

Overall, the incidence of CTCL was estimated at 6.4 cases per million between 1973 and 2002, and it has been increasing since the early 1970's. SS is a rare subtype of CTCL. Although data regarding the incidence of SS are limited, SS accounts for approximately 2.5% of the cases of CTCL, according to the U.S. National Cancer Institute's Surveillance, Epidemiology, and End Results (SEER) program. Men are generally affected twice as often as women. Whereas the black population has a higher overall incidence of CTCL, the incidence of SS, in particular, is higher among whites. The increased incidence is noted with increasing age; the average age at diagnosis is 50 to 60 years.

Few studies have examined the prognosis of SS. Available information indicates that the natural disease course of SS is more aggressive than that of mycosis fungoides (MF), and the prognosis for patients with MF is typically very poor. The median survival ranges from 2 to 4 years. Overall survival at 5 years is 26%, and disease-specific survival is 31% at 5 years. When extracutaneous involvement of the viscera is identified, median survival is typically 2.5 years or less. Prognostic factors associated with worse outcomes include advanced age (>60 yr), increased number of previous treatments, enlargement of peripheral lymph nodes, greater leukemic burden in the blood, male sex, increased lactate dehydrogenase levels, low percentage of CD8+ cells in lymph nodes, and large cell transformation.

In SS, the most common cause of death is complications from progressive disease, most frequently secondary infection resulting from breakdowns in the skin barrier and the immunosuppression that results from the hematologic involvement. The organisms tend to be *Staphylococcus aureus,* Enterobacteriaceae, and *Pseudomonas aeruginosa;* in advanced SS, opportunistic infections such as disseminated herpes and fungal infections can lead to death. Other common causes of death include cardiopulmonary disease and secondary malignancies because patients with SS have an overall increased risk of malignancies such as lung cancer, Hodgkin's lymphoma, and other types of non-Hodgkin's lymphoma.

Nevertheless, data are limited regarding the disease course itself and incorporation of the changes that have occurred since the early 2000s, including inclusion of new diagnostic criteria and use of immunomodulatory agents and monoclonal antibodies as treatment. As a result of the constantly evolving understanding of CTCL and the rarity of SS compared with the greater prevalence of MF, studies have frequently grouped relatively more indolent malignancies such as erythrodermic MF or advanced stage MF with SS, resulting in inaccurate data on the actual outcomes and survival of documented SS. Additional confounding factors in establishing clear epidemiologic data on survival and treatment include the frequent exclusion of patients with SS from clinical trials of CTCL treatment and the myriad definitions used as endpoints in various studies. Therefore, newer studies that use the revised international consensus definitions for SS and more uniform criteria for outcomes are urgently needed to develop a more accurate knowledge base for this aggressive malignancy.

A DIAGNOSIS IN EVOLUTION

Atypical circulating blood cells were first described in 1938 by Sézary,[1,2] when he observed large, abnormal cells with hyperconvoluted nuclei in the peripheral blood (*cellules monstreuses*) in the unique setting of generalized red skin. He came to the conclusion that patients with these findings were affected by a new, more aggressive hematologic malignancy, and the concept of SS took form. In 1961, Taswell and Winkelmann[3] at the Mayo Clinic identified a hallmark of the Sézary cell (the unique grooved nucleus that was shown to be serpentine, or cerebriform, on electron microscopy) and coined the term *Sézary syndrome.* Under the subsequent unifying term of CTCL, SS was originally regarded as an aggressive, leukemic form of MF and other primary T-cell lymphomas. Over time, the definition of SS has undergone progressive revisions, and the disease has become more well-defined. SS has remained a unique diagnostic entity separate from MF. In addition, scientific advances have allowed the incorporation of novel molecular techniques to more clearly define the leukemic component of the syndrome. Nevertheless, ambiguity persists

in fully quantifying the atypical lymphocytes in peripheral blood.

In the 1970s, the definition of SS included the classic triad of generalized erythroderma, lymphadenopathy, and blood involvement. Initial methods of measuring blood involvement focused on accounting for the percentage of leukocytes on a peripheral smear that were composed of atypical lymphocytes with the classic cerebriform nuclei. These cells, known as *Sézary cells,* became the standard hematologic benchmark of SS, with a cutoff of 1000 cells/mm^3 or more or greater than 5% of the total leukocytes needed for diagnosis. However, because this method of Sézary cell quantitation often involves a substantial degree of interobserver variability and requires considerable experience in interpretation, its clinical utility is limited. In addition, similar such cells were found in the blood of healthy persons and in patients with inflammatory skin diseases (so-called Sézary-like cells), a suggestion that the traditional Sézary cell may not, in fact, be specific to SS but may be simulated by any atypical lymphocytes with convoluted nuclei.

The leukemic criteria have thus evolved to incorporate more sophisticated diagnostic techniques, including polymerase chain reaction (PCR), Southern blot, immunohistochemistry, and flow cytometry, to provide a more specific diagnosis. The International Society for Cutaneous Lymphomas and the European Organization for Research and Treatment of Cancer published revised diagnostic criteria for CTCL and, more specifically, SS in 2007 (Table 7-1).[4] Staging based on this TNMB system is crucial at time of diagnosis because it helps guide therapy and can help glean information about prognosis. SS is defined as stages T4 (>80% of total body surface area [BSA] involved with erythroderma) and B2 (definitive leukemic involvement defined by molecular evidence of clonality by T-cell gene rearrangement in the blood, absolute Sézary cell count ≥ 1000/mm^3, CD4/CD8 ratio ≥ 10 by flow cytometry, and abnormal immunophenotype, including loss of CD7 [≥40%] or CD26 [≥30%]). In essence, SS is defined as T4N0-3M0-1B2. Importantly, no single test is consistently sufficient for diagnosis, and SS ultimately requires incorporation of all available clinical, pathologic, immunohistochemical, and cytogenetic findings.

TABLE 7-1 Tumor-Node-Metastasis-Blood Staging for Mycosis Fungoides and Sézary Syndrome

Stage	Description
T: Tumor	
T1	Patches, papules, or plaques < 10% body surface area
T2	Patches/plaques ≥ 10% body surface area
T3	One or more tumors (≥1 cm in diameter)
T4*	**Erythroderma (erythema ≥ 80% of body surface area)**
N: Nodal	
N0	No clinically abnormal peripheral lymph nodes
N1[†]	Clinically abnormal peripheral lymph nodes, histopathology Dutch grade 2 or NCI LN0-2
N2[†]	Clinically abnormal peripheral lymph nodes, histopathology Dutch grade 2 or NCI LN3
N3	Clinically abnormally peripheral lymph nodes, histopathology Dutch grade 3-4 or NCI LN4; clone-positive or -negative
NX	Clinically abnormal peripheral lymph nodes, no histopathologic information provided
M: Metastases/ Visceral Involvement	
M0	No visceral organ involvement
M1	Visceral organ involvement with pathologic confirmation
B: Peripheral Blood	
B0[†]	Absence of significant blood involvement: ≤5% of peripheral blood lymphocytes are Sézary cells
B1[†]	Low blood tumor burden: >5% of peripheral blood lymphocytes are Sézary cells
B2*	**High blood tumor burden: requires positive clonal rearrangement of T-cell receptor *plus* one of the following: absolute Sézary cell count ≥ 1,000 mm³; expanded CD4+ or CD3+ cells with CD4/CD8 ratio ≥ 10; expanded CD4+ cells with abnormal immunophenotype, including loss of CD7 (≥40%) or CD26 (≥30%)**

LN, lymph node; NCI, National Cancer Institute.

*Necessary criteria for Sézary syndrome.

[†]Can be divided into "a" and "b" types if information on clone is available from polymerase chain reaction or Southern blot analysis of T-cell receptor. "a" is clone-negative; "b" is clone-positive.

Adapted from Olsen E, Vonderheid E, Pimpinelli N, Willemze R, Kim Y, Knobler R, et al; ISCL/EORTC. Revisions to the staging and classification of mycosis fungoides and Sézary syndrome: a proposal of the International Society for Cutaneous Lymphomas (ISCL) and the cutaneous lymphoma task force of the European Organization of Research and Treatment of Cancer (EORTC). *Blood.* 2007;110:1713–1722. Epub 2007;May 31. Erratum in: *Blood.* 2008;111:4830. Used with permission.

PATHOGENESIS AND IMMUNOLOGY

Various theories have been postulated about the cause of SS, but no convincing evidence has delineated the cause of this malignancy. Environmental factors, such as industrial exposures, and cutaneous allergies to plants, metal, and insect bites have all been implicated in the pathogenesis, but no studies have supported this theory. Some studies have speculated that chronic antigenic stimulation with skin-associated bacteria, such as *S. aureus* and *Chlamydia,* could be linked to development of SS, a theory that follows similar associations such as gastric mucosal lymphoma with *Helicobacter pylori* or non-Hodgkin's lymphoma with hepatitis C. The finding of an increased frequency of particular human leukocyte antigen (HLA) class II alleles in patients with CTCL may support the notion of chronic antigenic stimulation, but further evidence is limited. Other associations have been made between SS and cytomegalovirus and Epstein-Barr virus; however, evidence for these associations is also scarce.

Because immunomodulatory agents such as interferon-alpha (IFN-α) have provided clinical benefit, the role of the immune system in SS has come into question. Over time, studies have uncovered the strong immunologic basis of this malignancy, which has in turn been the subject of novel immunomodulatory therapeutics research. The various facets of the pathogenesis and immunology are highlighted in the following sections.

Epidermotropism in Sézary Cells

The study of specific chemokine receptors (otherwise known as chemotactic cytokine receptors) has identified the unique development of skin-homing abilities of malignant T cells that typify CTCL. Because SS is classically associated with the proliferation of CD4+ malignant T cells, these cells have come into focus in research studies, especially in their variations of surface markers. In particular, CCR4 and CCR10 have been implicated in the affinity of these malignant T cells for skin. These two receptors have been noted on skin-homing common lymphocyte antigen–positive (CLA+) cells in SS and display CCL17 (a major ligand of the CCR4 compound) and CCL27 (a major ligand of the CCR10 compound). CCL17 and CCL27 have been found in increased quantities in SS, and evidence suggests their correlation with disease activity. These two chemokines facilitate T-cell migration to the skin and activate anti-apoptotic pathways to increase the survival of these cells.

To further promote this activity, malignant T cells often exhibit the loss of particular surface antigens, such as CD7, CD26, and CD49d. In particular, the loss of CD26 (otherwise known as dipeptidylpeptidase IV) promotes migration of Sézary cells into the skin in response to the ligand CXCL12, a process that thus assists in skin homing and enhanced survival of these malignant T cells. This pathway has been the target of immunologic therapeutic research; various fusion molecules are currently being studied to attempt to block both CCR4 and CCR10 and prevent the migration of malignant T cells into the skin.

Histopathologic studies have shown that the degree of epidermotropism is less marked in SS than in early CTCL or MF. This phenomenon has not been entirely explained, but it is believed to stem from altered chemokine gradients in patients with leukemic CTCL, unlike in those with skin-limited disease. In addition, new evidence indicates different markers in the malignant cells of SS versus MF. In malignant CD4+ cells of SS, CCR7 and L-selectin are co-expressed, and CD27 is expressed also—all markers of central memory T cells. CCR4 is also highly expressed. Alternatively, in MF, T cells from cutaneous lesions lack the CCR7–L-selectin and CD27 phenotype and instead express CCR4 in conjunction with CLA, thus representing an effector memory T cell. These fascinating results point to a clear difference between molecular characteristics of MF (a malignancy of skin-residing effector memory T cells) and SS (a malignancy of central memory T cells).

Loss of T-Cell Repertoire and Cellular Immunity

As with many hematologic malignancies, the predominance of a particular cellular clone can be a principal feature for both diagnosing the disease and mediating its pathogenesis. In SS, this results in major defects in cellular immunity, especially in advanced disease. PCR studies show a substantial reduction of T-cell receptor (TCR) diversity compared with that in the normal age-adjusted population, with the expansion of a malignant T-cell clone that exhibits a T-cell–receptor gene rearrangement. As the malignant T-cell population expands, cell-mediated immunity decreases as normal T-cell repertoires become restricted to make room for the malignant T-cell clone. Interestingly, in some cases of SS remission, normal T-cell repertoire recovers, an indication of reversibility with immunomodulatory therapies.

In addition to decreased diversity and number of cells, the function of natural killer (NK) cells and CD8+ cells is impaired. Normally, NK cells function as key players in cytotoxicity and IFN-γproduction, which typically serves the cellular response against viral and intrabacterial pathogens and the antitumor response. Furthermore, CD8+ T cells in the skin are associated with a favorable prognosis, possibly serving as an indication of a patient's antitumor response against malignant CD4+ T cells. In patients with SS, as the malignant T-cell load increases, the activation of normal NK and CD8+ cells decreases. Because both these cells are crucial in the direct antitumor response, this correlation is speculated to further exacerbate the growth of the malignant blood burden.

Tumor Microenvironment

As is common in many malignancies, patients with SS are immunocompromised, particularly those with more pronounced leukemic burden. Many factors contribute to this immunosuppression, but a major facet is the shift of immune response from Th1 to Th2 response. The Th2 response is linked to the development of tolerance and impaired antitumor immunity, as opposed to the Th1 response that leads to destruction of tumor cells.

This shift is promoted by the production of proinflammatory cytokines, such as interleukin-4 (IL-4) and IL-5. IL-4 is involved in differentiation of naïve helper T cells, and IL-5 stimulates B-cell growth, eosinophilic activation, and immunoglobulin production. Another prominent cytokine in this milieu, IL-10, acts along with IL-4 to stimulate the Th2 shift by blunting NK and CD8+ cell actions, suppressing Th1 response, and impairing normal differentiation of dendritic cells. IL-7

(a hematopoietic growth factor) and IL-18 (a proinflammatory cytokine involved in cell-mediated immunity) are also up-regulated in patients with SS, unlike in healthy persons. On a regulatory genetic level, a transcription factor associating with Th2 cell immunity, GATA-3, has been found to be overexpressed in Sézary cells. This cytokine imbalance, found in patients with both SS and advanced stage MF, shows the crucial role of the immune system in the pathogenesis of this unique malignancy. The Th2 shift is further evidenced by the therapeutic benefits that arise from use of IFN-α, IL-12, and tumor necrosis factor-alpha (TNF-α)—all agents that promote the Th1 response.

Dendritic Cells

Dendritic cells also play a central role in the pathogenesis of SS in a multifaceted manner. Some studies have noted that dendritic cells in the blood decrease as the tumor burden increases. Therefore, there is a decrease in the cumulative amounts of critical antitumor cytokines secreted by dendritic cells—IL-12, IL-15, and IFN-α. Another element of impaired dendritic cell production and function is the mutated form of CD40 ligand on malignant T cells. In the normal immunologic response, CD40 ligand (CD40L) on T cells is up-regulated and interacts with CD40 on antigen-presenting cells, which, in turn, activates the dendritic cells. In SS, the mutated or deficient CD40L prevents this normal interaction and, thus, decreases IL-12 production. Accordingly, as levels of dendritic cells decrease, there is a corresponding decrease in resistance against tumor growth and proliferation as the population of defective T cells that is unable to activate dendritic cells grows.

Infections

As a result of the decreased immune function in SS, for the reasons outlined previously, the number and severity of infections increase. In fact, this immunosuppression is frequently the cause of death in patients with SS. In many malignancies, chemotherapeutic agents typically create defects in immune function that result in worsening of infections, but in SS, such examples have been

BOX 7-1   Workup of a Patient with Sézary Syndrome

Laboratory	Hematologic	Procedures	Imaging
Routine chemistry tests Erythrocyte sedimentation rate Lactate dehydrogenase Protein electrophoresis Skin culture or scraping if infection (fungal, bacterial) is suspected	Complete blood count with differential Peripheral blood smear with Sézary cell count PCR or Southern blot analysis of TCR gene rearrangement Flow cytometry or immunophenotyping of peripheral blood (CD4, CD8, CD7, CD26, V beta)	Skin biopsy for routine histology with H&E, immunophenotyping, and TCR gene rearrangement analysis LN biopsy (target most accessible enlarged LN) BM biopsy or aspirate if needed to differentiate from other hematologic disorders	CT of chest, abdomen and pelvis (±PET) Routine chest radiography

BM, bone marrow; CT, computed tomography; H&E, hematoxylin-and-eosin; LN, lymph node; PCR, polymerase chain reaction; PET, positron emission tomography; TCR, T-cell receptor.

considered an inherent result of the malignancy itself. For example, studies have shown that herpesvirus is substantially worse in advanced SS, and others have associated SS with the development of JC-virus–linked progressive multifocal leukoencephalopathy, a condition that typically occurs only in severely immunocompromised patients. In addition, defects in neutrophil function and cytokine abnormalities are implicated in increased severity of bacterial infection and increased skin colonization of pathogens such as *S. aureus*.

should be noted; this information will assist in monitoring response to therapy or monitoring progression of disease in the case of pre-SS or MF. Further workup is outlined in Box 7-1. Of note in the hematologic workup, large Sézary cells frequently resemble the size of monocytes; therefore, monocytosis should raise a suspicion when noted in the clinical setting of erythroderma, and a peripheral smear should be more closely evaluated for Sézary cells. In addition, eosinophilia in patients with SS could be a contributing factor to the severe pruritus.

CLINICAL EVALUATION OF A PATIENT

In a patient suspected of having SS, the initial workup includes various hematologic, laboratory, imaging, and procedural evaluations. First and foremost, a careful and detailed history should be elicited to understand the time course and severity of symptoms, associated risk factors, and pertinent family, occupational, and social history and to provide a relevant review of systems. A thorough physical examination should be done that focuses on the dermatologic presentation, associated signs, and possible extracutaneous involvement in, for example, lymph nodes, spleen, and liver. For quantifying the extent of erythroderma or erythema, the percentage of total BSA involved

CLINICAL FINDINGS

SS typically is associated with a constellation of symptoms that, although profound and readily visible, introduce a wide range of conditions to be considered in the differential diagnosis. Most classically, patients with SS have a remarkable erythroderma—defined more precisely as erythema covering 80% or more of total BSA (although there is debate about the percentage involvement needed for diagnosis of erythroderma). In addition, lymphadenopathy is common, one indication of systemic involvement of the disease. Although lymphadenopathy is still a frequent finding in SS, it is no longer needed for the diagnosis of SS with the advent of new molecular techniques. The most

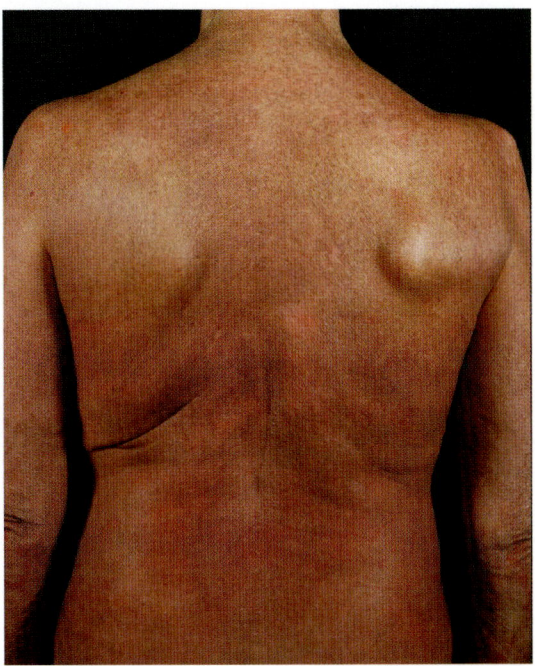

Figure 7-1 Erythroderma.

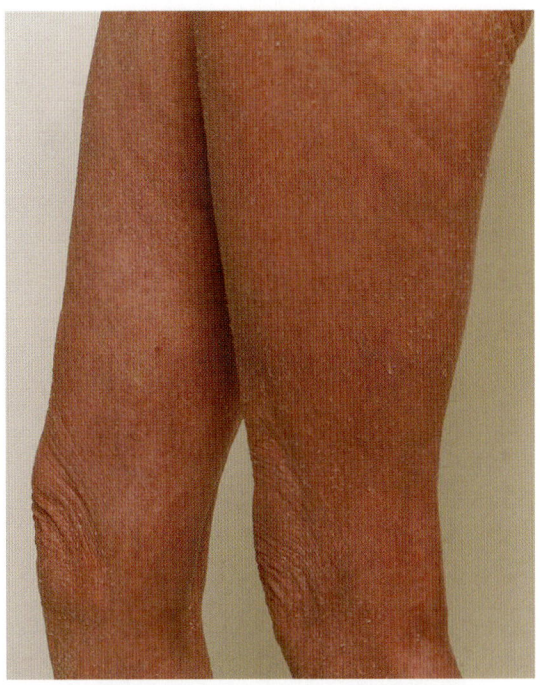

Figure 7-2 Erythroderma involving the lower extremities.

notable complaint of patients with SS is severe pruritus. This can be a devastating and debilitating symptom. Other common findings include palmoplantar keratoderma, scaling, fissuring of skin, lichenification, and ectropion. Some of these physical findings are shown in Figures 7-1 to 7-6. Bacterial or dermatophyte superinfection is frequent, especially in open skin wounds or areas of excoriation.

Although symptoms can progress over the course of years from a mild dermatitis to full-blown erythroderma and severe pruritus, the onset of symptoms occurs more typically over several months. Patients with SS may also present with or subsequently have development of patches, plaques, and tumors, as would be found in MF. Common signs and symptoms of SS are listed in Box 7-2.

In addition, SS may progress from a pre-SS state in which laboratory criteria are insufficient to meet the classic diagnosis of SS. Winkelmann originally described this phenomenon in 1984.[5] Similar to B-lymphocyte clonality and distinguishing monoclonal gammopathy of undetermined significance from multiple myeloma, studies have suggested the term *monoclonal T-cell dyscrasia of undetermined significance* to conceptualize the erythrodermic pre-SS state as a precursor to SS.

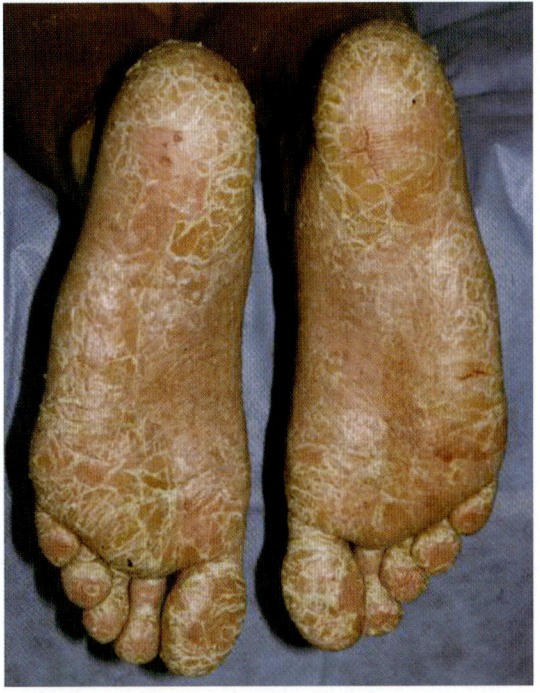

Figure 7-3 Plantar keratoderma.

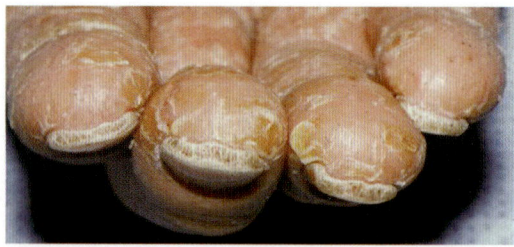

Figure 7-4 Onychodystrophy.

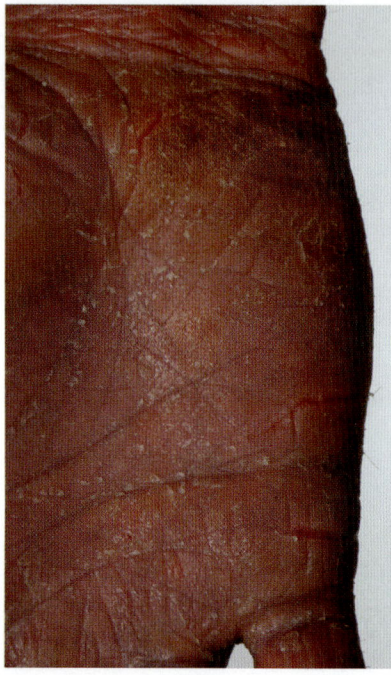

Figure 7-5 Hand with erythroderma and overlying scale and fissuring.

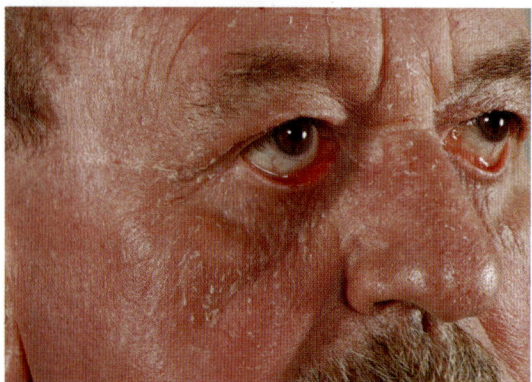

Figure 7-6 Ectropion.

BOX 7-2   Common Presenting Signs and Symptoms of Sézary Syndrome

Erythroderma	Pigmentary changes
Pruritus	Alopecia
Palmar and plantar keratoderma	Alopecia mucinosa
Lichenification	Onychodystrophy
Xerosis	Leonine facies
Exfoliation	Hepatosplenomegaly
Ectropion	Lymphadenopathy
Scaling or icythyosis-like changes	Systemic symptoms (fevers, chills, fatigue, weight loss)

Although erythroderma has always been a primary criterion in the diagnosis of SS, recent reports document existence of a non-erythrodermic SS picture. In a particular case report, a patient had hyperkeratosis, severe pruritus, and lymphadenopathy but lacked any patches, plaques, or erythema.[6] Nevertheless, skin biopsy showed a TCR clone identical to that identified in blood, lymph nodes, and bone marrow. In addition, a strong CD4+ cell predominance was identified and marked "sezaremia" was documented. Such cases illuminate atypical SS and offer broader insight into the requirements for the extent of erythroderma in the diagnosis of SS.

HISTOPATHOLOGIC FINDINGS

The histologic characteristics of skin biopsy specimens in SS may reflect the hematologic burden and confirm physical findings; however, only 60% of skin biopsy results in CTCL and SS are diagnostic. Repeat biopsies are frequently necessary because of nonspecific findings. Therefore, skin biopsies are not incorporated into the diagnostic criteria of SS, but they are almost always performed in patients suspected of having CTCL. In fact, skin biopsies are frequently more specific and diagnostic in cases of MF or skin-limited disease. Nevertheless, TCR clones found in the erythrodermic skin of patients with SS are particularly helpful when correlated with clones in the blood, lymph nodes, or bone marrow. Skin biopsy specimens designated for immunophenotyping and molecular genetic studies should be snap-frozen in liquid nitrogen and stored at −70°C to allow subsequent diagnostic analysis to be performed. Other skin biopsy tissue should be designated for hematoxylin-and-eosin staining.

The typical histopathologic findings on skin biopsy in patients with SS is a bandlike perivascular atypical lymphocytic infiltrate. However, epidermotropism is more commonly noted in MF than in SS. The finding of a perivascular infiltrate signifies the migration of atypical lymphocytes into the skin and is, thus, highly suspicious for SS, especially when correlated with appropriate laboratory and physical examination findings. Another classic finding, although more common in MF, is Pautrier microabscesses, or aggregated malignant T cells and Langerhans cells (epidermal dendritic cells) that exist within the epidermis. These microabscesses are fairly specific, but they are not always found on biopsy, especially in the majority of cases when SS arises de novo. A "string of pearls," or filing of malignant T cells along the basal layer of the epidermis, can also occur. The presence of large Sézary cells, large cell transformation, and other immunophenotypic abnormalities should be noted. Large cell transformations are associated with worse outcomes.

Within lymph nodes involved by SS, not only can a clone be identified using molecular methods but also histologic examination can show diffuse infiltration of Sézary cells and varied degrees of lymph node effacement. Similarly, bone marrow biopsies are performed in some instances, especially when other hematologic malignancies are part of the differential diagnosis. Imaging studies such as positron emission tomography (PET) or computed tomography (CT) are performed at initial staging to further assess visceral and nodal involvement. The role of CT is controversial in that it does not improve detection of advanced disease and typically provides only anatomic information. However, PET has increased sensitivity for detecting extracutaneous involvement by recognizing intensity of activity that correlates with histologic lymph node grade, and it is also used to monitor treatment response in patients with advanced disease.

METHODS OF ASSESSING HEMATOLOGIC INVOLVEMENT

With the lack of specificity or universality of histologic evaluation of skin and lymph nodes, the diagnostic shifts over the decades have come to focus on the hematologic aspects of SS, one of the key differentiators of SS from other CTCL variants. The spectrum of methods used to analyze peripheral blood involvement has expanded vastly in recent decades and has thus led to more accurate diagnosis. Nevertheless, the issue of false-negative and false-positive results persists.

Sézary Cell Counting

As outlined previously, this traditional method has been the foundation of measuring leukemic involvement of SS and involves enumerating atypical lymphocytes with convoluted nuclei—Sézary cells—in the peripheral blood smear. The result is reported as a percentage, and the absolute Sézary count is established by multiplying total leukocytes by this percentage to derive the number of Sézary cells per cubic millimeter. Absolute Sézary count was found to be a more reliable measure than percentage of total blood leukocytes; however, in some patients with benign dermatoses and reactive erythroderma, approximately 5% also may have absolute Sézary cell counts more than 1000/mm^3. New advances have incorporated other criteria into the diagnosis of SS, but the absolute Sézary cell count remains as a diagnostic criterion in the new diagnostic algorithms of the International Society of Cutaneous Lymphomas, in addition to the more objective molecular techniques. Sézary cells on peripheral blood smears are shown in Figure 7-7.

Immunophenotyping

With the use of flow cytometry, studies have been able to identify aberrations and particularly prevalent clonal populations in SS. This method, otherwise called *flow cytometric immunophenotyping*, uses antibodies directed against TCR beta chain variable region families and is able to provide both qualitative and quantitative estimates

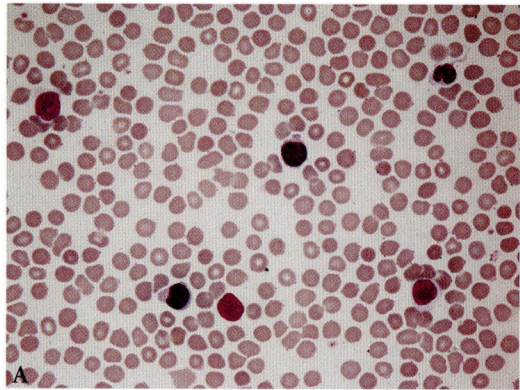
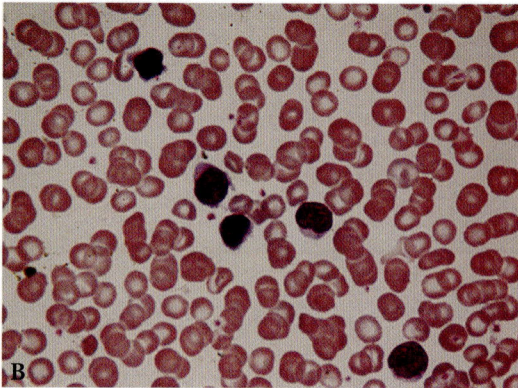

Figure 7-7 **A**, Peripheral blood smear Classic Sézary cells are visualized as large, dark, hyperconvoluted nuclei (Giemsa-Weight stain, high-power magnification). **B**, Peripheral blood smear. Sézary cells are seen with higher magnification.

of clonal activity. T-cell subsets are also analyzed quantitatively. The most commonly found immunophenotypic variant is CD4+CD7−; this variant is found in 60% to 70% of patients with SS. The CD4+CD26− and CD7−CD62L− subsets are of particular interest. In addition, the ratio of CD4 to CD8 cells is another criterion used in SS. A CD4/CD8 ratio of 10 or more is considered stage B2 and occurs in approximately 80% of patients with SS; such patients have a 5-year survival of 11%. Other common abnormalities include loss of pan–T-cell markers such as CD2, CD3, and CD5; absent expression of CD4 and CD8; or co-expression of CD4 and CD8.

Molecular Genetics

Leukemic involvement can also be measured using molecular genetic techniques, most notably Southern blot and PCR methods. Although these molecular techniques are not particularly quantitative, they are the most sensitive method of diagnosing SS by detection of clonal T-cell gene rearrangement. Southern blot has a clonal detection threshold of 1% to 5%; however, use of Southern blot has been overshadowed by the more precise use of PCR-based methods, which are at least 10 times more sensitive. However, this sensitivity even detects positive clones in precursors of SS, such as early CTCL or MF or parapsoriasis. Clonality by PCR in SS has been the focus of many studies in recent decades and has been validated as a prognostic factor for worse outcomes. In addition, the

identification of a circulating clone using PCR or Southern blot can be matched to clones found in the skin, lymph nodes, or bone marrow. However, as was noted in studies of Sézary cell counts, TCR gene rearrangements can also be found in benign inflammatory and autoimmune conditions, such as systemic sclerosis, and in the aged population; T-cell clonality has been reported in 6% to 24% of such benign skin conditions that also exhibit a lymphoid infiltrate. Alternatively, 10% to 15% of patients with SS test negative for TCR gene rearrangements. The use of these molecular techniques has revolutionized diagnosis and disease management, especially with the capacity to detect disease, relapse, and response to treatment more efficiently.

Cytogenetics

Cytogenetic abnormalities have also been identified in SS, likely resulting from a degree of chromosomal instability that is inherent in various malignancies. The most commonly noted aberrancy is the loss of the long arm of chromosome 10. Other translocations or deletions have been established on chromosomes 1, 6, 9, 11, 13, 14, and 17. Various tumor suppressor and apoptosis-related genes have been identified in patients with MF and SS, although the implications are still not clear. These include NAV3, *p53, p15, p16, JUNB*, and PTEN. Mutations in these genes tend to occur in later stage disease, a suggestion that they are secondary genetic events. Nevertheless, it is difficult to find recurring themes associated with poor prognosis because of the rarity of SS; however, new studies are being performed on larger cohorts based on recently revised diagnostic criteria and hold promise for a greater understanding of pathogenesis in the future.

DIFFERENTIAL DIAGNOSIS

Perhaps the most challenging diagnostic question arises in differentiating cases of erythrodermic MF, erythrodermic CTCL not otherwise specified (NOS), MF with leukemic components, SS, and the recently described nonerythrodermic SS (Table 7-2). Typically, erythrodermic MF is an evolution of preexisting MF (patch, plaque, or tumor CTCL); therefore, there is absent or minimal blood involvement (B0-B1). In erythrodermic CTCL NOS, preexisting MF is never seen, and blood involvement remains absent or minimal; in such cases, it would be rare to see a TCR clone. Current criteria indicate that patients with CTCL with B2 blood involvement lacking erythroderma should be designated as having "MF with leukemic involvement," but this categorization is in question because of convincing evidence of patients with so-called nonerythrodermic SS. In classic SS, preexisting MF can occur, but it is rare and might be associated with a different prognosis.

In addition, the marked clinical findings of SS, especially erythroderma, can mimic many benign conditions and several other neoplasias (Box 7-3). Most commonly, pityriasis rubra pilaris, parapsoriasis, drug-induced dermatitis, and contact dermatitis lead the top of the list on the clinical differential diagnosis of erythroderma.

TREATMENT

SS is an aggressive malignancy that is rarely curable; however, with early detection and implementation of proper treatment, the disease course can show improved response rate and the severe symptoms may be reduced. In cases of lymph node, bone marrow, and heavy leukemic involvement, the probability of sustained clinical remission is low, and relapses frequently occur within weeks to months of cessation of therapy. The spectrum of treatment ranges from topical agents to light therapy to systemic chemotherapies and typically needs to be administered for years. In theory, treatment for more limited disease, as in MF, begins with skin-targeted therapies, such as nitrogen mustard, topical corticosteroids, and ultraviolet light–based treatments. However, in the case of SS, in which systemic leukemic involvement is a main element of the disease, a more aggressive, systemic

TABLE 7-2   Variants of Cutaneous T-Cell Lymphoma in the Differential Diagnosis of Sézary Syndrome

CTCL Subtype	Erythroderma Present	Preexisting MF	Blood Findings	TNMB Designation
SS	Yes	Rarely	Leukemic	T4N0-3M0-1B2
Erythrodermic MF	Yes	Typically	Absent or minimal	T4N0-3M0-1B0-1
E-CTCL NOS	Yes	Absent	Absent or minimal	T4N0-3M0-1B0-1
MF with leukemic findings/ nonerythrodermic SS	No	Typically	Leukemic	T1-3N0-3M0-1B2

B, blood; CTCL, cutaneous T-cell lymphoma; E-CTCL NOS, erythrodermic CTCL not otherwise specified; M, metastasis; MF, mycosis fungoides; N, node; SS, Sézary syndrome; T, tumor.

Adapted from Vonderheid EC, Bernengo MG, Burg G, Duvic M, Heald P, Laroche L, et al; ISCL. Update on erythrodermic cutaneous T-cell lymphoma: report of the International Society for Cutaneous Lymphomas. *J Am Acad Dermatol.* 2002;46:95–106. Used with permission.

BOX 7-3   Differential Diagnosis of Erythroderma and Sézary Syndrome

	Benign	Malignant
Cutaneous drug reaction	Pityriasis rubra pilaris	Acute or chronic leukemia
Generalized anaphylaxis	Seborrheic dermatitis	CTCL spectrum disease
Urticaria/hives	Solar urticaria	Erythrodermic MF
Contact dermatitis	Bullous pemphigoid	Pre-Sézary syndrome
Eczema/atopic dermatitis	Graft-versus-host disease	
Purpura	Sarcoidosis	
Psoriasis	DRESS syndrome	
Parapsoriasis	Lupus erythematous	
Dermal reticulosis	Dermatomyositis	

CTCL, chronic T-cell lymphoma; DRESS, drug reaction with eosinophilia and systemic symptoms; MF, mycosis fungoides.

approach must be taken. This usually begins with single-agent therapies but can progress to a combination approach in the case of unresponsive disease or prior treatment failure. Combination approaches can be highly effective, approaching 90% overall response rates. However, when disease recurs despite systemic chemotherapeutic combination, outcomes are poor and the disease tends to be refractory to further interventions.

During the past several decades, considerable advances have allowed the development of innovative therapies to not only decrease severity of symptoms and increase survival time but also decrease the toxic effects of treatment. Because of the rarity of CTCL, particularly SS, randomized trials are difficult to perform, and thus establishment of evidence-based treatment algorithms is a conundrum. Nevertheless, the U.S. Cutaneous Lymphoma Consortium has recommended guidelines for therapy (Box 7-4).

It is important to consider the general health and age of a patient, availability of therapies, and the aggressiveness of disease when making management decisions. In addition, because of the complexities of the disease process and the interplay between hematologic and dermatologic manifestations, management is best handled by a multidisciplinary approach, including dermatologic, radiation oncologic, hematologic, and oncologic specialists.

The main therapeutic options are briefly described later. Overall treatment guidelines from the U.S. Cutaneous Lymphoma Consortium are presented in Table 7-3.

Immunomodulatory Agents

As mentioned previously, the first line of therapy in SS patients is a monotherapy systemic treatment with immunomodulatory agents, such as extracorporeal photophersis, interferons, retinoids, and denileukin diftitox. The immunologic defects described earlier have been observed to return to normal after clinical remission with such immunomodulatory therapies.

Extracorporeal Photopheresis

Extracorporeal photopheresis has been an effective and well-tolerated agent, acting as a systemic leukapheresis combined with photochemotherapy against malignant cells. This procedure typically occurs on 2 consecutive days every 4 weeks and involves injection of liquid 8-methoxypsoralen into a collection bag with enriched leukocytes. The exact mechanism of action remains unclear, but extracorporeal photopheresis is speculated to involve induction of apoptosis in malignant cells and conversion of monocytes into dendritic cells, effects that mount an improved immune response against the malignancy.

This therapy is effective and has been associated with increased survival time in patients with SS, although this continues to be in debate. Overall response rates for monotherapy range from 10% to 83% in patients with MF or SS treated with extracorporeal photopheresis for at least 3 months and from 18% to 90% for patients with SS in particular. Adjuvant therapy with IFN-α,

BOX 7-4 Treatment of Sézary Syndrome, as Recommended by the U.S. Cutaneous Lymphoma Consortium

Primary Treatment	Secondary Treatment (After Inadequate Response, Refractory Disease, or Progression Despite Primary Therapies)

Category A systemic therapies (monotherapies)
  ECP
  IFN-α
  Bexarotene
  Low-dose methotrexate (≤100 mg/wk)
  Denileukin diftitox (plus corticosteroid)
Category A combination therapies
  Systemic + SDT
    IFN-α or -γ + PUVA or topical nitrogen mustard
    Methotrexate (low-dose) + topical nitrogen mustard
    Bexarotene + PUVA
    Immunomodulators (ECP, IFN-α or -γ, bexarotene (singly or in combination) + TSEBT
  Systemic + systemic
    IFN-α + bexarotene
    ECP + other immunomodulators (bexarotene, IFN- α or -γ, low-dose methotrexate (singly or in combination)
    Methotrexate (low-dose) + IFN-α
	Category B systemic therapies (decision as to what order to use must take into account blood tumor burden, patient age, and overall health, prior therapies)
	Alemtuzumab
	Chlorambucil + corticosteroid
	Liposomal doxorubicin
	HDAC inhibitors
	  Vorinostat
	  Romidepsin
	Gemcitabine
	Deoxycoformycin
	High-dose methotrexate (>100 mg/wk)
	Fludarabine ± cyclophosphamide
	Mechlorethamine
	Consider allogeneic transplant as appropriate
	Clinical trial

ECP, extracorporeal photopheresis; HDAC, histone deacetylase; IFN, interferon; PUVA, psoralen plus ultraviolet A; SDT, skin-directed therapy; TSEBT, total skin electron beam therapy.
Adapted from Olsen EA, Rook AH, Zic J, Kim Y, Porcu P, Guerfeld C, et al. Sézary syndrome: immunopathogenesis, literature review of therapeutic options, and recommendations for therapy by the United States Cutaneous Lymphoma Consortium (USCLC). *J Am Acad Dermatol.* 2011;64:352–404. Epub 2010;December 9. Used with permission.

TABLE 7-3 Treatment Guidelines from the U.S. Cutaneous Lymphoma Consortium

Use disease burden and rapidity of progression as determinants of approach to therapy.
Preserve immune response whenever possible.
Use immunomodulatory therapy before chemotherapy unless burden of disease or failure of prior such therapies warrants otherwise.
Always consider combination therapy, particularly systemic immunomodulatory plus skin-directed treatments, which in general has greater efficacy than monotherapy.
Consider potential *Staphylococcus* infection as cause of worsening disease and maintain low threshold for use of systemic antibiotics to prevent life-threatening sepsis.
Preserve quality of life by aggressive treatment of pruritus.

Adapted from Olsen EA, Rook AH, Zic J, Kim Y, Porcu P, Guerfeld C, et al. Sézary syndrome: immunopathogenesis, literature review of therapeutic options, and recommendations for therapy by the United States Cutaneous Lymphoma Consortium (USCLC). *J Am Acad Dermatol.* 2011;64:352-404. Epub 2010;December 9. Used with permission.

granulocyte-macrophage colony-stimulating factor, bexarotene, or total body surface electron beam therapy provides even better response data; the overall response rate for CTCL in general was 55.7% and the complete response rate was 17.6% in an analysis of more than 400 patients.[7] In one comparative study, overall response rate was 40% in stages III and IV CTCL treated with extracorporeal photopheresis and 57% with extracorporeal photopheresis used in combination with an adjuvant immunomodulatory therapy.[8] Typically, therapy is recommended to be continued for 6 months after a response is attained before tapering the frequency. Complications are rare, but they include nausea, fever, hypotension during apheresis, or vascular-related injuries such as hematomas, superficial phlebitis, and catheter-related sepsis.

Interferons

IFNs are glycoproteins belonging to the group of cytokines that are released by lymphocytes in response to pathogens; therefore, they act as a central component of the immune response against viruses, bacteria, parasites, or tumor cells. In their function as immune system activators, IFNs, particularly IFN-α and IFN-γ, have been used to treat SS. Because the immune profile in patients with SS takes on a Th2 predominance, the use of IFNs can help restore a Th1 cytokine profile and bolster the immune system to fight the malignancy. Therefore, IFNs, IFN-α in particular, are first-line agents in treatment of SS. IFN-α is dosed as 3 to 10 million units daily or three times per week as intramuscular or subcutaneous injections; response time is in the order of weeks. IFN can be used as monotherapy or in combination with other agents such as psoralen plus ultraviolet A (PUVA), topical nitrogen mustard, or total skin electron beam therapy (TSEBT). Overall response rates of stages III and IV CTCL reach up to 70%, but no major studies have documented responses in SS alone. Nevertheless, positive responses have been obtained using IFN-α as part of a combination approach, with overall response rate ranging from 17% to 89%, especially when used in combination with extracorporeal photopheresis.

IFN-γ immunoregulates by enhancing CD8+ cytotoxicity and NK cell function, priming dendritic cells, and inhibiting regulatory T cells. Much less data exist on the use of IFN-γ in SS, but response to it has occurred in nonresponders to IFN-α. More data are needed about the efficacy of IFN-γ in SS in particular; however, use as an adjuvant therapy is recommended when monotherapy is insufficient.

In its primary biologic action, IFN-α creates a constellation of flulike symptoms, including fever, chills, myalgia, and fatigue; it is, therefore, not well tolerated by all patients. Other adverse effects include myelosuppression, anemia, thyroid dysfunction, and hepatotoxicity. IFN-γ has similar, but more mild, toxicities. Over time, resistance to IFN-α may develop in some patients because of the production of neutralizing antibodies and down-regulation of receptors.

Retinoids

Retinoids are vitamin A analogues that belong to the family of nuclear steroid receptors that bind to retinoid acid receptors and retinoid X receptors to modify transcription. They have been shown to assist the antitumor response by inhibiting malignant cell proliferation and induction of apoptosis and down-regulating the Th2 cell immunity. Non–retinoid X receptor selective retinoids, such as tretinoin, etretinate, and isotretinoin, have been used alone or in combination with other systemic treatments in treatment of CTCL with moderate success; however, because most studies grouped patients with MF and SS, efficacy data for SS are difficult to evaluate. Adverse effects of these retinoids include cheilitis, arthralgias, increased values on liver function tests, increased triglyceride values, and alopecia.

Bexarotene is a retinoid X receptor–specific synthetic agent approved by the U.S. Food and Drug Administration (FDA) in 1999 for treatment of relapsing or refractory CTCL in a dosing regimen of 300 mg/m². This agent has been studied in phase II and III clinical trials and has shown promising results in the treatment of SS; overall response rates of 24% to 78% have been reported when used as monotherapy. It has also been used in combination with other agents, and various case reports document success.

The most common adverse effects of bexarotene are hyperlipidemia and central hypothyroidism.

Patients with familial hypertriglyceridemia cannot tolerate this agent, but other patients can have reasonable control of hyperlipidemia by using lipid-lowering agents such as fenfibrate or atorvastatin. Hyperlipidemia, defined as more than 2.5 times the normal level of triglycerides, occurs in 70% of patients, and 60% have cholesterol levels of more than 300 mg/dL. Hypothyroidism is observed in 40% of patients in clinical trials and even more frequently in practice. Other adverse effects include cytopenia, fatigue, nausea, and peripheral edema. All retinoids are category X drugs and, thus, are contraindicated in pregnancy; women of childbearing age must take serious precautions, including responsible contraceptive use with two forms of contraception, while using retinoids.

Denileukin Diftitox

Approved by the FDA in 1999 for treatment of CTCL, denileukin diftitox (Ontak) is a recombinant fusion protein that combines IL-2 with a membrane translocation domain of diphtheria toxin; it thus targets and induces apoptosis in IL-2 receptor–bearing cells via inhibition of protein synthesis. In studies that have identified the subgroup of SS within the CTCL pool, overall response rates of 50% have been reported with corticosteroid premedication;[9,10] in other cases of stages I through IV CTCL, response rates have varied from 30% to 49% when denileukin diftitox was used as monotherapy.[11–13] When used in combination with bexarotene, it has been efficacious for treating CTCL—67% overall response rate. Again, no patients with SS were separately identified.

Acute toxic effects include hypersensitivity reaction with symptoms such as hypotension, tachycardia, fever, chills, flulike symptoms, nausea, and rarely, anaphylaxis. Delayed adverse effects include vascular leak syndrome with hypotension, edema, and hypoalbuminemia and other more rare complications such as vision changes, thromboses, and hyperthyroidism. Many of these effects can be minimized by using antihistamines, acetaminophen, and premedication with low-dose corticosteroids. The infusion should proceed over the course of at least an hour to diminish infusion reactions.

Chemotherapy

Chemotherapy can be used as a single agent or a combination therapy, especially when immunomodulatory monotherapy and combination approaches fail. Chemotherapy is also recommended in refractory disease and in cases of more aggressive transformation; multiagent chemotherapy can be helpful for abating severe leukemic burden and advanced disease when immunomodulatory therapies provide no response. As with many of the therapies for SS, large trials and multicenter studies are not available because of the rarity of the condition. Favorable responses have been noted, but results are usually short-lived and relapse is common. Because of the toxic effects of these agents, long-term use is not possible, and adverse effects can be fatal.

Methotrexate

Methotrexate has been a popular treatment option in SS, and a low-dose regimen of 100 mg/wk or less remains a first-line option for treatment. Methotrexate functions by inhibiting dihydrofolate reductase and thus blocking cell division in the S phase of replicating cells. It also has anti-inflammatory properties that are helpful in SS. Few studies report the efficacy of low-dose methotrexate monotherapy, but favorable results have been documented in various subtypes of CTCL.[14–16] In addition, methotrexate used in combination with other chemotherapeutics has shown benefit in individual cases of SS reported in large studies.[17-19] In high doses, it is very active against SS and can be given orally as a single agent.

Toxic effects of methotrexate include gastrointestinal upset, myelosuppression, hepatotoxicity, and other reactions such as oligospermia and anaphylaxis. Concomitant folic acid supplementation (1-5 mg daily) should be given, and leucovorin can be used to counter acute toxic reactions or high-dose therapy. As with bexarotene, methotrexate is teratogenic and contraception is necessary in female patients.

Purine Nucleoside Analogues

This group includes deoxycoformycin, fludarabine, cladribine, gemcitabine, and forodesine. Their use has been evaluated in several clinical trials, and they have been used as single-agent chemotherapy and in combination with other agents. Generally speaking, this class of drugs functions as antimetabolites by mimicking the function of purines and thus disturbing DNA synthesis in rapidly dividing cells. A varying degree of success has been noted with these agents, and they have been reported to induce complete response for years in case reports and among patients with SS within larger CTCL studies. However, on average, durations are relatively short, as is typical among chemotherapeutic agents.

Toxic effects of this class of chemotherapies reflect their mechanism of action in blocking DNA synthesis. These include gastrointestinal upset, myelosuppression, flulike symptoms, infection, and transient increased values on liver function tests. Other, more rare adverse effects include neurologic problems, renal syndromes such as hemolytic uremic syndrome, alopecia, and pulmonary toxicity.

Combination Chemotherapy

Multiagent chemotherapy is recommended to be used as an induction therapy that is subsequently followed with immunomodulatory therapy, which is far more sustainable and less toxic in the long run. Some intravenous combinations to keep in mind for induction include cyclophosphamide, doxorubicin, vincristine, and prednisone; methotrexate, cyclophosphamide, vincristine, and prednisone; and etoposide, idarubicin, cyclophosphamide, vincristine, prednisone, and bleomycin. A traditional combination used very commonly in the 1970s and 1980s was low-dose oral chlorambucil with prednisone; however, this is not used as commonly now as other immunomodulatory agents. Skin-directed therapies, such as nitrogen mustard or total electron beam radiation, are helpful adjuvants to systemic chemotherapy.

Stem Cell Transplant

Stem cell transplant is a novel and potentially curative therapy in patients with severe refractory SS; however, the risks are substantial, and this management plan is not for everyone. Allogeneic hematopoietic stem cell transplant

is particularly promising in that a durable clinical response is noted through a proposed graft-versus-lymphoma–mediated mechanism. A recent literature review identified 22 patients with SS who received allogeneic stem cell transplant and had a good response.[20] Of the 22 patients, 15 were alive and disease-free; the duration of follow-up ranged from 18 to 109 months; and chronic graft-versus-host disease was identified in 10 patients. Although this approach shows more long-lasting clinical remission, it is associated with a considerable set of risks, many of which are life-threatening, such as graft-versus-host disease and severe infection.

Experimental Therapies

Innovative new therapies are being explored to gain a better understanding of this aggressive malignancy, particularly in cases of refractory SS. These therapies include Toll-like receptor agonists, cytokine therapies, vaccines, histone deacetylase inhibitors, and various targeted antibodies. These agents show promise for treatment of SS, but evidence regarding outcomes and response is limited. Nevertheless, when other, more standard treatments fail, patients can be invited to participate in clinical trials with such new therapies. Exploration of these therapies could provide hope for the future in that impressive advancements in understanding CTCL have been made in recent decades.

Skin-directed Adjuvant Therapy

Because SS is a systemic disease with dangerous leukemic involvement, systemic immunomodulatory therapy and chemotherapy are essential components of management. Nevertheless, the use of skin-targeted adjuvant therapies provides much symptomatic relief and helps sooth the cutaneous aspect of SS.

Phototherapy

PUVA with the addition of orally administered 8-methoxypsoralen (0.6 mg/kg) 2 hours before treatment has been a key element of treatment for CTCL, especially for early stage disease. The activation of 8-methoxypsoralen by the UVA inhibits DNA synthesis, and thus, the number of circulating helper cells is decreased. Treatment is administered three times per week for 3 to 6 months. In SS, its efficacy as a cutaneous adjuvant therapy is highly valued. The properties of PUVA are also anti-inflammatory and cytotoxic. When used in combination with immunomodulatory therapy, there has been enhanced efficacy in many trials and retrospective studies.[21-24] It is particularly useful in assisting in clearance of erythroderma and pruritus.

Adverse effects include nausea, vomiting, xerosis, blistering, sunburn, and the increased risk of skin cancers. Ultraviolet B (UVB) phototherapy, although useful in early patch-stage CTCL, is not recommended for SS because of its tendency to exacerbate erythroderma.

Topical Nitrogen Mustard

Nitrogen mustard, otherwise known as mechlorethamine, was the first topical agent used to efficaciously treat CTCL, starting in the 1940s. It functions as an alkylating agent and helps control the symptoms and progression of cutaneous disease. It is useful therapy for MF and as adjuvant therapy in SS. Nitrogen mustard is applied to the entire skin surface in water or in an oil-water base twice a day for 6 to 12 months; it is gradually tapered into the maintenance phase.

The toxic effects of nitrogen mustard include allergic toxic contact dermatitis (occurring in 35-65% of patients), dry skin, hyperpigmentation, bullous reactions, urticaria, and Stevens-Johnson syndrome. Because it has carcinogenic properties, nitrogen mustard can increase the risk of nonmelanoma skin cancers. However, because this agent is limited to a cutaneous effect, it does not cause the dangerous effect of cytopenia as do other chemotherapeutic agents.

Total Skin Electron Beam Radiation

TSEBT has been used for more than 50 years in the treatment of CTCL, both limited and advanced disease. The powerful effect on relieving symptoms of pruritus, erythroderma, patches, plaques, and other lesions is impressive. Lymphoma cells are particularly vulnerable to the toxic effects of radiation. Typical dosing is 3000 to 3600 cGy administered over the course of 8 to 10 weeks.

Electron beam radiation should be administered as an adjuvant in SS, in a multifaceted attack on the various compartments of this malignancy. As with PUVA, the addition of electron beam radiation further amplifies the effects of immunomodulatory therapy, and it is recognized as the most likely skin-targeted therapy to induce a cutaneous complete response in all stages of MF.

Toxic effects include erythema, blistering, exfoliation, xerosis, initial alopecia, edema, nail dystrophy, and hyperpigmentation. In the long term, there is an increased risk of radiation dermatitis and nonmelanoma skin cancers.

General Skin Care and Symptomatic Relief

SS is a particularly disabling condition because of the severe pruritus. The management of pruritus is challenging, but addressing and treating this issue can provide a substantial increase in quality of life. Typically, the topical treatments used can minimize skin irritation, provide hydration, and relieve some of the erythema and inflammation associated with the pruritus of SS. Frequent use of moisturizers, creams, and antihistamines can also assist in relieving these symptoms. Soaking baths, avoidance of detergents, and liberal use of glycerin-based moisturizers help minimize xerosis and pruritus.

Gabapentin, at a starting dose of 300 mg three times daily and subsequently increasing the dose, can be used to treat pruritus and some of the pain, burning, tightness, and sharp pins-and-needles sensations experienced in SS. Low- to medium-potency topical corticosteroids are also helpful for decreasing the inflammatory response, but they should not be used for several weeks before skin biopsies because they can mask histopathologic characteristics. In severe cases, oral corticosteroids are effective, but they can cause rebound flares when tapered. Corticosteroid-induced adrenal insufficiency should be kept in mind in patients using chronic corticosteroids; findings could include hyperkalemia, hypotension, and eosinophilia.

Providing supportive skin care is particularly important in settings of exfoliation and damage to the protective barrier function, which is one of the main risks of infection. This is a major death risk, and in addition, the colonization of bacteria in the skin perpetuates the cycle of worsening erythroderma and leukemic burden. To address this, prompt treatment of infected areas of the skin, colonized ulcers, and fissures with antibiotic ointments helps prevent bacteremia and cellulitis. Other studies have shown the efficacy of continuous antistaphylococcal antibiotic coverage to control the erythroderma and pruritus and prevent severe sepsis.[25,26] In addition, dermatophytes frequently take hold in areas of keratoderma; therefore, such areas should be scraped and evaluated with potassium hydroxide preparation to assess for infection. Dermatophyte infection can be treated topically with antifungal gel or systemically with oral terbinafine if infection is widespread or severe. Considering the wide range of microbes that can take hold in the setting of immunocompromise, prophylaxis with trimethoprin-sulfamethoxazole, voriconazole, and acyclovir covers the majority of infectious agents and keeps the risk of serious infection low.

Recent clinical trials have highlighted additional agents that provide pruritic relief.[27-29] Such agents include vorinostat, romidepsin, and alemtuzumab. However, no studies have provided clear evidence that pruritic relief is associated with changes in overall survival. If all of these methods fail, outpatient or inpatient hospitalization with wet dressing treatments is highly efficacious for providing relief from recalcitrant erythroderma and pruritus. Nevertheless, aggressive treatment of pruritus is crucial in an attempt to improve quality of life in patients who have this aggressive malignancy.

CONCLUSION

SS is a distinctive, rare, and relatively aggressive variant of CTCL with unique molecular and immunologic qualities. Characterized by pruritic erythroderma and leukemic involvement with Sézary cells and a malignant CD4+ T-cell clone, SS is associated with a dismal prognosis, with median survival ranging from 2 to 4 years. The key to management of this disease is early diagnosis, proper workup, staging, and therapy. Because of the severity of symptoms that may occur in SS, not only survival but also quality of life must be

kept in mind, with a focus on palliative skin therapies. In recent years, groundbreaking research has paved the way for a greater understanding of the molecular and immunologic intricacies of SS. With this new understanding, the diagnostic criteria have evolved to more precisely delineate this complex malignancy. As a result, future studies will be able to more specifically target patients with SS and gain better insight into treatments, outcomes, and survival. The combination of classic topical treatments, novel chemotherapeutics, and immunomodulatory agents holds the greatest hope and promise for the future.

SUGGESTED READINGS

Agar NS, Wedgeworth E, Crichton S, Mitchell TJ, Cox M, Ferreira S, et al. Survival outcomes and prognostic factors in mycosis fungoides/Sézary syndrome: validation of the revised International Society for Cutaneous Lymphomas/European Organisation for Research and Treatment of Cancer staging proposal. *J Clin Oncol.* 2010;28:4730–4739. Epub 2010;September 20.

Abdul Samad K, Prasanna MK, Akhar AP. Sezary syndrome—without erythroderma. *Indian J Dermatol Venereol Leprol.* 2002 Jul-Aug;68(4):225–6.

Apisarnthanarax N, Talpur R, Duvic M. Treatment of cutaneous T-cell lymphoma: Current status and future directions. *Am J Clin Dermatol* 2002;3: 193–215.

Booken N, Weiss C, Utikal J, Felcht M, Goerdt S, Klemke CD. Combination therapy with extracorporeal photopheresis, interferon-alpha, PUVA and topical corticosteroids in the management of Sezary syndrome. *J Dtsch Dermatol Ges* 2010;8:428–38.

Chin KM, Foss FM. Biologic correlates of response and survival in patients with cutaneous T-cell lymphoma treated with denileukin diftitox. *Clin Lymphoma Myeloma* 2006;7: 199–204.

Duvic M, Chiao N, Talpur R. Extracorporeal photopheresis for the treatment of cutaneous T-cell lymphoma. *J Cutan Med Surg* 2003;7:3–7.

Foss FM, Bacha P, Osann KE, Demierre MF, Bell T, Kuzel T. Biological correlates of acute hypersensitivity events with DAB(389)IL-2 (denileukin diftitox, ONTAK) in cutaneous T-cell lymphoma: decreased frequency and severity with steroid premedication. *Clin Lymphoma* 2001;1:298–302.

Habermann TM, Pittelkow MR. Cutaneous T-cell lymphoma and cutaneous B-cell lymphoma. In: Abeloff MD, Armitage JO, Niederhuber JE, Kastan

MB, McKenna WG, eds. *Abeloff's Clinical Oncology.* 4th ed. Philadelphia: Churchill Livingstone/Elsevier; 2008:2405–2424.

Harrison AL, Duvic M. Diagnosis and treatment of Sézary syndrome. *J Dermatol* [Internet]. 2004 [cited 2011;April 19];2. Available at http://www.ispub.com/journal/the_internet_journal_of_dermatology/volume_2_number_2_11/article/diagnosis_and_treatment_of_sezary_syndrome.html

Hirayama Y, Nagai T, Ohta H, Koyama R, Matsunaga T, Sakamaki S, et al. Séezary syndrome showing a stable clinical course for more than four years after oral administration of etoposide and methotrexate [in Japanese]. *Rinsho Ketsueki* 2000;41:750–4.

Hwang ST, Janik JE, Jaffe ES, Wilson WH. Mycosis fungoides and Sézary syndrome. *Lancet.* 2008;371: 945–957.

Kim Y, Whittaker S, Demierre MF, Rook AH, Lerner A, Duvic M, et al. Clinically significant responses achieved with romidepsin in treatment-refractory cutaneous T-cell lymphoma: final results from a phase 2B, international, multicenter, registration study. *Blood* 2008;112:263.

Lundin J, Hagberg H, Repp R, Cavallin-Stahl E, Freden S, Juliusson G, et al. Phase 2 study of alemtuzumab (anti-CD52 monoclonal antibody) in patients with advanced mycosis fungoides/Sezary syndrome. *Blood* 2003;101:4267–72.

Matthias Lüftl, Martin Röcken, Gerd Plewig and Klaus Degitz. PUVA Inhibits DNA Replication, but not Gene Transcription at Nonlethal Dosages. *Journal of Investigative Dermatology* (1998) 111, 399 -405; doi:10.1046/j.1523–1747.1998.00316.x

McGinnis KS, Shapiro M, Vittorio CC, Rook AH, Junkins-Hopkins JM. Psoralen plus long-wave UV-A (PUVA) and bexarotene therapy: An effective and synergistic combined adjunct to therapy for patients with advanced cutaneous T-cell lymphoma. *Arch Dermatol.* 2003 Jun;139(6):771–5.

Olsen EA, Kim YH, Kuzel TM, Pacheco TR, Foss FM, Parker S, et al. Phase IIb multicenter trial of vorinostat in patients with persistent, progressive, or treatment refractory cutaneous Tcell lymphoma. *J Clin Oncol* 2007;25:3109–15.

Olsen EA, Rook AH, Zic J, Kim Y, Porcu P, Querfeld C, Wood G, Demierre MF, Pittelkow M, Wilson LD, Pinter-Brown L, Advani R, Parker S, Kim EJ, Junkins-Hopkins JM, Foss F, Cacchio P, Duvic M. Sézary syndrome: immunopathogenesis, literature review of therapeutic options, and recommendations for therapy by the United States Cutaneous Lymphoma Consortium (USCLC). *J Am Acad Dermatol.* 2011 Feb;64(2):352–404.

Olsen E, Duvic M, Frankel A, Kim Y, Martin A, Vonderheid E, et al. Pivotal phase III trial of two dose levels of denileukin diftitox for the treatment of cutaneous T-cell lymphoma. *J Clin Oncol* 2001;19: 376–88.

Olsen E, Vonderheid E, Pimpinelli N, Willemze R, Kim Y, Knobler R, Zackheim H, Duvic M, Estrach T, Lamberg S, Wood G, Dummer R, Ranki A, Burg G, Heald P, Pittelkow M, Bernengo MG, Sterry W, Laroche L, Trautinger F, Whittaker S; ISCL/EORTC. Revisions to the staging and classification of mycosis fungoides and Sezary syndrome: a proposal of the International Society for Cutaneous Lymphomas (ISCL) and the cutaneous lymphoma task force of the European Organization of Research and Treatment of Cancer (EORTC). *Blood.* 2007 Sep 15;110(6):1713–22.

Olsen E, Vonderheid E, Pimpinelli N, Willemze R, Kim Y, Knobler R, et al; ISCL/EORTC. Revisions to the staging and classification of mycosis fungoides and Sézary syndrome: a proposal of the International Society for Cutaneous Lymphomas (ISCL) and the cutaneous lymphoma task force of the European Organization of Research and Treatment of Cancer (EORTC). *Blood.* 2007;110:1713–1722. Epub 2007; May 31. Erratum in: *Blood* 2008;111:4830.

Olsen EA, Rook AH, Zic J, Kim Y, Porcu P, Guerfeld C, et al. Sézary syndrome: immunopathogenesis, literature review of therapeutic options, and recommendations for therapy by the United States Cutaneous Lymphoma Consortium (USCLC). *J Am Acad Dermatol.* 2011;64:352–404. Epub 2010; December 9.

Prince HM, Duvic M, Martin A, Sterry W, Assaf C, Sun Y, et al. Phase III placebo-controlled trial of denileukin diftitox for patients with cutaneous T-cell lymphoma. *J Clin Oncol* 2010; 28:1870–7.

Prince HM, Whittaker S, Hoppe RT. How I treat mycosis fungoides and Sézary syndrome. *Blood.* 2009;114:4337–4353. Epub 2009;August 20.

Saleh MN, LeMaistre CF, Kuzel TM, Foss F, Platanias LC, Schwartz G, et al. Antitumor activity of DAB389IL-2 fusion toxin in mycosis fungoides. *J Am Acad Dermatol* 1998;39: 63–73.

Schappell DL, Alper JC, McDonald CJ. Treatment of advanced mycosis fungoides and Sezary syndrome with continuous infusions of methotrexate followed by fluorouracil and leucovorin rescue. *Arch Dermatol* 1995;131:307–13.

Sezary A, Bouvrain Y. Erythrodermie avec pe´sence de cellules monstrueuses dans le derme et le sang circulant. *Bull Soc Fr Dermatol Syphiligr.* 1938;45: 254–260.

Sezary A, Horowitz A, Marchas H. Erythrodermie avec pre´sence de cellules monstrueuses dans le derme et dans le sang circulant (second cas). *Bull Soc Fr Dermatol Syphiligr.* 1938;45:395–400.

Shapiro M, Rook AH, Lehrer MS, Junkins Hopkins JM, French LE, Vittorio CC. Novel multimodality biologic response modifier therapy including bexarotene and long-wave ultraviolet A for a patient with refractory stage IVa cutaneous T-cell lymphoma. *J Am Acad Dermatol* 2002;47:956–61.

Talpur R, Bassett R, Duvic M. Prevalence and treatment of Staphylococcus aureus colonization in patients with mycosis fungoides and Sézary syndrome. *Br J Dermatol*. 2008 Jul;159(1):105–12. Epub 2008 Jul 1.

Taswell HF, Winkelmann RK. Sezary syndrome—a malignant reticulemic erythroderma. *JAMA*. 1961 Aug 19;177:465–72.

Vonderheid EC, Bernengo MG, Burg G, Duvic M, Heald P, Laroche L, et al; ISCL. Update on erythrodermic cutaneous T-cell lymphoma: report of the International Society for Cutaneous Lymphomas. *J Am Acad Dermatol*. 2002;46:95–106.

Vonderheid EC, Zhang Q, Lessin SR, Polansky M, Abrams JT, Bigler RD, et al. Use of serum soluble interleukin-2 receptor levels to monitor the progression of cutaneous T-cell lymphoma. *J Am Acad Dermatol* 1998;38:207–20.

Winkelmann RK, Buechner SA, Diaz-Perez JL. Pre-Sézary syndrome. *J Am Acad Dermatol*. 1984 Jun;10(6):992-9.

Wright JC, Lyons MM, Walker DG, Golomb FM, Gumport SL, Medrek TJ. Observations on the use of cancer chemotherapeutic agents in patients with mycosis fungoides. *Cancer* 1964;17:1045–62.

Zackheim HS, Kashani-Sabet M, Hwang ST. Low-dose methotrexate to treat erythrodermic cutaneous T-cell lymphoma: results in twenty-nine patients. *J Am Acad Dermatol* 1996;34: 626–31.

Zackheim HS, Kashani-Sabet M, McMillan A. Low-dose methotrexate to treat mycosis fungoides: a retrospective study in 69 patients. *J Am Acad Dermatol* 2003;49:873–8.

Zic JA. The treatment of cutaneous T-cell lymphoma with photopheresis. *Dermatol Ther* 2003;16:337–46.

ADULT T-CELL LEUKEMIA/LYMPHOMA

John P. Galvin, MD, MPH, and Timothy M. Kuzel, MD

INTRODUCTION

Adult T-cell leukemia/lymphoma (ATLL) is an aggressive T-cell leukemia that was first described in 1977 by Uchiyama and coworkers, who described the clinical and hematologic features in a group of patients in southwestern Japan. They observed that these patients shared unique peripheral malignant T cells with highly indented or lobulated nuclei. Patients frequently presented with involvement in the skin, liver, lung, spleen, and lymph nodes and with hypercalcemia. Another notable finding was the proximity of the patients' birthplaces. All of the affected patients originated from the same region of southern Japan. The unusual clustering of cases led many to theorize that ATLL was associated with an oncogenic virus. While investigating this theory, a unique retrovirus was isolated from patients with ATLL, which was called *human T-cell lymphotropic virus type-1 (HTLV-1)*. It is now accepted that HTLV-1 is the causative agent of ATLL. HTLV-1 also causes other diseases, including tropical spastic paraparesis/HTLV-1–associated myelopathy (TSP/HAM), uveitis, and infective dermatitis.

Since the identification of HTLV-1, seroepidemiologic surveys have shown that the virus exists in southwestern Japan and is also endemic in the Caribbean basin. HTLV-1 occurs sporadically in Africa, Central America, South America, the Middle East, and the southeastern United States. ATLL occurs in only 2% to 4% of HTLV-1–infected people. When it does occur, it is usually aggressive and difficult to treat, with most people surviving less than 1 year. Combination chemotherapy with cytotoxic agents has yielded complete response (CR) rates of 20% to 45%, but responses usually last only a few months. The combination of interferon-alpha (IFN-α) and zidovudine (AZT) has proved to be active in the treatment of patients with ATLL, with a small percentage of patients achieving long-lasting remissions. In specific types of ATLL, allogeneic hematopoietic cell transplantation (HCT) has also demonstrated a survival benefit.

EPIDEMIOLOGY

ATLL incidence varies according to the prevalence of HTLV-1 infection. Infection with HTLV-1 is endemic in several islands in southern Japan, the Caribbean basin, Western Africa, Peru, northeastern Iran, and the southeastern United States. In the Caribbean islands, 3% to 6% of the population is seropositive for HTLV-1, whereas fewer than 1% of people in affected areas of the United States and Europe are infected. In endemic regions of Japan, 6% to 37% of the population is infected with HTLV-1. Among these HTLV-1 carriers, 1.5 per 1000 men, and 0.5 per 1000 women will be diagnosed with ATLL each year. The overall risk is 2.5% in a carrier who lives to age 70. The median age at diagnosis is in the seventh decade. However, median age at diagnosis can vary with geographic location. For example, a study of 126 patients with ATLL from Jamaica reported a median age of 43 years. Seroprevalence increases with age and is also more common in females. In Jamaican people older than 70 years, 17.4% of women are HTLV-1–positive, compared with 9.1% of men. In Japanese people older than 80 years, 50% of women and 30% of men are seropositive.

HTLV-1 is transmitted through sexual intercourse, breast milk, shared needles among intravenous drug users, transfusion of blood products, and transplanted organs. Transmission of HTLV-1 occurs more efficiently from males to females, which may explain the increased seroprevalence among women. The rate of male-to-female transmission is correlated with the duration of relationship, increased antibody titer and viral load, increased male age, and a history of sexually transmitted disease in either partner. Female-to-male transmission of HTLV-1 is increased in men with genital ulcers.

Several studies in Japan and one in Africa have shown that the rate of mother-to-child transmission ranges from 15-25%, and is mostly through breast-feeding, although transplacental transmission can occur. In a study of 34 children born to seropositive women in Gabon, none of the children who became infected had detectable antibodies or virus before 18 months. Risk factors for mother-to-child transmission include high HTLV-1 antibody titer, prolonged ruptured membranes during delivery, low socioeconomic status, and prolonged breast-feeding.

Transfusion of HTLV-1–contaminated blood causes seroconversion 40% to 60% of the time, at a median of 51 days after the transfusion. Owing to the high efficiency of infection by contaminated blood, screening of blood and organ donors is important even in areas of low seroprevalence. The virus is transmitted by blood products that contain white blood cells, but it is not transmitted by transfusion of plasma alone. Screening of blood donors is the only way to prevent donor blood or organ transmission. Whereas screening for HTLV-1 is done in Japan, the Caribbean, and the United States, it is not performed in all areas with low seroprevalence.

The median age of onset for ATLL is approximately 55 years. The clinical features of ATLL can include lymphadenopathy (72%), hepatomegaly (47%), splenomegaly (25%), and skin lesions (53%) (Figure 8-1). Hypercalcemia occurs in 28% of cases. The white blood cell count ranges from normal to 500×10^9/L, and the leukemic cells have characteristic indented or lobulated nuclei. This appearance has led to the term *flower cells* to describe the leukemic cells (Figure 8-2). The typical phenotype of ATLL cells is CD3+, CD4+, CD8–, and CD25+. Suppression of the cellular immune system is a feature of HTLV-1 infection

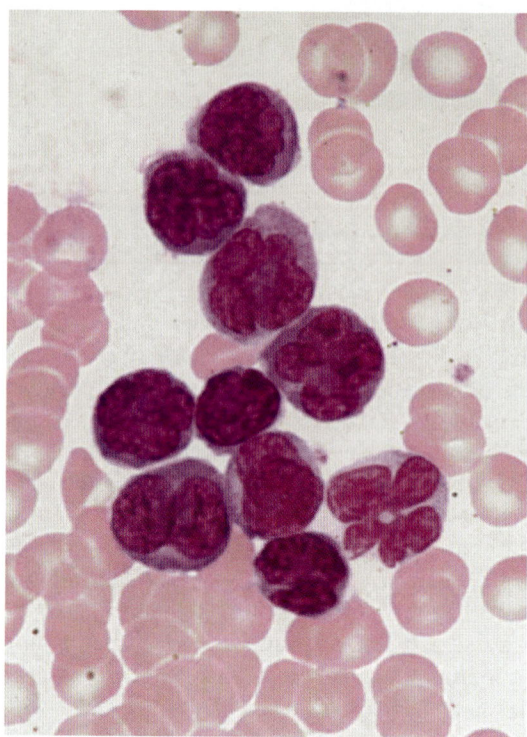

Figure 8-2 Characteristic "flower cells" in the peripheral blood of a patient with HTLV-1–associated leukemia/lymphoma. From ASH Image Bank. Isao Miyoshi. Adult T-cell Leukemia/Lymphoma. ASH Image Bank 2011; 2011–2098. © The American Society of Hematology.

and ATLL, and strongyloides and *Pneumocystis jiroveci* infection are seen relatively frequently.

DEVELOPMENT OF ADULT T-CELL LEUKEMIA/LYMPHOMA

HTLV was first described in 1979 in a patient with cutaneous T-cell lymphoma and was the first human retrovirus discovered. Two years later, HTLV-2 was discovered. More recently in 2005, HTLV-3 and HTLV-4 were discovered. Since its first discovery, HTLV-1 and HTLV-2 have been found to be involved in epidemics, affecting 15 to 20 million people worldwide. HTLV-1 is more clinically significant owing to its association with multiple disorders. At least 500,000 individuals infected with HTLV-1 will develop ATL, whereas others may develop HAM/TSP. HTLV-2

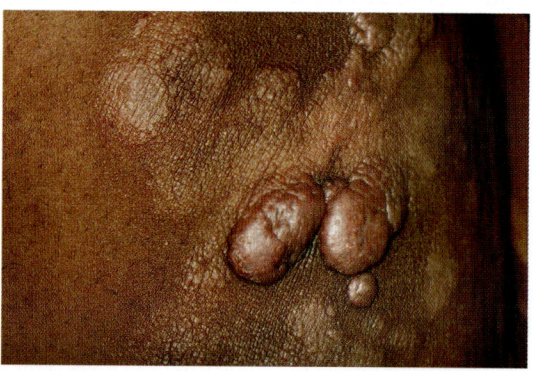

Figure 8-1 Skin lesion of a patient with human T-cell lymphotropic virus-1 (HTLV-1)–associated leukemia/lymphoma.

is associated with milder neurologic disorders and chronic pulmonary infections. No specific illnesses have yet been associated with HTLV-3 or HTLV-4.

HTLV-1 is an enveloped, single-stranded, diploid RNA retrovirus that is lymphotropic for T cells. HTLV-1 integrates into the host DNA randomly as a provirus. The HTLV-1 proviral genome is incorporated in the same location of the genome in all leukemic cells in an affected host. This suggests that the provirus infects an original malignant cell prior to clonal expansion. The HTLV-1 genome encodes three structural genes (*gag, pol,* and *env*) and two regulatory genes (*tax* and *rex*). HTLV-1 does not contain an onco-gene and most infected cells do not express any viral gene products. The only HTLV-1 gene prod-uct that is commonly expressed in tumor cells is the regulatory gene Tax (transactivating gene of the X region). The protein Tax induces cellu-lar proliferation, promotes cellular survival, and impairs DNA damage repair mechanisms. More specifically, Tax protein transactivates a host of cellular genes through transcription factors such as nuclear factor-kappaB (NF-κB). Expression of Tax protein in the cell results in migration of NF-κB from the cytoplasm to the nucleus, where it activates genes responsible for cellular prolifera-tion. In addition, tumor survival is promoted by inactivating the tumor suppressor p53. The irreg-ular expression of tax in ATLL cells suggests that Tax may be important in early transformation and not maintenance of the transformed state. Transformation of an HTLV-1–infected cell is a rare event and is likely dependent on heterogene-ous second, third, and fourth genetic hits.

Despite the high seroprevalence of HTLV-1, fewer than 5% of carriers will ever develop ATLL. The incubation period for the development of ATLL is 20 to 40 years. Therefore, HTLV-1 infec-tion early in life is likely necessary for the devel-opment of ATLL. In people infected before age 20, the lifetime risk of developing ATLL is about 5%. Owing to the long latency period and low incidence, it is difficult to study the progression from HTLV-1 to ATLL. Determining potential biomarkers as predictors for progression to ATLL in HTLV-1 carriers has revealed that a low or loss of Tax antibody titer and elevated HTLV-1 viral load are associated with progression to ATLL.

DIAGNOSIS

The criteria needed to make the diagnosis of ATLL are

- Histologically and/or cytologically proven lymphoid malignancy with T-cell surface antigens present.
- Abnormal T lymphocytes consistently pre-sent in the peripheral blood (except in the lymphoma type).
- Seropositivity for HTLV-1 demonstrated by indirect immunofluorescence, enzyme-linked immunosorbent assay (ELISA), passive hemagglutination, or Western blot. Infection with HTLV-1 can also be demonstrated by proviral DNA and clonal integration of the proviral DNA by Southern blot, polymerase chain reaction (PCR), or inverse PCR.

The sequence of antibody development to HTLV-1 has been determined. Initially, antibodies form to the core proteins encoded by *gag*. This is followed by antibodies to envelope proteins and, lastly, to the Tax-encoded regulatory protein. In the United States and Europe, ELISA is used as the initial screening test for HTLV-1 and it is confirmed by Western blot assay. The confirmatory Western blot also tests for reactivity to an HTLV-2 envelope protein. This distinction is necessary owing to the similar genome but different pathogenicity of these two viruses.

CLASSIFICATION/PROGNOSIS

ATLL is classified into four subtypes—acute, lymphoma, chronic, and smoldering—(Table 8-1) based on prognosis and clinicopathologic features. Patients with the acute type have the worst prog-nosis, with a median survival of 6.2 months. Those with lymphoma type have a median survival of 10.2 months, and those with chronic type lived a median of 24.3 months. Studies have shown that smolder-ing type can have a median time to transformation to a more aggressive variant of 38 months.

At least two major studies have evaluated the prognostic factors in ATLL. The major risk factors that confer a poor prognosis are poor perform-ance status, high serum lactic dehydrogenase (LDH), hypercalcemia, age older than 40 years,

TABLE 8-1   Description of the Subtypes of Adult T-Cell Leukemia/Lymphoma

Type	ACL	ALC (×10⁹)	TLC (×10⁹)	Lymph Nodes, Liver/Spleen	CNS, GI, Bone	Skin, Lung
Acute	>5%	>4.0	>4	Yes	Yes	Yes
Smoldering*	≥5%	<4.0		No	No	Yes or no
Chronic	≥5%	≥4.0	≥3.5	Yes or no	No	Yes or no
Lymphoma	≤1%	<4.0		Yes (lymph)	Yes or no	

*In case of less than 5% circulating abnormal lymphocytes in the smoldering type, at least one histologically proven lesion from the lung or skin should be present.
ACLs, abnormal circulating lymphocytes; ALC, absolute lymphocyte count; CNS, central nervous system; GI, gastrointestinal; TLC, T-cell lymphocyte count.

and increased number of total lesions. Several other markers may also be important predictors of shortened survival. These include microsatellite instability, Ki-67 positivity, atypical surface immunophenotype, serum thymidine kinase level, soluble interleukin-2 receptor (IL-2R) level, and a defective proviral integration pattern.

TREATMENT

Systemic Chemotherapy

The prognosis for the acute and lymphoma types of ATLL is poor, and chemotherapy with combinations of cytotoxic agents is not effective. Therapy is usually offered to patients only with poor prognosis ATLL (lymphoma-type, acute or unfavorable chronic type), whereas patients with smoldering or typical chronic ATLL are usually observed. This is primarily due to the fact that conventional chemotherapy does not affect the survival of patients with smoldering or typical chronic ATLL. The 5-year survival of patients with smoldering or typical chronic ATLL has been reported to be as high as 47%.

Treatment of poor-prognosis ATLL is a challenge owing to chemotherapy resistance and the existing immunocompromised state associated with HTLV-1 infection. Patients with poor-prognosis ATLL are, therefore, appropriate for a clinical trial. However, if patients are ineligible or there are no trials available, combination chemotherapy is the main treatment option. Allogeneic HCT may also be appropriate for patients with a good performance status and a matched related donor.

Many of the chemotherapy regimens used in aggressive non-Hodgkin's lymphoma have been investigated in ATLL. Unfortunately, these regimens have not offered ATLL patients durable responses. The median survival time for patients with poor-prognosis ATLL treated in prospective trials that employed combination chemotherapy ranges from 5 to 13 months. The combination regimen that have offered ATLL patients the best survival benefit is VCAP-AMP-VECP (vincristine, cyclophosphamide, doxorubicin, prednisone, ranimustine, vindesine, etoposide, and carboplatin).

A phase III randomized trial of 118 patients with poor-prognosis ATLL compared VCAP-AMP-VECP with CHOP (cyclophosphamide, doxorubicin, vincristine, and prednisone). Patients treated with VCAP-AMP-VECP had a significantly higher rate of CR (40%) compared with those treated with CHOP (25%). However, overall response did not differ between the two regimens (72% vs. 66%). Toxicities were more prevalent in the VCAP-AMP-VECP arm including grade 4 neutropenia (98% vs. 83%), grade 4 thrombocytopenia (74% vs. 17%), and grades 3 to 4 infections (32% vs. 15%).

The VCAP-AMP-VECP regimen (with prophylactic intrathecal chemotherapy and granulocyte colony–stimulating factor [G-CSF] support) involves 6 to 8 months of weekly chemotherapy and is associated with significant toxicity. Patients with a poor performance status would be less likely to tolerate this regimen and may benefit more from a CHOP-like regimen. For those without access to ranimustine, an alternative is hyperfractionated cyclophosphamide, vincristine, doxorubicin, and dexamethasone (hyper-CVAD).

Zidovudine/Interferon-alpha

The use of antivirals and interferon in ATLL is controversial. In patients with ATLL, the HTLV-1 virus is often not detectable and is thought to be in its latent state. Therefore, the activity of antiviral agents in ATLL would be expected to work through a mechanism other than its antiviral action. The antiviral agent AZT can terminate DNA replication, with cytostatic effects, and it can also block the transformation of lymphocytes that are co-cultured with HTLV-1–infected cell lines. IFN-a is known to have both antitumor and antiviral effects. Its antileukemic effect likely works by preventing proliferation by blocking protein synthesis and cell growth. It also induces the expression of major histocompatibility complex (MHC) molecules I and II on the surface of tumor cells and antigen-presenting cells, thus stimulating the cytotoxic T-cell response to tumor cells.

Small, prospective trials have evaluated the use of AZT plus IFN-a in the treatment of ATLL. The median survival with this combination ranged from 6 to 18 months. A 2010 meta-analysis of 245 patients with multiple subtypes of ATL (47% acute, 42% lymphoma-type 7% chronic and 4% smoldering) showed a five-year overall survival rate for AZT plus interferon alpha at 46%, chemotherapy at 20%, and chemotherapy followed by antiviral therapy at 12%. Patients with acute, chronic, and smoldering ATLL benefited from first-line antiviral therapy and patients with lymphoma-type ATLL did not benefit. For patients with smoldering or chronic ATLL, this regimen resulted in a 100% 5-year survival.

Owing to the poor prognosis of most patients with ATLL, novel therapies are continually being explored. An anti-CD52 antibody alemtuzumab has been reported to show benefit in preclinical studies and case reports of patients with ATLL. ATLL cells also can express CCR4. Anti-CCR4 antibody has been shown to be cytotoxic in preclinical studies and its use in a recent phase I study proved to be well tolerated and to have potential efficacy in ATLL. Arsenic trioxide and all-*trans*-retinoic acid (ATRA) are very active in the treatment of acute promyleocytic leukemia and have also been shown to be active against ATLL cells in preclinical studies. They have also proved to be antileukemic in phase II studies in poor-prognosis ATLL patients. Additional agents being investigated for the treatment of ATLL include histone deacetylase inhibitors, lenalidomide, pralatrexate, and bortezomib.

Hematopoietic Cell Transplantation

Autologous and allogeneic HCT have been investigated to treat patients with ATLL. Autologous HCT has not shown any benefit. However, allogeneic HCT offers a graft-versus-leukemia effect and should be considered in poor-prognosis ATLL.

A number of studies have investigated the role of allogeneic HCT in ATLL. An overall survival benefit can be achieved in some patients, with evidence of a graft-versus-virus and a graft-versus-leukemia effect; however, treatment-related mortality is high. Allogeneic HCT has been shown to significantly decrease viral load, suggesting an enhancement of HTLV–specific immune response. A small retrospective analysis of 40 patients with acute or lymphoma-type ATLL who underwent an allogeneic HCT reported 15 patients in CR, 13 in partial remission (PR), 3 with stable disease, and 9 with progression of disease. The overall median survival time after HCT was 9.6 months. There were 16 treatment-related deaths. The 3-year relapse-free survival rate was 34%. In a larger retrospective study of 386 patients with ATLL who underwent allogeneic HCT from matched related donors (154 patients), mismatched related donors (43 patients), matched unrelated donors (99 patients), or unrelated cord blood donors (90 patients), the 3-year survival rate was 33%. The most significant risk factors were age older than 50 years, male gender, having an unrelated donor, and not being in a complete remission at the time of HCT.

CONCLUSIONS

ATLL is an aggressive form of leukemia that is diagnosed in 2% to 4% of patients who are infected with the HTLV-1 retrovirus. HTLV-1 is an enveloped, single-stranded RNA retrovirus that has tropism for T lymphocytes. Infection with this virus is endemic in southern Japan and the Caribbean basin and may occur sporadically in the southeastern United States and other regions. The prevalence of seropositivity to HTLV-1 virus in endemic regions ranges from

3% to 6% in the Caribbean basin to as high as 6% to 37% in Japan. The virus is transmitted principally by sexual intercourse and breast-feeding. Infection is associated with an increased risk of specific lymphoproliferative disorders, including ATLL. ATLL is classified into four subtypes: acute, lymphoma, chronic, and smoldering. The acute and lymphoma forms have a very poor prognosis: 6-month median survival for the acute form, and 10 months median survival for the lymphoma form. Patients may also be prone to the development of opportunistic infections and often die from infectious complications including *P. jirovecii* pneumonia, cryptococcus meningitis, and disseminated herpes zoster. Treatment of ATLL with combination chemotherapy may be effective, but relapses are common, and survival has generally been poor. In addition to systemic chemotherapy, patients with acute, chronic, and smoldering ATLL have been shown to benefit from antivirals and immunomodulators (AZT and IFN-α). Also, allogeneic HCT offers a graft-versus-leukemia effect and should be considered in poor-prognosis ATLL.

SUGGESTED READINGS

Bazarbachi A, Plumelle Y, Carlos Ramos J, et al. Meta-analysis on the use of zidovudine and interferon-alfa in adult T-cell leukemia/lymphoma showing improved survival in the leukemic subtypes. *J Clin Oncol*. Sep 20 2010;28(27):4177–4183.

Brennan M, Runganga J, Barbara JA, Contreras M, Tedder RS, Garson JA, et al. Prevalence of antibodies to human T cell leukaemia/lymphoma virus in blood donors in north London. *BMJ*. 1993;307:1235–1239.

Brito-Babapulle F, Arya R, Griffiths T, Pagliuca A, Mufti GJ. BEAM regimen and G-CSF in HTLV-I-associated T-cell lymphoma. *Lancet*. 1992;339:133–134.

Bunn PA Jr, Schechter GP, Jaffe E, Blayney D, Young RC, Matthews MJ. Clinical course of retrovirus-associated adult T-cell lymphoma in the United States. *N Engl J Med*. 1983;309:257–264.

Chen YC, Wang CH, Su IJ, Hu CY, Chou MJ, Lee Th, et al. Infection of human T-cell leukemia virus type I and development of human T-cell leukemia lymphoma in patients with hematologic neoplasms: a possible linkage to blood transfusion. *Blood*. 1989; 74:388–394.

Coste J, Lemaire JM, Barin F, Courouce AM. HTLV-I/II antibodies in French blood donors. *Lancet*. 1990; 335:1167–1168.

Dalgleish AG. Human T cell leukaemia/lymphoma virus and blood donation. *BMJ*. 1993;307:1224–1225.

Gibbs WN, Lofters WS, Campbell M, Hanchard B, LaGrande L, Cranston B, et al. Non-Hodgkin lymphoma in Jamaica and its relation to adult T-cell leukemia-lymphoma. *Ann Intern Med*. 1987;106: 361–368.

Grassmann R, Dengler C, Müller-Fleckenstein I, Fleckenstein B, McGuire K, Dokhelar MC, et al. Transformation to continuous growth of primary human T lymphocytes by human T-cell leukemia virus type I X-region genes transduced by a Herpesvirus saimiri vector. *Proc Natl Acad Sci U S A*. 1989;86:3351–3355.

Gross DJ, Kavanaugh A. HTLV-I. *Int J Dermatol*. 1990; 29:161–165.

Jaffe ES, Blattner WA, Blayney DW, Bunn PA Jr, Cossmann J, Roert-Guroff M, et al. The pathologic spectrum of adult T-cell leukemia/lymphoma in the United States. Human T-cell leukemia/lymphoma virus-associated lymphoid malignancies. *Am J Surg Pathol*. 1984;8:263–275.

Kalyanaraman VS, Sarngadharan MG, Robert-Guroff M, Miyoshi I, Golde D, Gallo RC. A new subtype of human T-cell leukemia virus (HTLV-II) associated with a T-cell variant of hairy cell leukemia. *Science*. 1982;218:571–573.

Kamihira S, Sohda H, Atogami S, Toriya K, Yamada Y, Tsukazaki K, et al. Phenotypic diversity and prognosis of adult T-cell leukemia. *Leuk Res*. 1992;16: 435–441.

Kawano F, Yamaguchi K, Nishimura H, Tsuda H, Takatsuki K. Variation in the clinical courses of adult T-cell leukemia. *Cancer*. 1985;55:851–856.

Komuro A, Hayami M, Fujii H, Miyahara S, Hirayama M. Vertical transmission of adult T-cell leukaemia virus. *Lancet*. 1983;1:240.

Kuwazuru Y, Hanada S, Furukawa T, Yoshimura A, Sumizawa T, Utsunomiya A, et al. Expression of P-glycoprotein in adult T-cell leukemia cells. *Blood*. 1990;76:2065–2071.

Lofters W, Campbell M, Gibbs WN, Cheson BD. 2'-Deoxycoformycin therapy in adult T-cell leukemia/lymphoma. *Cancer*. 1987;60:2605–2608.

Major prognostic factors of patients with adult T-cell leukemia-lymphoma: a cooperative study. Lymphoma Study Group (1984-1987). *Leuk Res*. 1991; 15:81–90.

Nagafuji K, Harada M, Teshima T, Eto T, Takamatsu Y, Okamura T, et al. Hematopoietic progenitor cells from patients with adult T-cell leukemia-lymphoma are not infected with human T-cell leukemia virus type 1. *Blood*. 1993;82:2823–2828.

Osame M, Izumo S, Igata A, Matsumoto M, Matsumoto T, Sonoda S, et al. Blood transfusion and HTLV-I associated myelopathy. *Lancet*. 1986;2:104–105.

Pagliuca A, Layton DM, Allen S, Mufti GJ. Hyper-infection with strongyloides after treatment for adult T cell leukaemia-lymphoma in an African immigrant. *BMJ.* 1988;297:1456–1457.

Poiesz BJ, Ruscetti FW, Gazdar AF, Bunn PA, Minna JD, Gallo RC. Detection and isolation of type C retrovirus particles from fresh and cultured lymphocytes of a patient with cutaneous T-cell lymphoma. *Proc Natl Acad Sci U S A.* 1980;77:7415–7419.

Sadamori N, Ikeda S, Yamaguchi K, Mine K, Hakariya S, Kinoshita H, et al. Serum deoxythymidine kinase in adult T-cell leukemia-lymphoma and its related disorders. *Leuk Res.* 1991;15:99–103.

Shimoyama M, Ota K, Kikuchi M, Yunoki K, Konda S, Takatsuki K, et al. Chemotherapeutic results and prognostic factors of patients with advanced non-Hodgkin's lymphoma treated with VEPA or VEPA-M. *J Clin Oncol.* 1988;6:128–141.

Shimoyama M, Ota K, Kikuchi M, Yunoki K, Kondi S, Takatsuki K, et al. Major prognostic factors of adult patients with advanced T-cell lymphoma/leukemia. *J Clin Oncol.* 1988;6:1088–1097.

Shimoyama M. Diagnostic criteria and classification of clinical subtypes of adult T-cell leukaemia-lymphoma. A report from the Lymphoma Study Group (1984-87). *Br J Haematol.* 1991;79:428–437.

T-lymphoma associated with HTLV-I outside the Caribbean and Japan. *Lancet.* 1985;2:337–338.

Uchiyama T, Yodoi J, Sagawa K, Takatsuki K, Uchino H. Adult T-cell leukemia: clinical and hematologic features of 16 cases. *Blood.* 1977;50:481–492.

Yamada Y, Kamihira S, Amagasaki T, Kinoshita K, Kusano M, Chiyoda S, et al. Adult T cell leukemia with atypical surface phenotypes: clinical correlation. *J Clin Oncol.* 1985;3:782–788.

Yamada Y, Murata K, Kamihira S, Atogumi S, Tsukasaki K, Sohda H, et al. Prognostic significance of the proportion of Ki-67-positive cells in adult T-cell leukemia. *Cancer.* 1991;67:2605–2609.

Yamaguchi K, Yul LS, Oda T, Maeda Y, Ishii M, Fujita K, et al. Clinical consequences of 2'-deoxycoformycin treatment in patients with refractory adult T-cell leukaemia. *Leuk Res.* 1986;10:989–993.

CD30+ LYMPHOPROLIFERATIVE DISORDERS

William A. Kanner, MD, Katherine L. Craven, MD, and James W. Patterson, MD

In 1985, Stein and his coworkers described a tumor composed of sheets of large, atypical, cohesive lymphocytes that expressed the Ki-1 antigen, also known as *CD30*. This description paved the way for recognition of a new group of cutaneous lymphoproliferative disorders (CLPDs) that included both lymphomatoid papulosis (LyP) and the tumor Stein described, cutaneous anaplastic large cell lymphoma (ALCL). CLPDs represent about 25% of all cutaneous T-cell lymphomas, making them the second most common behind mycosis fungoides (MF) in incidence.

LyP had been previously described by Dupont in 1956 and, then, more definitively, by Macauly in 1968. It was thought to be a clinically benign, histologically malignant condition, but occasional evolution to lymphoma eventually led to its classification together with ALCL by the World Health Organization (WHO) and the European Organization for Research and Treatment of Cancer (EORTC). LyP is now recognized to be a lymphoproliferative disorder with a predominance of clonal CD30+ T cells.

At our institution, we have diagnosed 80 cases of CD30+ CLPD since the early 2000s. Fifty of these cases were received in consultation, and 30 represented "in-house" cases. Of the 80 cases, 24 were diagnosed as LyP and 13 cases as primary cutaneous anaplastic large cell lymphoma (PCALCL). Of the remaining 43 cases, 2 represented systemic ALCL, 5 represented transformed MF, and in the rest of the cases, it was not possible to definitively classify the type of CD30+ CLPD.

Other entities that may fall within the CD30+ lymphoproliferative category include borderline cases, Hodgkin's lymphoma (HL), and transformed MF. Borderline cases are those that exhibit features of both LyP and PCALCL and, thus, cannot be assigned to either category. Finally, there are numerous reactive conditions that must be distinguished from CD30+ CLPDs. The aim of this chapter is to address the clinicopathologic features of CD30+ CLPDs as well as the main differential diagnoses.

The definitions and discussions incorporate the WHO and EORTC classifications and definitions.

THE CD30 ANTIGEN

The CD30 antigen is a transmembrane glycoprotein that belongs to the tumor necrosis factor (TNF) superfamily. The most widely known monoclonal antibody to CD30 is Ki-1. However, Ber-H2 is another monoclonal antibody that is thought to bind to a different region of the CD30 antigen. Expression of CD30 antigen has been shown to be present on the cell membrane, cytoplasm, and, in the case of Ber-H2, the Golgi apparatus (with dotlike positivity). The Golgi staining seen with Ber-H2 is possibly the result of antibody recognition to a precursor molecule.

CD30 is expressed on numerous cells including activated T and B cells, some plasma cells, dendritic cells, and histiocytes. In a normal lymph node, CD30 can be expressed on activated B and T cells in the paracortical region and in germinal centers. Neoplasms expressing CD30 include ALCL (cutaneous and systemic), T-cell neoplasms, HL, embryonal carcinoma, some mesotheliomas, and some vascular tumors. There are also numerous inflammatory and infectious diseases that express CD30. The clinical, microscopic, immunophenotypic, and molecular features of LyP and PCALCL are summarized in Table 9-1.

LYMPHOMATOID PAPULOSIS

Epidemiology

The incidence of LyP peaks in the fifth decade and there is a 2:1 male-to-female preponderance. However, females outnumber males in the patient population younger than 19 years of age. LyP has also been well described in children and adolescents.

TABLE 9-1   The Clinical, Microscopic, Immunophenotypic, and Molecular Features of Lymphomatoid Papulosis and Anaplastic Large Cell Lymphoma

	LyP	Primary Cutaneous ALCL
Clinical presentation	Fifth decade Dome shaped necrotic and crusted papules that are recurrent and self-limiting Torso, extremities, other	Sixth decade Violaceous to red nodule, tumor or plaque Solitary lesion Head, extremities
Histology	Classic wedge-shaped dermal infiltrate Type A: Scattered large atypical cells (resemble Reed-Sternberg cells), background mixed inflammatory infiltrate Type B: Scattered small atypical cells resembling cells seen in MF, epidermotropism Type C: Clusters or sheets of large atypical cells, frequent mitotic figures	Dermal infiltrate with no epidermotropism Large atypical cells with anaplastic features
Immunophenotype	Positive (usually): CD30, CD2, CD3, CD4, TIA-1, granzyme, perforin, HLA-DR, CD25, Ki-67 Negative: ALK-1, CD8 (usually), CD7, CD15 Positive (rare): CD56 (does not portend a bad prognosis)	Positive (usually): CD30 (>75% of neoplastic cells by definition), CD2, CD3, CD4, CD5, CD8, TIA-1, granzyme, perforin, CD25, Ki-67 Negative: ALK-1, EMA, CD8, CD7, CD15, cytokeratin Positive (rare): CD56 (does not portend a bad prognosis)
Clonal T-cell gene rearrangements	Found in half of cases	Often
Treatment	Observation Methotrexate PUVA or UVB Tetracycline or bexarotene	Observation Excision Methotrexate Chemotherapy
Prognosis	Excellent but may be associated with ALCL, HL, MF	Excellent

ALCL, anaplastic large cell lymphoma; HL, Hodgkin's lymphoma; HLA, human leukocyte antigen; LyP, lymphomatoid papulosis; MF, mycosis fungoides; PUVA, psoralen plus ultraviolet A; UVB, ultraviolet B.

Clinical Presentation

LyP classically presents as dome-shaped necrotic and crusted papules that occur in clusters or groups on the trunk and extremities, but it may occur anywhere (Figures 9-1 and 9-2). It has a chronic progressing, resolving, and recurring course, with an episode of active lesions lasting anywhere from 3 to 12 weeks before spontaneously involuting. Commonly, atrophic scars remain at the site of healing papules. The frequency of episodes is variable, as is the overall duration of the condition. It typically follows this relapsing-remitting course for two to three decades, but may resolve completely with no sequelae other than mild scarring.

LyP can present atypically with pustular or vesicular lesions, lesions resembling pyogenic granuloma, follicular-based papules, or plaques. When involvement is focal or restricted to one area, lesions tend to persist longer than usual.

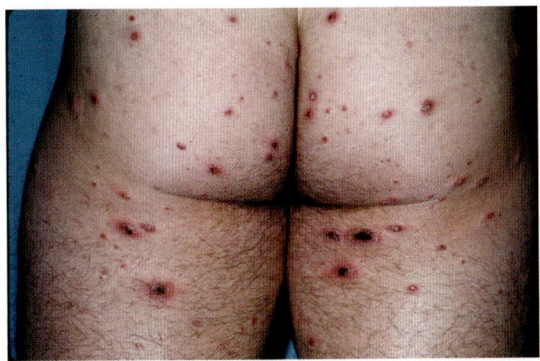

Figure 9-1 Clinical photograph of lymphomatoid papulosis (LyP). Courtesy of Dr. Kenneth Greer, University of Virginia Department of Dermatology.

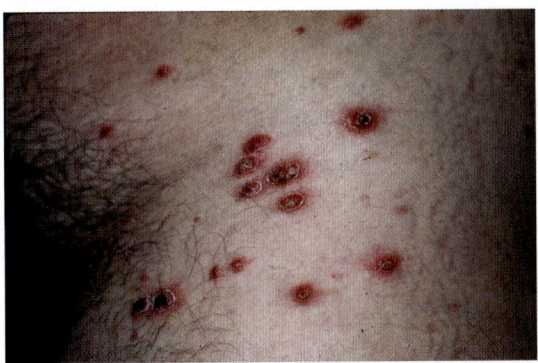

Figure 9-2 Clinical photograph of LyP. Courtesy of Dr. Kenneth Greer, University of Virginia Department of Dermatology.

Clinical Course

For the majority of patients, LyP is chronic but has no impact on overall health. Disease-specific survival at 5 years is 100% and overall survival at 5 years is 92%. In 10% to 20% of cases, LyP is associated with malignancy. MF is the most common associated malignancy and can develop before, after, or concurrently with LyP. ALCL is the second most commonly associated malignancy; when accompanying LyP, it always develops in existing LyP lesions. HL can also occur before, after, or at anytime during the course of LyP. When limited to the skin, these malignancies do not portend a poor prognosis. However, ALCL will occasionally become systemic, significantly reducing 5-year survival. It is thought that there is an associated mutation in lymphocyte growth factor receptors, leading to increased activity of transforming growth factor-beta (TGF-β) and up-regulation of CD30 expression and proliferation of lymphoblastic cells. Recent studies have shown an association between LyP and nonhematologic malignancies as well.

Histopathologic Features

Histologic diagnosis of LyP is truly a challenge because the features vary significantly. In fact, in many respects, it is the clinical features that truly make the diagnosis. Classically, there are three subtypes of LyP: A, B, and C.

In type A, low-power examination demonstrates a classic wedge-shaped dermal infiltrate (Figure 9-3). However, it is important to recognize that the histologic features vary according to the stage of the lesion. Thus, one may find epidermal changes such as ulceration, spongiosis, or exocytosis. Within a mixed inflammatory infiltrate, there are scattered single or clustered large atypical lymphoid cells (Figure 9-4). The neoplastic cells have vesicular nuclei with clumped chromatin and prominent nucleoli. There is abundant cytoplasm, and these cells may resemble the neoplastic cells seen in HL (Reed-Sternberg cells) or ALCL.

In type B, the low-power appearance is of a dense dermal infiltrate that may be bandlike. On high-power examination, there is an MF-type appearance in which there is epidermotropism consisting of small atypical lymphoid cells with hyperchromatic, convoluted, or cerebriform nuclei.

In type C, there is a more monotonous population of large atypical cells and, compared with type A, there is a less prominent associated inflammatory infiltrate (Figures 9-5 and 9-6). It is here that borderline cases fall, in that there are cases that cannot be differentiated between type C LyP and PCALCL. Unfortunately, there are no good clinicopathologic criteria to distinguish between the two. However, one interesting study demonstrated that MUM-1 positivity was found more often in LyP cases than in ALCL.

Histologic variants of LyP include those cases with folliculotropic infiltrates and follicular mucinosis, myxoid variants, and those having angiocentric or angiodestructive features.

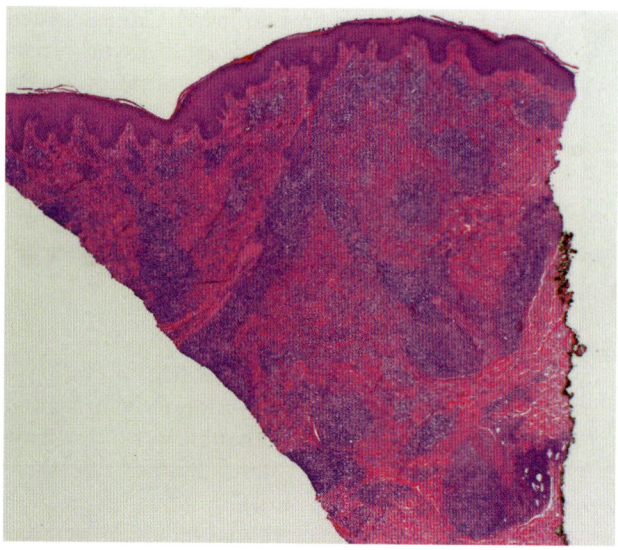

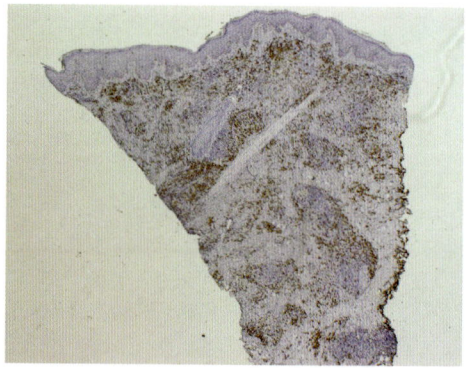

Figure 9-3 LyP, low-power magnification, hematoxylin-and eosin (H&E). The inflammatory infiltrate has a vague wedge-shaped configuration with the base of the wedge at the dermal-epidermal junction and the point of the wedge in the dermis. **Inset,** LyP, low-power magnification from the same case, H&E. There are scattered CD30 positive neoplastic cells throughout the infiltrate.

Immunophenotype

The neoplastic cell in LyP is an activated T-helper cell. In types A and C, the neoplastic cells stain with CD30 (see Figures 9-3 and 9-4 insets). In type B, the neoplastic cells do not always express CD30, but they stain positive for CD3 and CD4. CD8 staining is not usually observed, although it has been reported in pediatric patients. The cytotoxic granule protein markers granzyme B, perforin,

or most frequently, TIA-1 may be positive. Other activation markers such as human leukocyte antigen (HLA)-DR, CD25, and Ki-67 are expressed. Important markers such as ALK-1, CD7, and CD15 are usually, but not always, negative in LyP. Although CD56 may be positive in some cases, it is not associated with a worse prognosis.

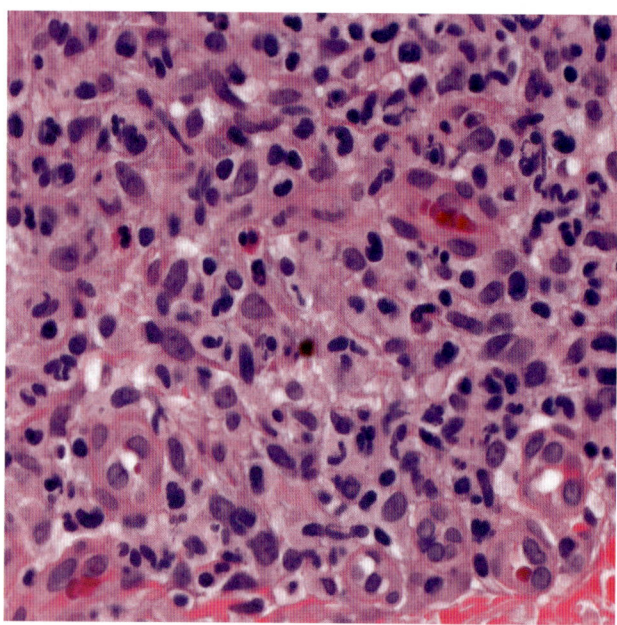

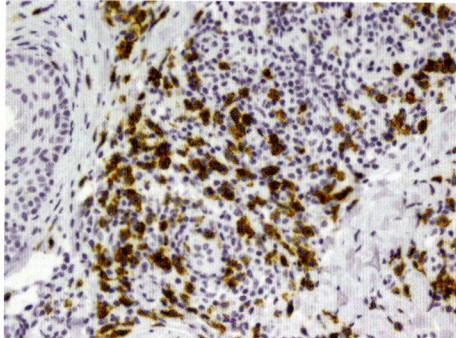

Figure 9-4 LyP, high-power magnification from the same case, H&E. There are scattered, large neoplastic cells with clumped and marginated chromatin with prominent nucleoli. The cytoplasm is pale with indistinct borders. There is an associated mixed inflammatory infiltrate consisting of small lymphocytes, neutrophils, and eosinophils. **Inset,** LyP, low-power magnification from the same case. A CD30 stain highlights the neoplastic cells, which are scattered throughout the inflammatory infiltrate.

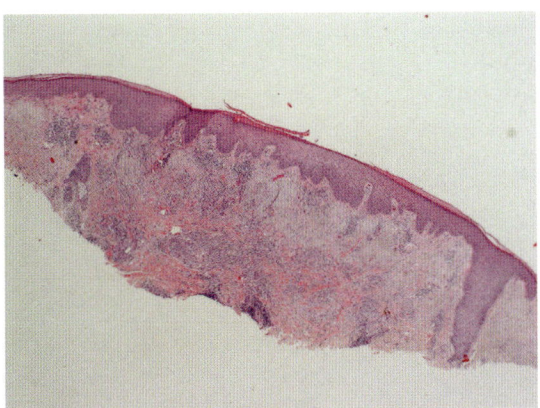

Figure 9-5 LyP type C, low-power magnification, H&E. There is prominent solar elastosis and overlying scale crust present. The inflammatory infiltrate is scattered throughout the specimen with extensive involvement of the dermis.

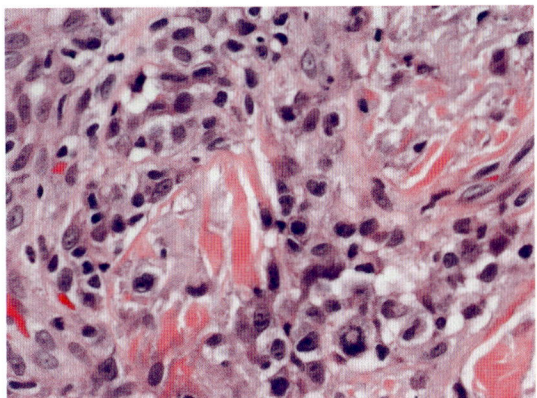

Figure 9-6 LyP type C, high-power magnification from the same case, H&E. The infiltrate consists of a sheet of neoplastic cells with large atypical nuclei, prominent nucleoli, and abundant cytoplasm. Some of the cells demonstrate anaplastic morphology. This appearance is identical to primary cutaneous anaplastic large cell lymphoma (PCALCL).

Genetics

Although there are no consistent genetic markers in LyP, T-cell rearrangements demonstrate a clonal rearrangement more than half of the time.

Differential Diagnosis

LyP can clinically and pathologically resemble benign, reactive conditions; therefore, accurate history and observation of the clinical course are often imperative for correct diagnosis. Diagnosis is often delayed 1 to 3 years when LyP is mistaken for arthropod bites. Indeed, arthropod bites can resemble LyP both clinically and histologically. History of onset, duration, and recurrence can be helpful in these cases. If onset is seasonal without recurrence during winter months, arthropod bite is more likely. In addition, the CD30+ cells found in scabies are both T and B lymphocytes. However, it must be kept in mind that nodular scabies can persist longer than most arthropod reactions, lasting up to 2 to 3 months. Cutaneous leishmaniasis, which can be difficult to distinguish from LyP based on clinical picture and hematoxylin-and-eosin (H&E)–stained sections, can sometimes be diagnosed by finding organisms with special stains when prompted by a history of recent travel to an endemic area.

Pityriasis lichenoides et varioliformis acuta (PLEVA) is the condition most frequently confused with LyP. Clinically, patients with PLEVA will present with an acute onset of multiple erythematous, crusted papules on trunk and extremities. It spontaneously resolves in a few weeks to months and may heal with small, atrophic scars. It typically does not recur. It is seen most frequently in children and has no association with hematologic or nonhematologic malignancies. Given the prognostic difference, it is critical to distinguish these two conditions. Often, simple observation is adequate to differentiate these two conditions. If the eruption does not recur, PLEVA is the more likely diagnosis. By histology, both may have a similar low-power histologic appearance of a wedge-shaped lesion with epidermal necrosis. Furthermore, PLEVA does not have significant cytologic atypia, does not express CD30, and does not display clonality in the majority of cases.

Other clinical masqueraders of LyP include folliculitis, prurigo nodularis, various cutaneous viral infections, and myelodysplastic syndromes. Although these conditions can often be ruled out based on histologic examination, it is always important to correlate the microscopic findings with other clinical and laboratory data.

Treatment

Observation is the first step in the approach to treatment of LyP. Not only is observation important in establishing a correct diagnosis, but also it often is the only treatment required. When lesions are asymptomatic and not cosmetically disfiguring, patients can be monitored through the course of the disease for development of malignancy. Although treatment of LyP does not influence the risk of developing lymphoma, treatment is sometimes desired in severe or persistent cases.

Low-dose methotrexate is a preferred treatment for LyP. Generally, doses start at 15 to 20 mg/wk, with maintenance doses given every 10 to 14 days. On this regimen, the condition is controlled in 90% of patients and induces complete remission in 20%. Patients are often free of active lesions in 4 weeks.

In cases unresponsive to methotrexate, or in patients who cannot take the medication, psoralen plus ultraviolet A (PUVA) and ultraviolet B (UVB) are useful alternatives. PUVA at 50 to 480 J/cm twice-weekly has resulted in complete clearance. Tetracycline has anecdotally been effective and, although there are no good supportive data, it is a reasonable treatment option for children over the age of 8 years (to avoid mottling of dental enamel). It is thought the efficacy in treating LyP is related to tetracycline's anti-inflammatory effects rather than its antibacterial effects. Interferon-alpha (IFN-α) and IFN-β administered as local injections have also been used with success in some patients. It is postulated that CD30+ cells have features of Th2 cells and, as such, can be suppressed by these Th1 cytokines.

Systemic and topical bexarotene has been used with moderate success. Oral bexarotene in doses of 10 mg/kg resulted in a 54% overall response rate in one study. Topical treatment with bexarotene 1% gel led to remission of individual lesions and an overall response rate of 68%.

Liu and coworkers have expressed the view that there is no role for chemotherapy in this disease because recurrence is the norm following this form of therapy.

PRIMARY CUTANEOUS ANAPLASTIC LARGE CELL LYMPHOMA

Epidemiology

ALCL is predominantly a primary cutaneous neoplasm. Worldwide, there is a 1.5 to 2:1

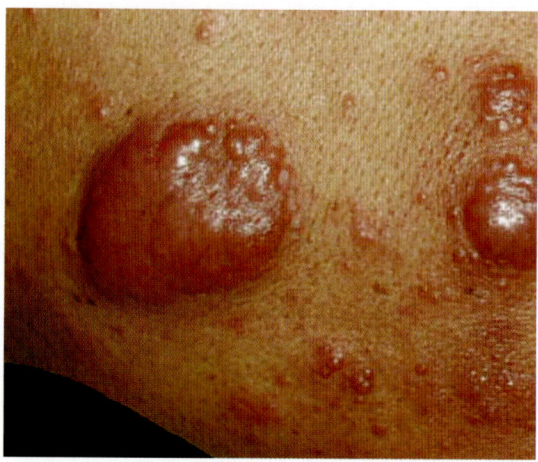

Figure 9-7 Clinical photograph of PCALCL. Courtesy of Dr. Mark Wick, University of Virginia, Department of Pathology.

male-to-female predominance, although there is no significant gender difference in the United States. Peak age is the sixth decade.

Clinical Presentation

In contrast with lymphomatoid papulosis, PCALCL typically presents as a solitary lesion (Figure 9-7). It may be a violaceous to red nodule, tumor, or plaque. Lesions may ulcerate, but they are most often asymptomatic. The most common sites of involvement are the head and extremities. In 20% of cases, cutaneous ALCL may be generalized or multifocal, and in 20%, there may be extracutaneous involvement, with lymph nodes the most frequently involved site.

Clinical Course

Despite the concerning histologic picture, PCALCL has a good prognosis. Twenty-five percent will spontaneously regress. The remaining cases are indolent, and if dissemination occurs, it does so late in the disease. Disease-specific survival at 5 years is 85% to 90%.

Histopathologic Features

On low-power examination, the lesion usually appears diffuse and cohesive and does not involve the epidermis (Figure 9-8). In fact, the epidermis may notably show pseudoepitheliomatous hyperplasia. Although confined mainly to the dermis, the

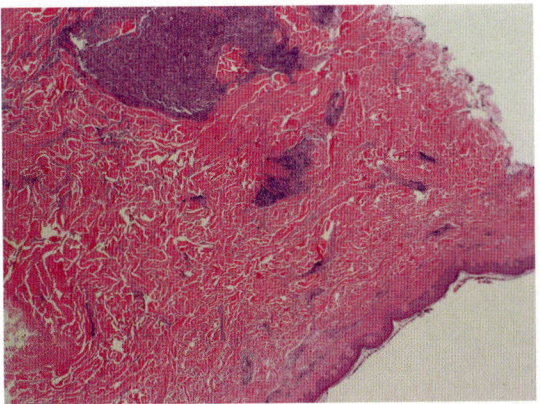

Figure 9-8 PCALCL, low-power magnification, H&E. The dense inflammatory infiltrate is located in the dermis and does not extend into the epidermis.

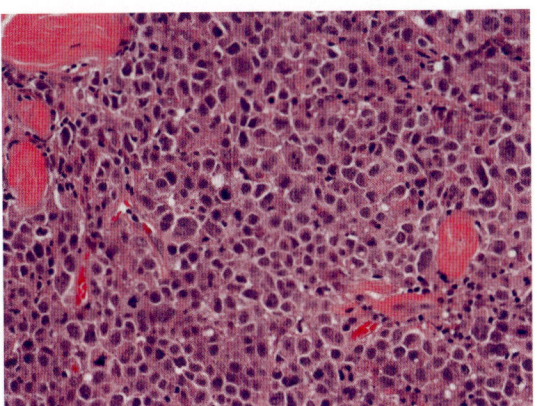

Figure 9-9 PCALCL, high-power magnification from the same case as in Figure 9-8, H&E. The infiltrate consists of a sheet of neoplastic cells with large atypical nuclei, prominent nucleoli, and abundant cytoplasm. Some of the cells demonstrate anaplastic morphology. Mitotic figures are easily appreciated. Neutrophils are also present.

infiltrate may extend into the subcutis. Ulceration may be present, and at times, geographic necrosis may exist. High-power examination demonstrates confluent sheets of neoplastic cells with a so-called anaplastic morphology (Figure 9-9). This includes pleomorphic nuclei, sometimes multiple, in a variety of configurations, prominent nucleoli, and abundant eosinophilic cytoplasm. Although often abundant, these large cells may at times be few in number. Mitotic figures may be numerous and atypical-appearing. The tumor environment may include a significant population of reactive lymphocytes, often at the periphery of the lesion. However, at times, there may be a more mixed infiltrate consisting of lymphocytes, neutrophils, macrophages, and eosinophils. In fact, there is a neutrophil-rich variant, which is also referred to as *pyogenic large cell lymphoma*. Other histologic types include a keratoacanthoma-like and a sarcomatoid variant.

Immunophenotype

The neoplastic cell in PCALCL is an activated T cell. As an initial determination of the lymphoid nature of this neoplasm, the majority of cases stain positively for CD45 and lack cytokeratin staining. By definition (WHO/EORTC), greater than 75% of the neoplastic cells in cutaneous ALCL must be CD30+ (Figure 9-10). These cells also often stain positively for CD4, indicating a T-cell phenotype. Other T-cell markers are variably positive and include CD2, CD3, CD5, and CD45RO. Cytotoxic

granule proteins including TIA-1, granzyme B, and perforin are frequently positive. Whereas the systemic form of ALCL may stain with EMA and/or ALK-1, most cutaneous cases do not stain with either of these markers (Figure 9-10 insert). CD15 is often negative in these lesions.

Genetics

Most cases demonstrate clonal T-cell receptor gene rearrangements. However, the ALK translocation is not present, in contrast to systemic ALCL.

Differential Diagnosis

The most important differential diagnostic consideration to exclude in a patient with PCALCL is systemic ALCL with cutaneous involvement. This can be difficult because skin involvement occurs in 40% to 60% of cases of systemic ALCL and clinically can look very similar, although lesions are more frequently multiple. Systemic ALCL has the t(2;5)(p23;q35) translocation with corresponding expression of the ALK-1 gene. Primary cutaneous ALCL will be ALK-1−. The importance of differentiating these two conditions lies mainly in their prognostic differences: whereas PCALCL generally has a good prognosis, cutaneous involvement of systemic ALCL is indicative of a poor prognosis.

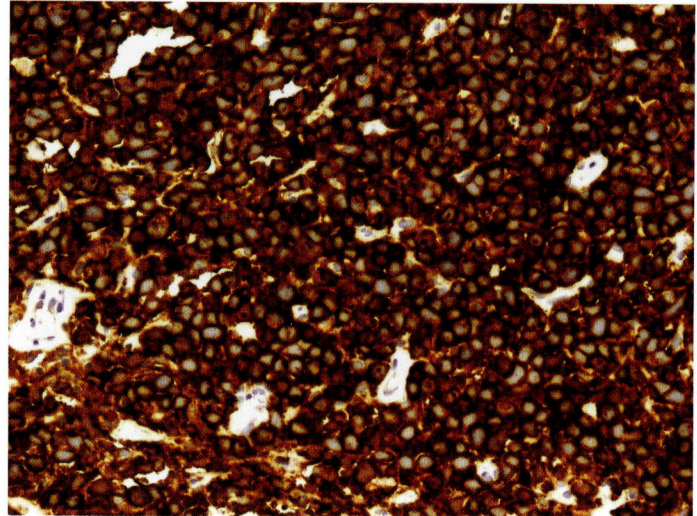

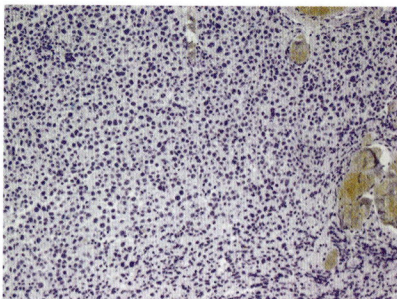

Figure 9-10 PCALCL, high-power magnification from the same case as in Figure 9-8. CD30 immunostaining is strongly and diffusely positive in essentially all the neoplastic cells. **Inset,** PCALCL, high-power magnification from the same case as in Figure 9-8. ALK-1 staining is negative in the neoplastic cells.

LyP and PCALCL share many clinical and histopathologic features. It is believed by some that these entities exist on a spectrum, rather than being two distinct conditions, and any lesions that resolve spontaneously should be considered to be LyP rather than ALCL. Cases that cannot be differentiated on clinical or histologic examination are considered borderline cases. In such cases, it is recommended that treatment for an unclear case of ALCL be delayed for 6 to 8 weeks because it may resolve spontaneously. If this occurs, a retrospective diagnosis of LyP may be appropriate. As previously mentioned, MUM1 has been found to be a possible discriminator between LyP and PCALCL.

Cutaneous HL is another tumor comprised of atypical CD30+ lymphocytes. The incidence is rare and has been decreasing in the last 50 years with most recent data ranging from 0.85% to 3.4% in patients with known HL. There is some controversy over the possible existence of primary cutaneous HL. However, Kaden and colleagues reported an eruption of papules and nodules that closely resembled LyP clinically but contained Reed-Sternberg cells that, like HL cells, were CD30+, CD15+, CD45R–. This is in contrast to the immunoprofile of similar cells in LyP, which are typically CD30+, CD15–, CD45R+. On clinical follow-up, two of their five patients developed mixed-cellularity HL in lymph nodes. However, most often, cutaneous lesions specific to HL occur when malignant cells in a patient with nodal disease invade the skin. Clinically, the lesions are multiple, erythematous, painless papules and nodules that may progress to ulceration. Typically, distribution is on the chest wall, axillae, or other area that drains the affected lymph nodes. Cutaneous involvement typically indicates advanced disease and portends a poor prognosis. The combined clinical and histologic picture is usually adequate to distinguish among the entities.

As with any tumor consisting of large atypical cells forming clusters, one must consider carcinoma and melanoma. Thus, cytokeratin staining and a melanocytic marker may be helpful.

Transformed MF often expresses CD30. This presents a diagnostic challenge because MF in association with other CLPDs can look identical. Differentiating the two is important because transformed MF has a disease-specific 5-year survival of 44% compared with the 87% to 100% 5-year survival of patients with primary cutaneous CLPD. Most frequently, the histopathologic pictures of the two tumors are distinct if MF occurs in conjunction with primary cutaneous CLPD. In transformed MF, pleomorphic cerebriform T-cells are mixed with fewer than 75% CD30+ large lymphocytes. The patient's clinical course and evolution is also revealing, and a diagnosis of transformed MF is more certain if the tumor arises in an existing MF lesion.

Treatment

The first step in approach to treatment of ALCL is 4 to 8 weeks of observation because 25% of diagnosed cases will regress. A minority of cases will not recur, but most patients require observation and follow-up to monitor for recurrence.

Excision has been used for treatment of solitary lesions and is a good option. However, margins are often found to be positive and require further treatment. Radiation is the treatment of choice for solitary lesions. Electron beam irradiation is used, at 4 to 10 million eV. Penetration of the electron beam does not go deeper than the dermis, so there are no systemic effects. However, it is not practical for multiple non-regressing lesions. In addition, there are local side effects, including alopecia, atrophy of sweat glands and skin, radiation dermatitis, and edema. Most frequently, excision and radiation are used in conjunction for single, non-resolving lesions.

Systemic therapies have also been used to treat PCALCL, and typically single-agent therapy is preferred because multiple agents have not been shown to be more effective at inducing long-term remission. Methotrexate is commonly used in higher weekly doses than that used to treat LyP. Other systemic medications used are etoposide, imiquimod, interferon, bexarotene, and doxarubacin. The combination of cyclophosphamide, doxorubicin, vincristine, and prednisone (CHOP) has been used for patients that develop systemic involvement. For systemic, recalcitrant disease, bone marrow transplant has been moderately successful.

OTHER LYMPHOPROLIFERATIVE DISORDERS WITH CD30+ EXPRESSION

As mentioned previously, CD30 expression may be present in HL, transformed MF, and Sézary syndrome. Pagetoid reticulosis is another condition with CD30+ cells. This entity presents as a psoriasiform lesion and histologically is notable for prominent epidermotropism of atypical CD30+ cells. Adult T-cell lymphoma/leukemia may also present with skin lesions with a variety of clinical and histologic presentations. The clinical features and human T-cell lymphotropic virus (HTLV) testing are crucial to this diagnosis. Two other rare conditions are associated with CD30 expression. The first consists of "hydroa vacciniforme-like" lesions that are associated with Ebstein-Barr virus (EBV). The second has been termed *lymphoma and leukemia-associated cutaneous atypical CD30+ T-cell reactions*. Su and Duncan reported two examples of the latter, one in a patient with B-cell lymphoma and another with myeloid leukemia. In both cases, skin lesions developed after chemotherapy, and in both instances, the lesions spontaneously resolved. Microscopic findings included perivascular CD30+ lymphoid cells.

REACTIVE CONDITIONS WITH CD30+ LYMPHOCYTES (CD30+ PSEUDOLYMPHOMAS)

Arthropod bite reactions and PLEVA, as previously discussed, are examples of inflammatory conditions that express CD30 positivity. These reactive conditions can clinically resemble either ALCL or, more commonly, LyP. Type A LyP frequently has a prominent eosinophilic component, closely mimicking arthropod bite reactions.

Viral infections activate T cells and initiate a blastic response, which leads to up-regulation of expression of CD30. Clinically, molluscum contagiosum can appear as multiple self-resolving papules and commonly occurs in children. Typically, the flesh-colored umbilicated appearance and the classic viral change on histologic examination are sufficient to differentiate this entity from LyP. Milker's nodule, caused by cutaneous infection with paravaccinia virus, can be diagnosed by its distribution primarily on the hands and a history of direct exposure to sheep or goats. There are two case reports of CD30+ herpes simplex virus/varicella-zoster virus (HSV/VZV) infection, which was distinguished from LyP by viral inclusions found deep in the follicular unit and a history of tinnitus and neuralgic pain in a patient with trigeminal distribution of lesions. CD30+ lymphocytes are extremely rare in human papillomavirus (HPV) infections. EBV+ lymphoproliferative diseases often express CD30, especially in immunosuppressed patients. These cases can be differentiated from LyP and ALCL by the presence of both T- and B-cell CD30 positivity.

Drug reactions can mimic ALCL pathologically with large, atypical CD30+ lymphocytes. However, the clinical pattern is usually distinct, described as urticarial plaques or a typical morbilliform rash. The key to this diagnosis is recent exposure to a medication. The most likely medications associated with a CD30+ lymphoid infiltrate are sulfa derivatives and antiepileptics, especially carbamazepine.

There have been several case reports of recurrent pruritic papules in patients with myelodysplastic syndrome. The papules occur on the face, trunk, and extremities. They worsen with time, resolve spontaneously, and recur. These patients also present with anemia and leukopenia. Many cases go on to become predominantly neutrophilic infiltrates, consistent with Sweet's syndrome, and it is believed that this CD30+ lymphocytic lesion represents a chronic, recurrent lymphocytic variant of Sweet's syndrome.

SUGGESTED READINGS

Barnadas MA, Lopez D, Pujol RM, Garcia-Patos V, Curell R, de Moragas JM. Pustular lymphomatoid papulosis in childhood. *J Am Acad Dermatol.* 1992;27:627–628.

Beljaards RC, Willemze R. The prognosis of patients with lymphomatoid papulosis associated with malignant lymphomas. *Br J Dermatol.* 1992;126:596–602.

Bekkenk MW, Geelen FA, van Voorst Vader PC, et al. Primary and secondary cutaneous CD30(+) lymphoproliferative disorders: A report from the dutch cutaneous lymphoma group on the long-term follow-up data of 219 patients and guidelines for diagnosis and treatment. *Blood.* 2000;95:3653–3661.

Calzado-Villarreal L, Polo-Rodriguez I, OrtizRomero PL. Primary cutaneous CD30+ lymphoproliferative disorders. *Actas Dermosifiliogr.* 2010;101:119–128.

El Shabrawi-Caelen L, Kerl H, Cerroni L. Lymphomatoid papulosis: Reappraisal of clinicopathologic presentation and classification into subtypes A, B, and C. *Arch Dermatol.* 2004;140:441–447.

Falini B, Pileri S, Pizzolo G, et al. CD30 (ki-1) molecule: A new cytokine receptor of the tumor necrosis factor receptor superfamily as a tool for diagnosis and immunotherapy. *Blood.* 1995;85:1–14.

Guitart J, Querfeld C. Cutaneous CD30 lymphoproliferative disorders and similar conditions: A clinical and pathologic prospective on a complex issue. *Semin Diagn Pathol.* 2009;26:131–140.

Heald P, Subtil A, Breneman D, Wilson LD. Persistent agmination of lymphomatoid papulosis: An equivalent of limited plaque mycosis fungoides type of cutaneous T-cell lymphoma. *J Am Acad Dermatol.* 2007;57:1005–1011.

Hsu YJ, Su LH, Hsu YL, Tsai TH, Hsiao CH. Localized lymphomatoid papulosis. *J Am Acad Dermatol.* 2010;62:353–356.

Introcaso CE, Kantor J, Porter DL, Junkins-Hopkins JM. Cutaneous hodgkin's disease. *J Am Acad Dermatol.* 2008;58:295–298.

Kato N, Matsue K. Follicular lymphomatoid papulosis. *Am J Dermatopathol.* 1997;19:189–196.

Kempf W. CD30+ lymphoproliferative disorders: Histopathology, differential diagnosis, new variants, and simulators. *J Cutan Pathol.* 2006;33 Suppl 1:58–70.

Kempf W, Kutzner H, Cozzio A, et al. MUM1 expression in cutaneous CD30+ lymphoproliferative disorders: A valuable tool for the distinction between lymphomatoid papulosis and primary cutaneous anaplastic large-cell lymphoma. *Br J Dermatol.* 2008;158:1280–1287.

Knaus PI, Lindemann D, DeCoteau JF, et al. A dominant inhibitory mutant of the type II transforming growth factor beta receptor in the malignant progression of a cutaneous T-cell lymphoma. *Mol Cell Biol.* 1996;16:3480–3489.

Liu HL, Hoppe RT, Kohler S, Harvell JD, Reddy S, Kim YH. CD30+ cutaneous lymphoproliferative disorders: The stanford experience in lymphomatoid papulosis and primary cutaneous anaplastic large cell lymphoma. *J Am Acad Dermatol.* 2003;49:1049–1058.

Macaulay WL. Lymphomatoid papulosis. A continuing self-healing eruption, clinically benign—histologically malignant. *Arch Dermatol.* 1968;97:23–30.

Nijsten T, Curiel-Lewandrowski C, Kadin ME. Lymphomatoid papulosis in children: A retrospective cohort study of 35 cases. *Arch Dermatol.* 2004;140:306–312.

Patterson JW, Wick MR. *Nonmelanocytic Tumors of the Skin.* Vol 4. Washington, DC: American Registry of Pathology; 2006.

Patterson JW, White RM. Lymphomatoid papulosis. *South Med. J* 1986;79:850–856.

Scarisbrick JJ, Calonje E, Orchard G, Child FJ, Russell-Jones R. Pseudocarcinomatous change in lymphomatoid papulosis and primary cutaneous CD30+ lymphoma: A clinicopathologic and immunohistochemical study of 6 patients. *J Am Acad Dermatol.* 2001;44:239–247.

Schiemann WP, Pfeifer WM, Levi E, Kadin ME, Lodish HF. A deletion in the gene for transforming growth factor beta type I receptor abolishes growth regulation by transforming growth factor beta in a cutaneous T-cell lymphoma. *Blood.* 1999;94:2854–2861.

Schwab U, Stein H, Gerdes J, et al. Production of a monoclonal antibody specific for hodgkin and sternberg-reed cells of hodgkin's disease and a subset of normal lymphoid cells. *Nature.* 1982;299:65–67.

Stein H, Mason DY, Gerdes J, et al. The expression of the hodgkin's disease associated antigen ki-1 in reactive and neoplastic lymphoid tissue: Evidence that reed-sternberg cells and histiocytic malignancies are derived from activated lymphoid cells. *Blood.* 1985;66:848–858.

Swerdlow SH, Campos E, Harris NL, et al. *World Health Organization Classification of Haematopoietic and Lymphoid Tissues.* 4th ed. Lyon: IARC Press; 2008.

Vergier B, de Muret A, Beylot-Barry M, et al. Transformation of mycosis fungoides: Clinicopathological and prognostic features of 45 cases. french study group of cutaneious lymphomas. *Blood.* 2000;95:2212–2218.

Wang HH, Lach L, Kadin ME. Epidemiology of lymphomatoid papulosis. *Cancer.* 1992;70:2951–2957.

Wang HH, Myers T, Lach LJ, Hsieh CC, Kadin ME. Increased risk of lymphoid and nonlymphoid malignancies in patients with lymphomatoid papulosis. *Cancer.* 1999;86:1240–1245.

Willemze R, Jaffe ES, Burg G, et al. WHO-EORTC classification for cutaneous lymphomas. *Blood.* 2005;105:3768–3785.

Willemze R, Kerl H, Sterry W, et al. EORTC classification for primary cutaneous lymphomas: A proposal from the cutaneous lymphoma study group of the european organization for research and treatment of cancer. *Blood.* 1997;90:354–371.

Wu WM, Tsai HJ. Lymphomatoid papulosis histopathologically simulating angiocentric and cytotoxic T-cell lymphoma: A case report. *Am J Dermatopathol.* 2004;26:133–135.

SUBCUTANEOUS PANNICULITIS-LIKE T-CELL LYMPHOMA

Abhinav B. Chandra, MD, MSc, FACP, Yiqing Xu, MD, PhD, and Yiwu Jim Huang MD, PhD

BACKGROUND

Subcutaneous panniculitis-like T-cell lymphoma (SPTCL) is a rare entity of non-Hodgkin's lymphoma, first described in 1991 by Gonzalez and coworkers in a series of eight patients. It is characterized by panniculitis-like skin lesions, with infiltration of the skin by neoplastic T cells derived from post-thymic cytotoxic T cells. It is a disease of the young with average age of presentation in the mid-30s. The clinical course is mostly indolent characterized by recurrent panniculitis; it also could be aggressive, especially when it is complicated with hemophagocytic syndrome (HPS).

T-cell receptors (TCRs) have two phenotypes—α/β and γ/δ—both of which express CD3. α/β T cells are divided into CD4+ cells, which are responsible for cytokine secretion, and CD8+ cells, which are mainly the cytotoxic subset. γ/δ T cells express γ/δ TCRs and can display one or more natural killer (NK)–associated markers such as CD16 and CD56. They constitute less than 5% of T cells in the peripheral blood and are found in the red pulp of the spleen and in the epithelium, where they are involved in mucosal immunity.

SPTCLs can be divided into two subtypes based on their TCR phenotype: SPTCL, α/β subtype and γ/δ subtype. These two subtypes are not only different in surface markers but also very different in clinical courses. SPTCL with α/β T-cell phenotype are CD4–, CD8+, CD56– and usually have an indolent course as opposed to that of TCR γ/δ origin expressing CD4–, CD8–, CD56+ phenotype, which mimics the clinical course of other γ/δ cutaneous T-cell lymphomas. They are much more aggressive and have a significantly worse prognosis than that with α/β phenotype (Table 10-1).

SPTCL was initially classified as a provisional entity in the Revised European-American

TABLE 10-1 Differentiating Features between the α/β and the γ/δ T-Cell Phenotypes

	α/β	γ/δ
Frequency	62-75%	25-38%
Median age	36	59
Clinical course	Indolent and recurrent	Aggressive
Skin ulceration	Rare	Common
HPS	Uncommon	Common
Immunophenotype	CD3+, CD4–, CD8+, CD56–, TCR-βF1+	CD3+. CD4–. CD8–, TCR-δ–1+ usually CD56+
EBV	Negative	Negative
Treatment	Local radiation, immunosuppressants, single-agent chemotherapy or polychemotherapy	As other γ/δ cutaneous lymphomas, polychemotherapy, with or without HSCT
Survival	Favorable	Poor

EBV, Ebstein-Barr virus; HPS, hemophagocytic syndrome; HSCT, hematopoietic stem cell transplantation; TCR, T-cell receptor.

Lymphoma (REAL) classification and in the European Organization for Research and Treatment of Cancer (EORTC) classification in 1997. It was reclassified as a distinct entity by the World Health Organization (WHO)/EORTC in 2005. Particularly, the definition of SPTCL is now restricted to those with α/β TCR phenotype only; cases with TCR γ/δ phenotype are now placed in a new provisional category of cutaneous γ/δ T-cell lymphoma.

Of note, most of the SPTCL cases reported in the literatures before the WHO/EORTC classification included both subtypes, in which approximately 62% to 75% were of α/β phenotype and 25% to 38% were of γ/δ phenotype (see Table 10-1).

ETIOLOGY/PATHOGENESIS

The etiology and pathogenesis of SPTCL remain unclear. It is a disease frequently associated with autoimmune disorders. The associated autoimmune phenomena span a wide spectrum from laboratory abnormalities only (positive antinuclear antibody or Coombs test) to well-established autoimmune diseases. Treatment of lymphoma has led to resolution of autoimmune diseases as well in some cases. Interestingly, there were also reports of new development or progression of SPTCL during immunosuppressive therapy for autoimmune diseases, pregnancy, or human immunodeficiency virus (HIV) infection. Therefore, it seems that dysregulation of the immune system plays a role in this malignancy. Further investigation to clarify this association is warranted.

Epstein-Barr virus (EBV) does not seem to play an important role in the pathogenesis of SPTCL. Using in situ hybridization, EBV was almost always negative in SPTCL neoplastic cells in the majority of the reported cases occurring in Western countries. However, positive EBV detection was reported in a few cases from Asia and Middle East. The relationship of EBV and SPTCL needs further evaluation.

EPIDEMIOLOGY

SPTCL is very rare. Worldwide, it accounts for approximately 0.2% of all primary cutaneous lymphomas and 0.9% of T-cell and NK-cell lymphomas. In North America, it represents 1.3% of all T-cell and NK-cell lymphomas; in Europe, it is 0.5%; and in Asia, it is 1.3%. Because only the α/β phenotype is now considered SPTCL, the incidence could even be lower. The median age at presentation is 36 years, and approximately 20% of patients are younger than 20. In contrast, other T-cell and NK-cell lymphomas have a median age of 62 years. Willemze and colleagues reported that SPTCL affects females more than males with a male to female ratio of 0.5, but Go and associates observed roughly equal number of male and female patients.

CLINICAL FINDINGS

Patients usually present with multiple, recurrent erythematous to violaceous indurated subcutaneous nodules or plaques predominantly involving the extremities and the trunk (Figure 10-1). Facial involvement is less common, but occasionally periorbital involvement can be observed (Figure 10-2). Skin ulceration is uncommon (<10%). In early stages, nodules may regress spontaneously and nodules at various stages of healing may be seen. Lipoatrophy may be present after regression of the nodules. Although dissemination to lymph nodes and other organs on initial presentation is very unusual, constitutional symptoms such as fever, chills, malaise, anorexia, and weight loss are present in up to 40% of patients. More than 50% of patients have

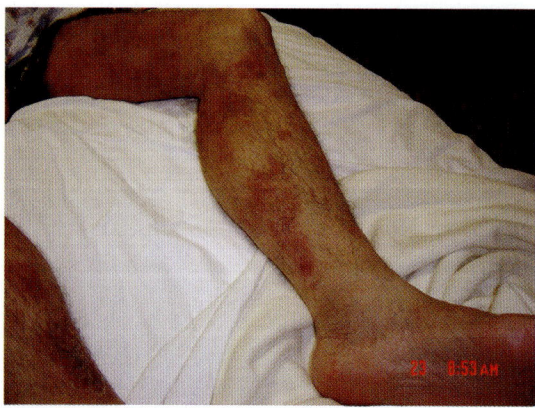

Figure 10-1 Subcutaneous nodules on the lower extremities.

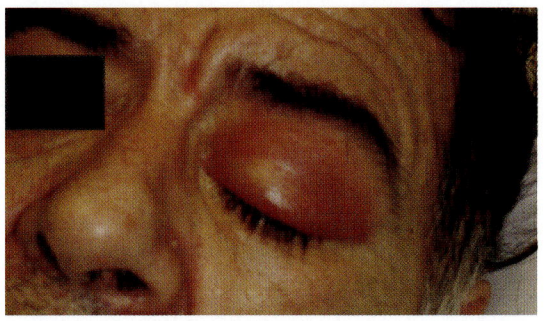

Figure 10-2 Periorbital involvement of the left eye.

laboratory abnormalities such as anemia, leukopenia, thrombocytopenia, and elevated liver function tests; some may also have laboratory abnormalities indicating autoimmune conditions. Approximately 20% of SPTCL patients have documented autoimmune conditions; those reported conditions include systemic lupus erythematosus (SLE), psoriatic arthritis, idiopathic thrombocytopenic purpura, juvenile rheumatoid arthritis, Sjögren's disease, multiple sclerosis, Raynaud's disease, and Kikuch's disease.

The 5-year overall survival (OS) in patients with SPTCL is more than 80%. Patients without HPS appear to have a significant better 5-year OS (91%) than those with HPS (46%).

Differential Diagnosis for Clinical Findings

SPTCL is difficult to diagnose based on cutaneous findings alone. For some patients, longer follow-up with multiple biopsies is needed to make an accurate diagnosis of SPTCL.

The typical rash, which is composed of erythematous or violaceous indurated nodules or plaques, can be confused with rashes in patients with SLE, psoriatic arthritis, and juvenile rheumatoid arthritis, as well as other cutaneous lymphomas. Other conditions that exhibit a similar pattern of rash include reactive panniculitis, Weber-Christian disease (idiopathic lobular panniculitis), atypical lymphocytic lobular panniculitis, and to some extent, even erythema nodosum, pseudolymphoma, and venous stasis.

Atypical lymphocytic lobular panniculitis, a new provisional entity described in the recent literature, warrants some further discussion here.

Its clinical course is characterized by waxing and waning plaques and the presence of systemic symptoms of fever and fatigue. Laboratory abnormalities such as cytopenias can also occur in this disorder. However, this condition is self-limited, is usually not progressive, and never involves lymph nodes.

HISTOPATHOLOGIC FINDINGS

The accurate diagnosis of SPTCL, as with other cutaneous lymphomas, is not easy owing to reactive tissue response that masks the identification of neoplastic T cells. It relies on a combination of a typical histologic presentation, appropriate immunohistochemical evaluation, and molecular analysis.

Histologically, neoplastic cells are usually of intermediate size with round to oval hyperchromatic nuclei with inconspicuous nucleoli and abundant pale cytoplasm. The tumor infiltrates extend diffusely through the subcutaneous tissues with relative sparing of dermis and epidermis. A helpful diagnostic feature is the rimming of the neoplastic T cells with surrounding individual fat cells in a wreathlike manner (Figures 10-3

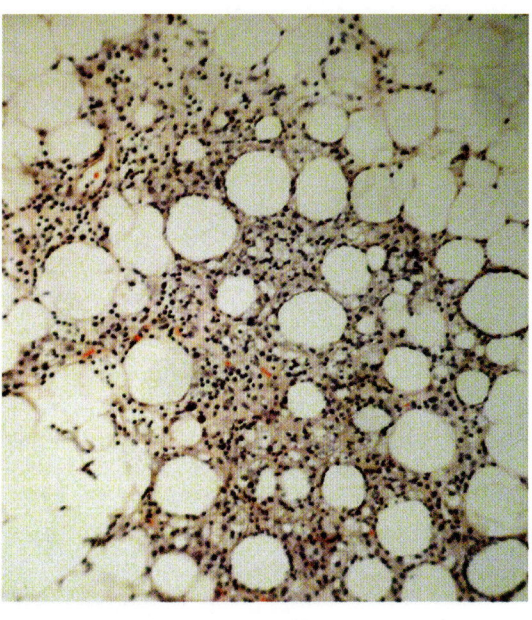

Figure 10-3 Tumor infiltrate extend diffusely through the subcutaneous tissue from skin biopsy (hematoxylin-and-eosin [H&E] stain, 100× original magnification).

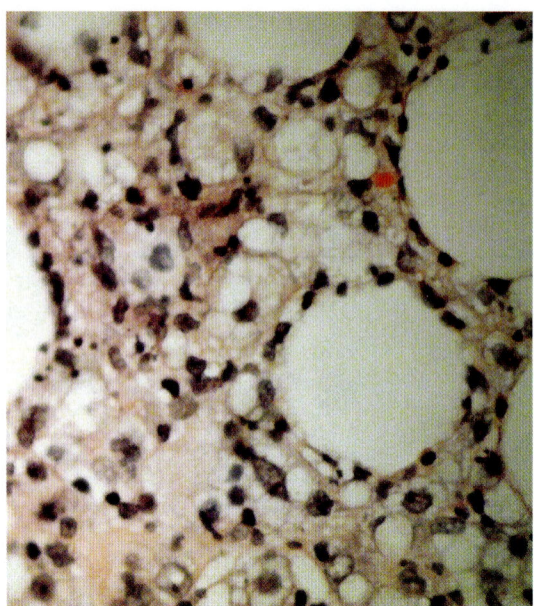

Figure 10-4 The rimming of the neoplastic cells surrounding individual fat cells, which is the helpful classic diagnostic feature for subcutaneous panniculitis-like T-cell lymphoma (H&E stain, 400× original magnification).

and 10-4). Small reactive lymphocytes and many histiocytes are also typically present. Nuclear fragmentation (karyorrhexis) of lymphoid cells, fat necrosis, and cytophagocytosis are frequently seen. Leukocytoclasia can also be observed. Angioinvasion may occur but not as a primary event and usually without angiodestruction.

Immunophenotypically, the neoplastic cells (α/β SPTCL) express common cytotoxic T-cell markers CD3+, CD8+, and cytotoxic granular proteins: TIA-1, perforin, and granzyme A. CD4, CD30, and CD56 are absent in lymphoma cells. All α/β SPTCL cases are positive for T-cell receptor (TCR) βF1 and negative for TCR δ-1. The γ/δ TCR SPTCLs, which were included in previous studies but are now a new category of cutaneous γ/δ T-cell lymphoma, are CD56+, CD4–, CD8– (see Table 10-1). TCR gene rearrangement study is also helpful to determine the clonality of the neoplastic cells. In most cases, clonal rearrangements of TCR genes can be detected.

It is rare for SPTCL to be present in the bone marrow or lymph nodes, but hemophagocytosis may be detected in the bone marrow, lymph nodes, spleen, and liver without direct infiltration by neoplastic lymphocytes.

Differential Diagnosis for Histology

Although there is a characteristic histologic feature in SPTCL (i.e., the presence of neoplastic T cells forming a rim around individual fat cells in the subcutaneous lobules, or so-called rimming of adipocytes), the presence of this feature alone is not enough for accurate diagnosis. A similar histologic feature has been described in several other types of cutaneous lymphomas, including cutaneous γ/δ T-cell lymphoma, mycosis fungoides (MF), aggressive epidermotropic CD8+ T-cell lymphoma, extranodal NK-cell lymphoma, blastic NK-cell lymphoma, and secondary cutaneous large B-cell lymphoma. This feature has also been described in some cases of lupus erythematosus panniculitis (LEP). However, the neoplastic cells in MF are usually CD4+, whereas CD8+ epidermotropic lymphoma has epidermotropic infiltrates and involvement of subcutaneous tissues. Other lymphomas have their distinct immunophenotypes and clinical features, described in other chapters in this book. Therefore, patients presenting with this histopathologic feature should be classified only upon precise correlation of clinicopathologic, immunophenotypic, and molecular analysis.

SPTCL should also be distinguished from malignant histiocytosis if histocyte infiltration in the tumor is seen. Histologically, malignant histiocytosis is associated with large atypical histiocytes primarily involving the reticuloendothelial system with secondary cutaneous involvement. It lacks the features of atypical lymphoid cells, karyorrhexis, cytophagia, or the detection of a clonal population of T cells as seen in SPTCL.

SPTCL also shares similarities with extranodal NK-cell lymphoma. Occasionally, "rimming" of adipocytes is also present in extranodal NK-cell lymphoma, and it may have clonal TCR gene rearrangement and express T-cell–associated markers as well. Histiocytic component can be present in the infiltrate. Clinically, it also can present with cutaneous nodules or ulcers and can be associated with the HPS. However, angioinvasion with angiodestruction, predominant dermal infiltrate, granulomatous inflammation, CD56+, and detection of tumoral EBV are more characteristic of extranodal NK-cell lymphoma. Particularly, all extranodal NK-cell lymphoma cases are positive for the detection of EBV in neoplastic cells, which is best demonstrated by in situ hybridization.

Benign panniculitis should be differentiated from SPTCL. Histologically, it is characterized by the presence of a mixed inflammatory infiltrate comprising lymphohistiocytic cells, plasma cells, and neutrophils. In addition, the lymphoid infiltrate is usually without overt atypia. There is usually lymphocyte infiltrates of CD20+ B cells mixed with CD3+ T cells, CD4+, and CD8+ T cells in equal proportions. The T cells in this case rarely express TIA-1.

LEP can be difficult to differentiate from SPTCL. Rimming of fat lobules has been reported in LEP, and the infiltrate is composed of a mixture of lymphocytes, histiocytes, and plasma cells. It primarily involves the epidermis and forms lymphoid follicles with reactive germinal centers. The cellular infiltrate is composed of prominent plasma cells and clusters of B cells. The TCRγ gene rearrangement is typically polyclonal.

Atypical lymphocytic lobular panniculitis, characterized by recurrent infiltrative plaque-like lesions, is thought to be a morphologic and biologic continuum with SPTCL. It shares with SPTCL an infiltration of the panniculus by small to intermediate-sized atypical lymphocytes with extension into the dermis primarily in an epidermotropic and eccrinotropic array, but it is largely unaccompanied by significant necrosis.

and 19 is common in MF and Sézary's syndrome (SS), the gains of 5q and 13q appear to be more unique in SPTCL. In addition, fluorescence in situ hybridization (FISH) analysis showed deletion of NAV3 (neuron navigator 3), which has also been described in MF and SS.

Other Ancillary Studies

SPTCL is gallium-avid. Whole body gallium-67 scintigraphy is able to show positive uptake at the lymphomatous infiltrations of the skin, and a negative conversion after successful treatment is correlated with good clinical response. One report described the application of a high-resolution ultrasonography, showing thickening of the subcutaneous fat layer with homogeneous hyperechoic infiltration and poorly defined margin over the skin lesions. The hyperechogenicity was suspected to be due to the increased numbers of the fat–soft tissue interfaces and the amount of sound beam reflected. Computed tomography (CT) scan and magnetic resonance imaging (MRI) can be helpful for identification of the subcutaneous lesions and lymph nodes.

Most cases of SPTCL have been shown to have positive uptake in ^{18}F fluoro-2-deoxyglucose (FDG) positron emission tomography/computed tomography (PET/CT) scan. It has been utilized for detecting skin lesions, initial staging, quantifying disease burden, and monitoring treatment response in a few case reports. Larger studies are required to define the role of PET/CT in this disease.

CYTOGENETICS/MOLECULAR

The immunophenotype of neoplastic cells in SPTCL is CD3+, CD4–, CD8+, and CD56– with strong expression of proteins normally seen in cytotoxic T cells, such as granzyme B, TIA-1, and perforin. These malignant cells are positive for βF1 demonstrating an α/β T-cell phenotype.

DNA copy number aberrations in multiple chromosomes have been described using single-cell comparative genomic hybridization (CGH). Commonly observed are loss of chromosomes in chromosomes 1p, 2p, 2q, 5p, 7q, 9q, 10q, 11q, 12q, 16, 17q, 19, 20, and 22; and gains of chromosomes 2q, 4q, 5q, 6q, and 13q. Whereas the loss of 10q

TREATMENT

The treatment of SPTCL is challenging owing to the rarity of this disease and the lack of large randomized clinical trials. Data available to date are based on retrospective analysis of case reports, case series, or single-institution experiences. It is important to know that most of the case series included both subtypes of SPTCL, and some of the aggressive treatment used may have been applied to the γ/δ subtype, which is now known as *γ/δ cutaneous T-cell lymphoma*. The γ/δ cutaneous T-cell lymphoma carries an aggressive clinical course and poor prognosis (see Table 10-1).

So far, no single chemotherapy regimen has been established as a standard treatment for this disease. It is important to note that spontaneous resolution of skin lesions without treatment has been reported. Local radiation therapy, immunosuppressive therapy, and single or combination chemotherapy all have been used with various success. In general, patients who present with indolent or localized disease appear to respond to single-agent chemotherapy or immunosuppressive therapy alone, whereas anthracycline-based combination regimens and autologous or allogeneic stem cell transplant are required in advanced disease and in recurrent or refractory patients.

Radiation Therapy and Surgery

SPTCL is a radiation-sensitive disease. For patients with solitary or localized skin lesions only, radiation can lead to high local control rate. Willemze showed that, in four patients presenting with solitary or localized skin lesions who were treated with radiotherapy alone, all of them achieved complete response (CR). Only one relapsed and was successfully re-treated with radiotherapy. However, radiation alone may not achieve durable remissions. In a case series reported by Go and coworkers, upfront radiation treatment alone was given to 11 patients with 4 CRs (36%), 5 partial responses (PRs; 45%), and an overall response (OR) rate of 81%. Of the patients who achieved CR, 2 had durable remissions for more than 12 months, all other patients who were not in CR or developed recurrent disease required further chemotherapy. Radiation therapy can also be used as a palliative measure to relieve pain and improve quality of life in patients with widespread disease who are not candidates for aggressive chemotherapy or are resistant to chemotherapy. Surgical excision is used only for limited local disease.

Chemotherapy

In patients with indolent disease, single-agent chemotherapy has been frequently utilized as first-line treatment with a high response rate. In the EORTC Group Study, 24 out of 76 patients were initially treated with either single agent of prednisone, cyclosporine, chlorambucil, methotrexate, cyclophosphamide, gemcitabine, or inferferon-alpha, or combination of prednisone with one of these agents. Among them, 67% achieved CR and 21% achieved PR whereas only 12.5% did not respond to this less aggressive treatment. However, 56% of those complete responders relapsed. Some of them achieved sustained remission after re-treatment with prednisone or other immunosuppressive agents. Fludarabine has also been shown to result in long-term response in a single case report.

Anthracycline-based chemotherapy regimens such as CHOP (cyclophosphamide, doxorubicin, vincristine, prednisone) or CHOP-like regimens have been the most widely used. It has proved to be highly effective, leading to durable remissions for most patients who require aggressive treatment. In the EORTC Group Study, 31 out of 76 patients received first-line CHOP regimen; 61% achieved CR and 10% achieved PR. In those complete responders, only 10% relapsed.

In the relapse and refractory setting, many other combination chemotherapy regimens, such as cisplatin-based, melphalan-based, ifosfamide-based, and purine nucleoside analogue–based regimens, have also been used as salvage treatment with various success.

Immunosuppressive treatment is also effective. Systemic steroids alone can achieve long-term remission in some patients. Three out of 12 patients without CR after CHOP treatment in the EORTC series went into CR with prednisone alone, prednisone combined with methotrexate, or allogeneic stem cell transplant (SCT). Cyclosporine A (CsA) has shown impressive activity in chemotherapy-resistant SPTCL. In one case series, 9 of 11 cases demonstrated response to CsA, with 8 CRs. Time to first response to CsA was usually within 2 weeks, regardless of what the prior treatment regimens were. Patients who presented with HPS also showed good response. Hence, CsA should also be considered an active agent in this disease.

Biologic Agents

Denileukin Diftitox (Ontak), a recombinant fusion protein linking human interleukin-2 and diphtheria toxin, had been used as an initial treatment for SPTCL with some success, one out of two patients in Alpdogan and associates' report achieved PR. Furthermore, McGinnis and colleagues also showed evidence that this agent resulted in durable responses in refractory patients.

Alemtuzumab, an anti-CD52 chimeric monoclonal antibody, in combination with CHOP chemotherapy has been shown to be an effective initial treatment for a few patients in several small case series. However, toxicities, particularly reactivation of herpes zoster and development of EBV-related lymphoproliferative disorders were reported. Toxicity, especially the high percentage of herpes viral reactivation including EBV-related lymphoproliferation requires careful monitoring.

Hematopoietic Stem Cell Transplantation

Autologous hematopoietic stem cell transplantation (HSCT) and a few cases of allogeneic HSCT following high-dose chemotherapy have been attempted in refractory cases. A very high CR rate has been reported, but case numbers are small and duration of follow-up is limited. Go and associates reviewed 13 cases in the literature, 92% achieved CR after autologous HSCT with median response duration of more than 14 months. Willemze and coworkers reported three CRs out of four patients who underwent autologous SCT or allogenic SCT. Another case report described a teenage patient with primary refractory disease who was treated with alemtuzumab followed by allogeneic bone marrow transplantation (BMT). She remained in CR 31 months later.

Subcutaneous Pannicullitis-like T-Cell Lymphoma with Hemophagocytic Syndrome

HPS in SPTCL represents one of the most important prognostic factors. Weenig and colleagues found that the mortality rate was as high as 81%, whereas others reported a 5-year survival rate of 46%. HPS is thought to be the result of severe uncontrolled hyperinflammatory response, leading to prolonged and excessive activation of macrophages, histiocytes, and CD8+ T cells. The predominant clinical features include fever, cytopenias, hepatitis, coagulopathy, and splenomegaly. The optimal management of these patients remains unclear. Anthracycline-based polychemotherapy has been the mainstay of treatment.

Long-term remissions have been reported. However, for patients with relapsed or refractory disease, high-dose chemotherapy followed with autologous or allogenic HSCT seems to be the most effective salvage treatment. CsA with or without steroids also has been showed to induce long-term remission in some case reports.

SUMMARY

SPTCL is a rare T-cell non-Hodgkin's lymphoma characterized by panniculitis-like skin lesions, with infiltration of the skin by neoplastic T cells (CD3+, CD4–, CD8+, and CD56–). HPS can be present in up to 20% of cases and is associated with a poor prognosis. There is no definitive standard of care at present. Patients with early stage or indolent disease can be treated with immunosuppressants, single-agent chemotherapy, or local radiation therapy. For aggressive or advanced stage disease, combination chemotherapy appears to be the most appropriate treatment. Salvage chemotherapy with or without HSCT has been used for refractory disease. Large prospective studies and long-term follow-up of patients are required to better characterize this rare entity.

SUGGESTED READINGS

Alpdogan O, Ornstein D, Subtil T, Seropian S, et al. Outcomes in subcutaneous panniculitis-like T-cell lymphoma (STCL). *Blood (ASH Annual Meeting Abstracts)*. 2008;112:3750.

Dores GM, Anderson WF, Devesa SS. Cutaneous lymphomas reported to the National Cancer Institute's Surveillance, Epidemiology, and End Results program: applying the new WHO-European Organization for Research and Treatment of Cancer Classification System. *J Clin Oncol*. 2005;23:7246–7248.

Ghobrial IM, Weenig RH, Pittlekow MR, Qu G, Kurten PJ, Ristow K, et al. Clinical outcome of patients with subcutaneous panniculitis-like T-cell lymphoma. *Leuk Lymphoma*. 2005;46:703–708.

Go RS, Gazelka H, Hogan, JD, Westen SM. Subcutaneous panniculitis-like T-cell lymphoma: complete remission with fludarabine. *Ann Hematol*. 2003;82:247–250.

Go RS, Wester SM. Immunophenotypic and molecular features, clinical outcomes, treatments, and prognostic factors associated with subcutaneous panniculitis-like T-cell lymphoma: a systematic analysis of 156 patients reported in the literature. *Cancer.* 2004;101: 1404–1413.

Goldschmidt N, Amir G, Krieger M, Gilead L, Paltiel O. Fatal hemophagocytic syndrome in a patient with panniculitis-like T-cell lymphoma and no clinical evidence of disease. *Leuk Lymphoma.* 2003;44: 1803–1806.

Gonzalez CL, Medeiros LJ, Braziel RM, Jaffe ES. T-cell lymphoma involving subcutaneous tissue: a clinicopathologic entity commonly associated with hemophagocytic syndrome. *Am J Surg Pathol.* 1991;15: 17–27.

Hahtola S, Burghart E, Jeskanen L, Karenko L, Abdel-Rahman WM, Polzer B, et al. Clinicopathological characterization and genomic aberrations in subcutaneous panniculitis-like T-cell lymphoma. *J Invest Dermatol.* 2008;128:2304–2309.

Harris NL, Jaffe ES, Stein H, Banks PM, Chan JK, Cleary ML, et al. A revised European-American classifcation of lymphoid neoplasms: a proposal from the International Lymphoma Study group. *Blood.* 1994;84:1361–1392.

Hashimoto H, Sawada K, Koizumi K, Nishio M, Endo T, Takashima T, et al. Effective CD34– selected autologous peripheral blood stem cell transplantation in a patient with subcutaneous panniculitic T cell lymphoma (SPTCL) transformed into leukemia. *Bone Marrow Transplant.* 1999;24:1369–1371.

Hung GD, Chen YH, Chen DY, Lan JL. Subcutaneous panniculitis-like T-cell lymphoma presenting with hemophagocytic lympho-histiocytosis and skin lesions with characteristic high-resolution ultrasonographicfindings. *Clin Rheumatol.* 2007;26:775–778.

Ichii M, Hatanaka K, Imakita M, Ueda Y, Kachino B, Toamki T. Successful treatment of refractory subcutaneous panniculitis-like T-cell lymphoma with allogeneic peripheral blood stem cell transplantation from HLA-mismatched sibling donor. *Leuk Lymphoma.* 2006;47:2250–2252.

Jaffe E, Harris NL, Stein H, et al. *The World Health Organization Classification of Tumours: Tumours of the Hematopoietic and Lymphoid Tissues.* Lyon, France: IARC Press; 2001:212–213.

Jassal DS, Kasper K, Morales C, Rubinger M. Autologous peripheral stem cell transplantation for aggressive hemophagocytic syndrome associated with T-cell lymphoma: Case study and review. *Am J Hematol.* 2002;69:64–66.

Kako S, Izutsu K, Ota Y, Nguyen D, Bui C. FDG-PET in T-cell and NK-cell neoplasms. *Anal Oncol.* 2007;18:1685–1690.

Lozzi GP, Massone C, Citarella L, Kerl H, Cerroni L. Rimming of adipocytes by neoplastic lymphocytes:

a histopathologic feature not restricted to subcutaneous T-cell lymphoma. *Am J Dermatopathol.* 2006;28:9–12.

Magro CM, Crowson AN, Byrd JC, Soleymani AD, Shendrick I. Atypical lymphocytic lobular panniculitis. *J Cutan Pathol.* 2004;31:300–306.

Magro CM, Schaefer JT, Morrison C, Parcu P. Atypical lymphocytic lobular panniculitis: a clonal subcutaneous T cell dyscrasis. *J Cutan Pathol.* 2008;35: 947–954.

McGinnis KS, Shapiro M, Junkins-Hopkins JM, Smith M, Lessin SR, Vittorio CC, et al. Denileulin diftitox for the treatment of panniculitic lymphoma. *Arch Dermatol.* 2002;138:740–742.

Mukai HY, Okoshi Y, Shimizu S, Katsawa Y, Takei N, Hasegawa T, et al. Successful treatment of a patient with subcutaneous panniculitis-like T-cell lymphoma with high-dose chemotherapy and total body irradiation. *Eur J Haematol.* 2003;70:413–416.

Parveen Z, Thompson K. Subcutaneous panniculitis-like T-cell lymphoma: redefinition of diagnostic criteria in the recent World Health Organization-European Organization for Research and Treatment of Cancer classification for cutaneous lymphomas. *Arch Pathol Lab Med.* 2009;133:303–308.

Perez-Persona E, Mateos-Mazon JJ, Lopez-Villar O, Areos MJ, Encinas C, Graciani IF, et al. Complete remission of subcutaneous panniculitic T cell lymphoma after allogenic transplantation. *Bone Marrow Transplant.* 2006;38:821–822.

Rojnuckarin P, Nakorn TN, Assanasen T, Wannakrairot P, Intraqumtornchai T. Cyclosporin in subcutaneous panniculitis-like T cell lymphoma. *Leuk Lymphoma.* 2007;48:560–563.

Shen L, Alam-Fotias S, Mansberg R, et al. Subcutaneous panniculitis-like T cell lymphoma demonstrated on Gallium-67 scintigraphy. *Clin Nucl Med.* 2005; 30:500–502.

Swerdlow SH, Campo E, Harris NL, et al. *WHO Classification of Tumours of Haematopoietic and Lymphoid Tissues.* Vol. 2. IARC WHO Classification of Tumours, No. 2. Lyon, France: IARC Press; 2008.

Vose J, Armitage J, Weisenburger D. International peripheral T-cell and natural killer/T-cell lymphoma study: pathologyfindings and clinical outcomes. *J Clin Oncol.* 2008;26:4124–4130.

Weenig RH, Ng CS, Perniciaro C. Subcutaneous panniculitis-like T-cell lymphoma: an elusive case presenting as lipomembranous panniculitis and a review of 72 cases in the literature. *Am J Dermatopathol.* 2001;23:206–215.

Willemze R, Jansen PM, Cerroni L, Berti E, Santucci M, Assaf C, et al. Subcutaneous panniculitis-like T-cell lymphoma: defnition, classifcation, and prognostic factors: an EORTC Cutaneous Lymphoma Group Study of 83 cases. *Blood.* 2008;111:838–845.

Willemze R, Kerl H, Sterry W, Berti E, cerroni L, Chimenti S, et al. EORTC classifcation for primary cutaneous lymphomas: a proposal from the Cutaneous Lymphoma Study Group of the European Organization for Research and Treatment of Cancer. *Blood.* 1997;90:354–371.

Zhang H, Gupta R, Wang JC, Lipton JF, Huang JW. Subcutaneous panniculitis-like T-cell lymphoma in a patient with long-term remission with standard chemotherapy. *J Natl Med Assoc.* 2007;99:1190–1192.

CUTANEOUS EXTRANODAL NATURAL KILLER/T-CELL LYMPHOMA

Won Seog Kim, MD, and Young-Hyeh Ko, MD

BACKGROUND

Extranodal natural killer (NK)/T-cell lymphoma (ENKL) is a distinct entity, according to the World Health Organization (WHO) classification and represents 5% to 10% of non-Hodgkin's lymphomas (NHLs). Previously, it was termed "angiocentric lymphoma" because of the presence of angioinvasion or angiocentric infiltration of tumor cells with necrosis. Currently, this type of lymphoma is termed *extranodal NK/T-cell lymphoma of nasal type* because, in most cases, the disease arises in the upper aerodigestive tract, mainly the nasal and paranasal areas, whereas only 20% of ENKLs arise outside the aerodigestive tract. The skin is one of the sites involved most commonly, followed by the gastrointestinal tract, testis, etc., in decreasing order of frequency. Therefore, primary cutaneous ENKL is a disease that is quite rare, even in ENKL-common areas. Although the natural history and clinical features of cutaneous ENKL are not well known, most ENKLs are aggressive, with a high rate of mortality. Meticulous examinations of the nasal area are essential for the exclusion of the possible secondary involvement of nasal ENKL.

ETIOLOGY/PATHOGENESIS

The underlying cause of cutaneous ENKL is largely unknown. Moreover, most of the knowledge on this condition stems from nasal ENKL, because of its rarity. Some studies are comparing the clinicopathologic features of nasal and extranasal ENKLs; however, their results are not conclusive yet. Therefore, the ideas are just following those derived from the study of nasal ENKL.

ENKL itself is strongly associated with Epstein-Barr virus (EBV) infection, which manifests type II latency. EBV integration occurs directly in malignant T and NK cells. EBV infection is thought to be an early event in lymphomagenesis. However, the role of the EBV-transforming gene remains unknown.

The geographic distribution of ENKL can provide some clues on genetic predisposition to this disease. Regarding T-cell immunity, the low frequency of the human leukocyte antigen (HLA)-A*0201 allele suggests an important role for EBV-specific cytotoxic T-lymphocyte (CTL) activity in ENKL lymphomagenesis.

Environmental factors for cutaneous ENKL lymphomagenesis are not known. Exposure to pesticides and chemical solvents is suggested as a possible cause of nasal ENKL. Long-standing EBV infection, such as hydroa vacciniforme and mosquito bite hypersensitivity, can be a cause of ENKL.

EPIDEMIOLOGY

It is quite difficult to establish the true incidence of cutaneous ENKL. No population-based studies are available on the incidence and prevalence of cutaneous ENKL. Moreover, most cases of ENKL arise in the nasal and paranasal areas. Therefore, although cutaneous ENKL is the most common extranasal ENKL, its incidence is rarely reported.

ENKL is more common in Asian countries and among Native Americans of Latin America. It represents approximately 5% to 8% of all cases of lymphoma and up to 30% of cases of mature T-cell lymphoma in Asian countries. In contrast, the incidence of ENKL in Europe and North America is only approximately1%. Within this disease entity, cutaneous ENKL represents less than 10% of all ENKL cases. Therefore, cutaneous ENKL itself is a quite rare disease. Even in Asian countries, the incidence is less than 1% of all lymphomas.

CLINICAL FINDINGS

The clinical features of cutaneous ENKL are not well known. In most reports, this entity is analyzed as part of non-nasal ENKL. The median age of onset of ENKL is 40 to 50 years and the disease is quite uncommon among children and young adults. There is male predominance in ENKL as a whole; however, this remains controversial in extranasal ENKL, including cutaneous disease. Compared with nasal ENKL, non-nasal ENKL usually exhibits a more aggressive clinical behavior, presenting with more advanced-stage disease, presence of B symptoms(fever, weight loss, night sweating), poor performance status, higher IPI (International Prognostic Index) score, and inferior response to chemotherapy. There are no reports comparing clinical presentation between cutaneous ENKL and other extranasal ENKLs.

Early lesions of cutaneous ENKL may present as a skin nodule. However, the most typical lesion is a nonhealing skin ulceration because its histology is characterized by angioinvasion and necrosis (Figure 11-1). Patients often also present with fever caused by hemophagocytic syndrome and/ or superinfection. Some of the cases can represent the secondary involvement of upper airway ENKL. Therefore, nasal examination is necessary (Figure 11-2).

The Ann Arbor system is not satisfactory for the staging of ENKL because ENKL itself is an extranodal lymphoma and approximately 80% of the patients would have stage I/II disease according to Ann Arbor staging, especially in nasal cases. Some reports demonstrate the importance of local tumor invasiveness and regional lymph node involvement. Unlike the situation in other lymphomas, EBV in situ hybridization is strongly

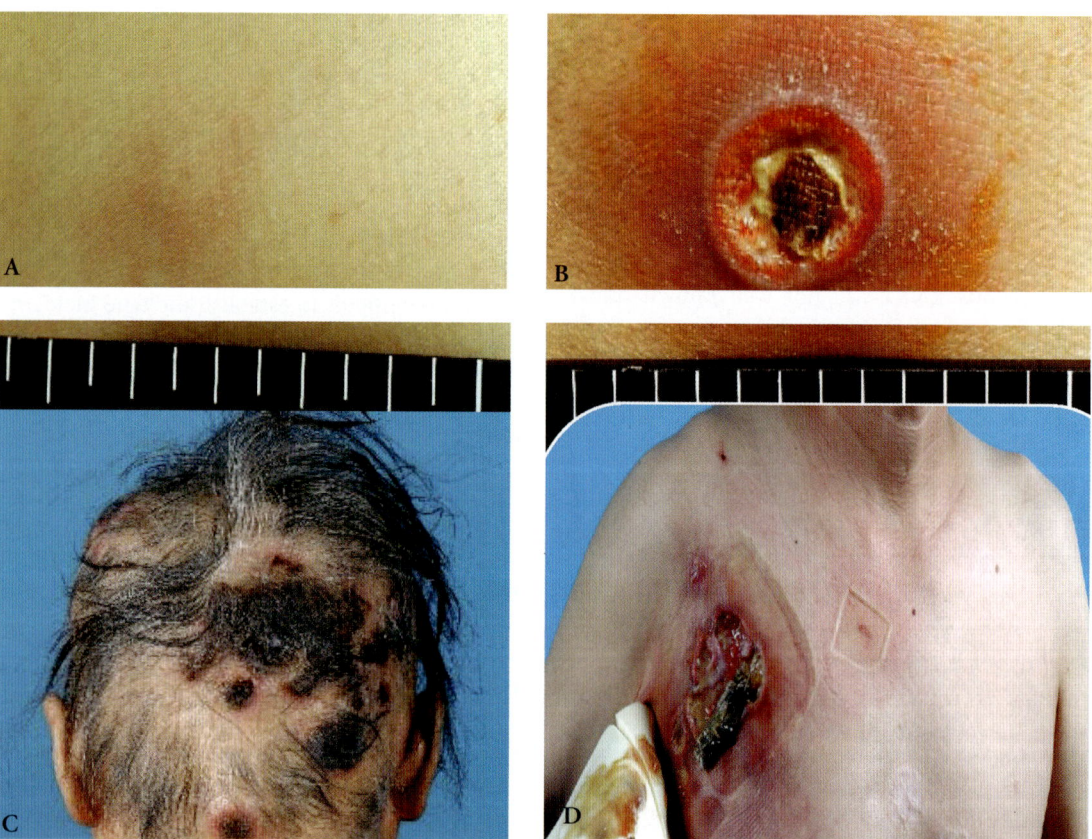

Figure 11-1 **A,** An early skin lesion that presented as a small skin nodule. **B,** Evolution of a skin lesion into a nonhealing ulceration. **C,** Advanced skin lesions in the scalp. **D,** Big ulceration and previous scar from skin lesion.

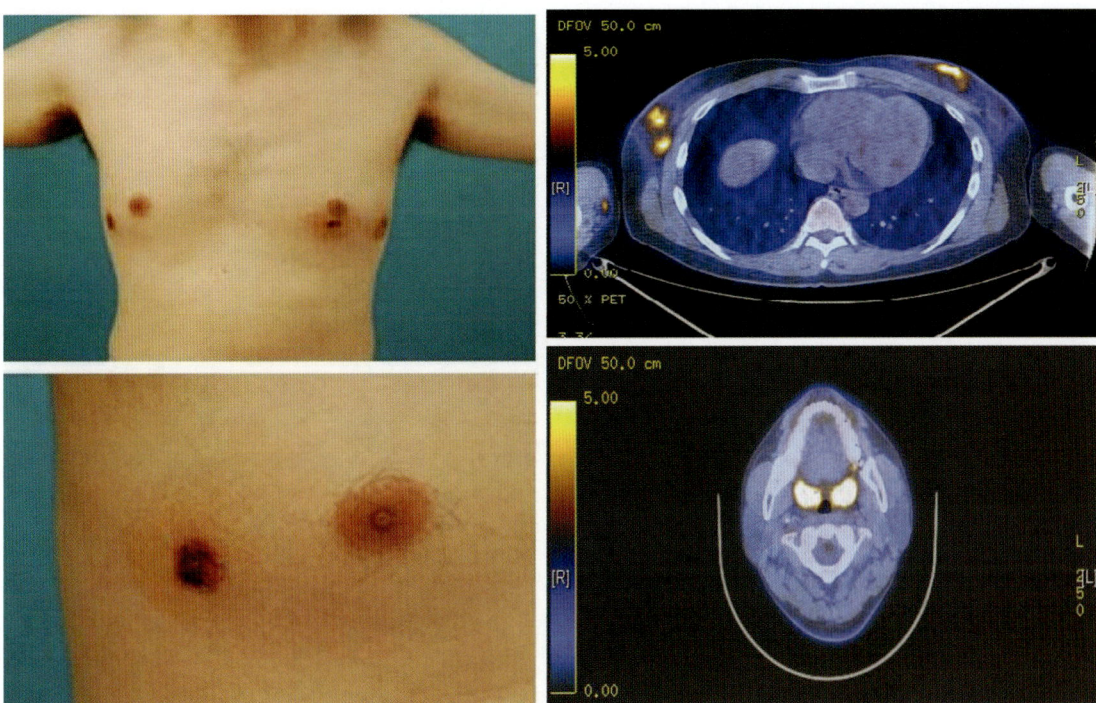

Figure 11-2 Secondary involvement form upper airway lesion. Positron emission tomography/computed tomography (PET/CT) scan showed skin lesions from primary and tonsil extranodal natural killer/T-cell lymphoma (ENKL).

recommended for the detection of bone marrow involvement in ENKL. The role of positron emission tomography (PET) remains controversial. Previous reports show that ENKL is generally fluorodeoxyglucose (FDG)–avid but exhibits significantly lower metabolic activity compared with aggressive B-cell lymphoma because of the necrosis and inflammatory components of this type of tumor. Moreover, PET has limitations regarding the evaluation of cutaneous lesions.

Because ENKL is an EBV-associated neoplasm, EBV DNA can be released from apoptotic tumor cells during proliferation. Serial quantification of EBV DNA from plasma or whole blood revealed the presence of a correlation between this parameter and disease status. Therefore, circulating EBV DNA can be a useful tumor marker for the prediction of prognosis and evaluation of treatment response in ENKL.

As is the case in other lymphomas, the IPI age/stage/extranodal/lactate dehydrogenase (LDH)/performance status (PS) has predictive value

for the prognosis of ENKL. However, an excessive number of cases are classified as having low and low/intermediate risk based on the IPI. The Korean prognostic index for NK/T-cell lymphoma (B symptom/stage/regional lymph node/LDH) is a prognostic model that is specific for ENKL. This index has a predictive power that is much stronger than that of the IPI, even though the extranasal status itself implies poor prognosis.

HISTOPATHOLOGIC FINDINGS

The histologic changes that occur in cutaneous ENKL are similar to those that are observed in nasal ENKL. Usually, these tumors involve the entire cutaneous layer, with perivascular, periadnexal, or diffuse infiltration of neoplastic cells. Sometimes, neoplastic infiltration is confined to the subcutaneous adipose tissue, which mimics subcutaneous panniculitis-like T-cell lymphoma. Prominent angiocentricity and angiodestruction

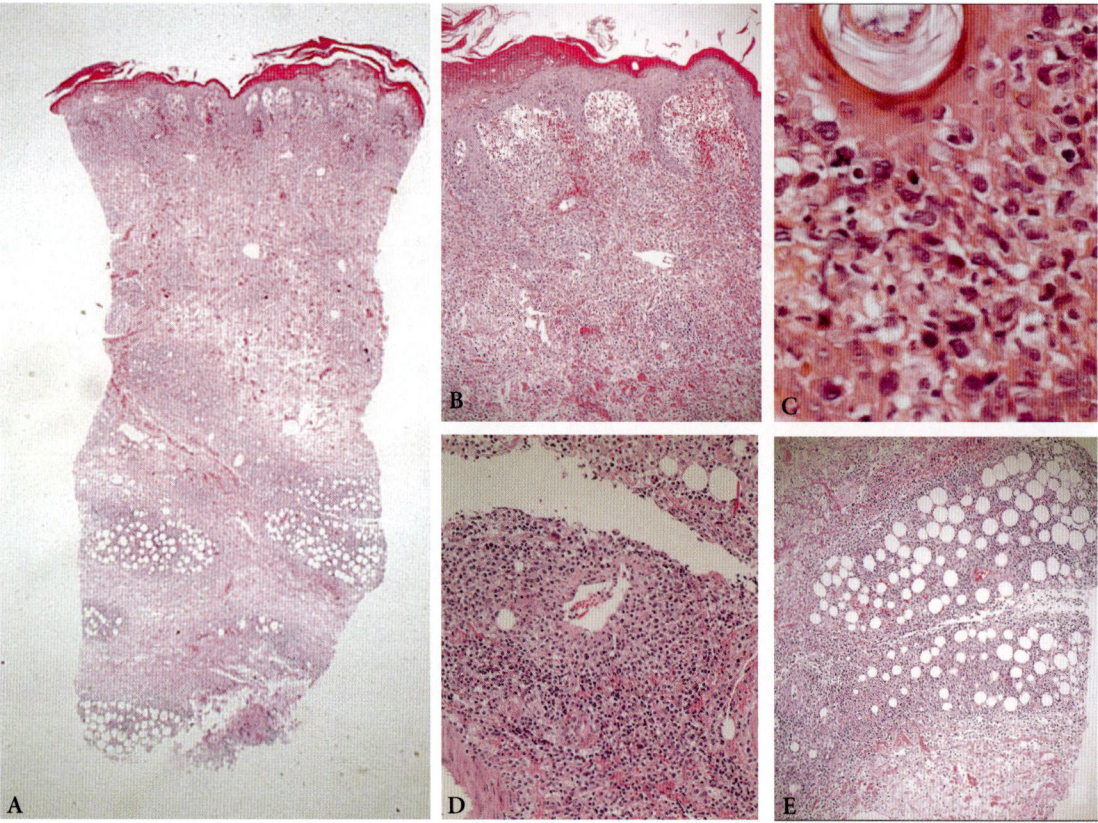

Figure 11-3 An ENKL involving the entire cutaneous layer as well as the subcutis **A**. The dermis shows diffuse infiltration of tumor cells **B**, which are large and pleomorphic **C**, with angiocentricity **D**. **E**, Extensive infiltration of subcutaneous adipose tissue is present.

are often accompanied by extensive necrosis. Histiocytic infiltration with active hemophago-cytosis is common. NK/T-cell lymphoma has a broad cytologic spectrum, ranging from small to large cells, with most cases consisting of medium-sized cells with irregular or oval nuclei, moderately dense chromatin, and pale cytoplasms (Figure 11-3). The immunophenotype of typical ENKL is positive for CD2, CD56, and cytoplas-mic CD3ε and negative for surface CD3. It is also positive for cytotoxic granules, granzyme B, perforin, and TIA. Occasionally, it is also posi-tive for CD30 and CD7. Some cases are negative for CD56. Cases that are negative for CD56 and positive for cytoplasmic CD3ε are also classified as ENKL if they are positive for both cytotoxic granules and EBV, as detected using EBV-encoded small RNA (EBER) in situ hybridization (Figure 11-4).

Differential Diagnosis for Histology

Predominant involvement of subcutaneous fat tissue is observed in various cutaneous diseases, including panniculitis, subcutaneous panniculitis-like T-cell lymphoma, primary cutaneous γ/δ T-cell lymphoma, and ENKL.

The infiltration of fat lobules by neoplastic ENKL cells results in a lobular panniculitis-like reaction with granulomas. The recognition of atypical lymphoid cells exhibiting angiocentricity, together with immunohistochemistry and EBER in situ hybridization, is crucial for the correct diagnosis of ENKL (Table 11-1).

Subcutaneous panniculitis-like T-cell lym-phoma consists of small, medium-sized, or some-times large pleomorphic T cells with an α/β+, CD3+, CD4–, and CD8+ T-cell phenotype and expression of cytotoxic proteins. The overlying

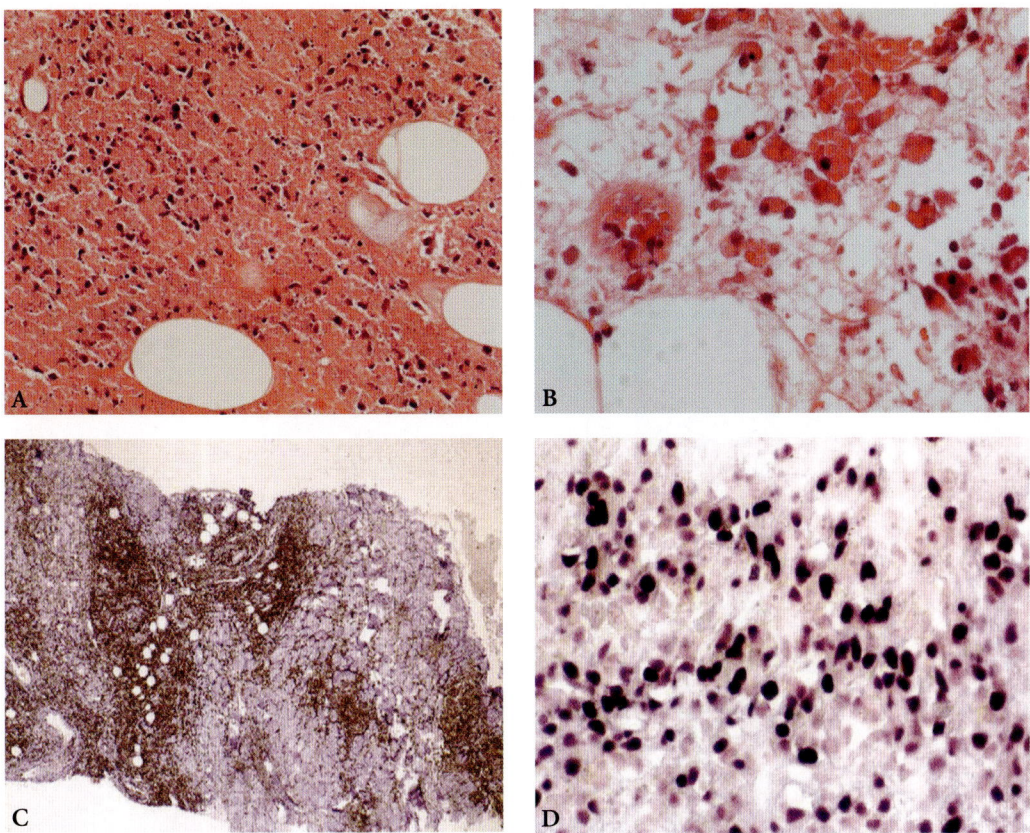

Figure 11-4 Diffuse necrosis of the skin **A**, with hemophagocytic histiocytes **B**, is common in ENKL. Tumor cells express CD56 **C**, and are also positive for EBER in situ hybridization **E**.

epidermis and dermis are typically uninvolved. Rimming of individual fat cells by neoplastic T cells is a helpful, although not completely specific, diagnostic feature. Necrosis, karyorrhexis, and cytophagocytosis are common findings. Such histologic changes are very similar to those found in cutaneous ENKL and involve predominantly the subcutis; however, cutaneous ENKL usually exhibits small nodular infiltrates in the dermis. In addition, immunohistochemical analysis and EBER in situ hybridization can clearly differentiate these two types of tumor.

Primary cutaneous γ/δ T-cell lymphoma is a lymphoma composed of a clonal proliferation of mature, activated γ/δ T cells with a cytotoxic phenotype. This group includes cases previously known as "subcutaneous panniculitis-like T-cell lymphoma of γ/δ phenotype." These γ/δ+ cases often are not confined to the subcutis and may extend into

the dermis. In such cases, differentiation between cutaneous γ/δ T-cell lymphoma and nasal-type ENKL extending into the subcutis may be difficult. The immunophenotype of primary cutaneous γ/δ T-cell lymphoma is βF1−, CD3+, CD2+, CD5+/−, CD56+ and presence of cytotoxic granules. Most cases lack CD4 and CD8. EBV is negative.

The literature rarely describes cases of primary cutaneous EBV-associated T-cell lymphoproliferative disorder. These cases present with skin ulcers and mass lesions confined to the extremities, without systemic involvement. Skin biopsy reveals the presence of dense superficial and deep perivascular and periappendageal lymphoid infiltrates expressing CD3 and CD8, but not CD56. Tumor cells are EBV+ and clonal for T-cell receptor (*TCR*) gene rearrangement. The tumors localize in the skin of the extremities and exhibit an indolent clinical course. These cases should be

TABLE 11-1   Differential Diagnosis of Primary Cutaneous T- or Natural Killer–Cell Lymphomas

Lymphoma	Extranodal NK/T-Cell Lymphoma	Subcutaneous Panniculitis-like T-Cell Lymphoma	γ/δ T-Cell Lymphoma	CD4+ Small/Medium T-Cell Lymphoma	CD8+ Aggressive Epidermotropic Cytotoxic T-Cell Lymphoma	Anaplastic Large Cell Lymphoma
Histologic findings	Involves entire cutaneous layer with angiocentricity, necrosis and hemophagocytosis	Confined to subcutaneous adipose tissue with rimming the fat cells	Involves the dermis and subcutis with rimming the fat cells	Mainly involves the dermis with no involvement of the epidermis	Pagetoid epidermal involvement	Diffuse involvement of the dermis
Immunophenotype	cCD3+sCD3-CD4- CD8-/+CD56+ TIA1+granzyme B+perforin+	sCD3+CD4- CD8+βF1+	sCD3+CD4- CD8- CD56+βF1-	sCD3+CD4+ CD8-βF1+ CD56-	sCD3+CD4- CD8+CD56-	sCD3+CD4+ CD8-CD30+
EBER	+	–	–	–	–	–
TCR rearrangement	Germline	Clonal	Clonal	Clonal	Clonal	Clonal

NK, natural killer; TCR, T-cell receptor.

distinguished from ENKLs, which usually exhibit an aggressive clinical course.

CYTOGENETIC/MOLECULAR ASPECTS

Genetic changes in ENKL have been studied in nasal lesions and in some cases of extranasal lesions. Studies confined to cutaneous lesions are scarce.

Most cases of ENKL are of NK lineage, with some cases of T-cell lineage. Therefore, gene rearrangement studies for the *TCR* and *Ig* genes are in a germline configuration in the majority of cases. A small proportion of cases show rearrangements of the *TCR* gene (=27%, which probably represents neoplasms of cytotoxic T cells). Cutaneous ENKL may be of "T" lineage more commonly than nasal lymphoma.

Few studies have investigated ENKL lymphomagenesis. Genetic alterations were detected in tumor suppressor genes and several oncogenes. Mutations of *p53* were detected in 24% to 60% of cases and their frequency varies according to region. Mutations in *c-kit* were observed in 20% to 70% of cases; almost half of the cases also harbor a *Fas* gene mutation. Deletion of 6q is the cytogenetic alteration reported most commonly. Recently, genomic alterations of cutaneous ENKL were detected using array-based comparative genomic hybridization, which showed gain of 1q and 7q and loss of 17p in cases of cutaneous ENKL and gain of 7q and loss of 9p, 12p, and 12q in nasal ENKL.

A microarray study showed the overexpression of several genes associated with vascular biology, EBV-induced genes, and Platelet derived growth factor receptor(PDGFR)-α in ENKL, which provided evidence of the deregulation of the tumor suppressor *HACE1* in the frequently deleted 6q21 region. Another microarray study revealed that gene signatures (e.g., angiogenesis, genotoxic stress, and proliferation) and signaling pathways, including the transforming growth factor-beta (TGF-β), Notch, and Wnt pathways, were significantly enriched in ENKL compared with interleukin-2 (IL-2)-activated normal NK cells. NK/T-cell lymphoma cells of NK lineage have a very similar molecular profile to that of ENKL or peripheral T-cell lymphoma cells of γ/δ T lineage.

TREATMENT

The optimal treatment for cutaneous ENKL has not been fully defined because of the rarity of this disease. Most of the knowledge available on this subject stems from the experience of nasal ENKL.

In cases of localized nasal ENKL, the role of radiotherapy is critical regarding both radiotherapy alone and radiotherapy concurrent with chemotherapy. However, approximately 25% of the patients experience systemic relapse after the use of radiotherapy alone. Most cases of cutaneous ENKL are diagnosed as advanced stage disease. Therefore, the role of radiotherapy in ENKL remains controversial, even though anecdotal experiences show that this treatment seems to have some efficacy.

Chemotherapy should be the main treatment for advanced cases of ENKL. Unlike what is observed in other lymphomas, anthracycline-containing chemotherapies, such as cyclophosphamide, hydroxydaunoimycin, Oncovin, prednisone (CHOP), are not effective for ENKL, yielding a response less than 20%, because of high expression of multidrug-resistant (MDR) gene. Recently, the combination of chemotherapy regimens with MDR-nonaffected agents, such as methotrexate with L-asparaginase, led to a significant improvement in outcome. In particular, L-asparaginase seems to be efficient as a single agent and, as a part of a chemotherapy regimen, it can yield a response rate of 50% to 60%.

Some reports demonstrated promising results for high-dose chemotherapy with autologous hematopoietic stem cell transplantation (auto-HSCT). The long-term survival of patients with complete remission (CR) was 65% to 80%. These results seem to be superior to those of historical control experiments; however, these patients were highly selected. A recent multinational study showed benefits of auto-HSCT only in high-risk patients using the Korean prognostic index. As a whole, the role of auto-HSCT remains controversial. However, it seems to be beneficial for advanced stage and/or high-risk cutaneous ENKL, especially in the first CR.

A graft-versus-lymphoma effect is possible in allogeneic HSCT (allo-HSCT). A successful outcome of this approach was reported, including a 2-year survival of 40%. However, allo-HSCT cannot be recommended as a front-line treatment because of its association with a treatment-related mortality of approximately 40%.

SUMMARY

Cutaneous ENKL is a disease that is quite uncommon. Nonhealing ulceration is its most typical skin lesion, even though early lesions can be skin nodules. Examination of the nasal area is essential for the exclusion of the secondary involvement of nasal ENKL. Subcutaneous panniculitis-like T-cell lymphoma, cutaneous γ/δ T-cell lymphoma, and cutaneous EBV-associated T-cell lymphoproliferative disorder should be excluded to confirm the diagnosis of cutaneous ENKL. This lymphoma is quite resistant to anthracycline-based chemotherapy. The role of radiation and L-asparaginase–containing chemotherapy in the treatment of ENKL needs to be explored.

SUGGESTED READINGS

Au WY, Pang A, Choy C, Chim CS, Kwong YL. Quantification of circulating Epstein-Barr virus (EBV) DNA in the diagnosis and monitoring of natural killer cell and EBV-positive lymphomas in immunocompetent patients. *Blood.* 2004;104:243–249.

Au WY, Weisenburger DD, Intragumtornchai T, Nakamura S, Kim WS, Sng I, et al. Clinical differences between nasal and extranasal natural killer/T-cell lymphoma: a study of 136 cases from the International Peripheral T-Cell Lymphoma Project. *Blood.* 2009;113:3931–3937.

Ham MF, Ko YH. Natural killer cell neoplasm: biology and pathology. *Int J Hematol.* 2010;92:681–689.

Kim SJ, Kim K, Kim BS, Kim CY, Suh C, Huh J, et al. Phase II trial of concurrent radiation and weekly cisplatin followed by VIPD chemotherapy in newly diagnosed, stage IE to IIE, nasal, extranodal NK/T-Cell Lymphoma: Consortium for Improving Survival of Lymphoma study. *J Clin Oncol.* 2009;27:6027–6032.

Kwong YL, Anderson BO, Advani R, Kim WS, Levine AM, Lim ST. Management of T-cell and natural-killer-cell neoplasms in Asia: consensus statement from the Asian Oncology Summit 2009. *Lancet Oncol.* 2009;10:1093–1101.

Kwong YL. Natural killer-cell malignancies: diagnosis and treatment. *Leukemia.* 2005;19:2186–2194.

Lee J, Kim WS, Park YH, Park SH, Park KW, Kang JH, et al. Nasal-type NK/T cell lymphoma: clinical features and treatment outcome. *Br J Cancer.* 2005;92:1226–1230.

Lee J, Park YH, Kim WS, Lee SS, Ryoo BY, Yang SH, et al. Extranodal nasal type NK/T-cell lymphoma: elucidating clinical prognostic factors for risk-based stratification of therapy. *Eur J Cancer.* 2005;41:1402–1408.

Lee J, Suh C, Park YH, Ko YH, Bang SM, Lee JH, et al. Extranodal natural killer T-cell lymphoma, nasal-type: a prognostic model from a retrospective multicenter study. *J Clin Oncol.* 2006;24:612–618.

Vose J, Armitage J, Weisenburger D. International peripheral T-cell and natural killer/T-cell lymphoma study: pathology findings and clinical outcomes. *J Clin Oncol.* 2008;26:4124–4130.

PRIMARY CUTANEOUS PERIPHERAL T-CELL LYMPHOMA, UNSPECIFIED

Dana S. Ward, MD, and Kara Braudis, MD

Primary cutaneous peripheral T-cell lymphoma (PCPTCLs), unspecified, represents a heterogeneous group of rare neoplasms, which include all primary cutaneous T-cell lymphomas not classified into a more well-defined subtype (Table 12-1). These neoplasms represent only 2% of all primary cutaneous lymphomas. Peripheral T-cell lymphomas in general may lack one or more T-cell–associated antigens and may express molecules resembling a subset of stem cell from which

TABLE 12-1   Summary of PCPTC Lymphomas

Provisional Classification	Histologic Characteristics	Immunohisto-chemical Profile	Clinical Findings	5-Year Survival (%)
CD4+ small/ medium pleomorphic TCL	Small to medium-sized pleomorphic cells Dermis and subcutis Periadnexal	CD4+, CD3+, CD30–, CD8–	Solitary plaque or tumor Predilection for head, neck, torso, arms	60–80
CD+ aggressive epider-motropic TCL	Marked epider-motropism Adnexa involved Large pleomorphic or blastic cells	CD3+, CD8+, CD56+, granzyme B–positive, perforin-positive, TIA-1+, CD45RA+, CD45RO–, CD2–, CD4–, CD5–, CD7±	Patches, plaques, papulonodules, tumors Metastasis common	18
Cutaneous γ/δ TCL	Epidermotropism, dermal aggregate, panniculitis-like, or diffuse Apoptosis, necrosis, angioinvasion	CD2+, CD3+, CD56± CD7+, granzyme-positive, perforin-positive, TIA-1+, CD4–, CD8–, βF1–	Disseminated plaques or ulcerated, necrotic nodules/tumors, or panniculitis-like; predilection for extremities Mucosal presentation or involvement common Hemophagocytic syndrome may be present	<10
Cutaneous TCL, unspecified	Large neoplastic cells > 30%	Variable; CD30– or scattered, rare expression of CD56	Multiple presentations	<20

TCL, T-cell lymphoma.

they are derived. PCPTCLs typically show clonal rearrangement of T-cell receptor (TCR) genes. With a few notable exceptions, these lymphomas are aggressive, as evidenced by a disease-specific overall survival rate of 16%. Some cases of peripheral T-cell lymphomas previously unspecified may now represent specific entities, owing to improved classification with recent studies.

The more clearly defined cases of PCPTCL have been given provisional entries in the World Health Organization/European Organization for Research and Treatment of Cancer (WHO/EORTC) classification, and include (1) primary cutaneous CD4+ small/medium-sized pleomorphic T-cell lymphoma (PCSMTCL), (2) primary cutaneous aggressive epidermotropic CD8+ T-cell lymphoma (PCAECTL), and (3) cutaneous γ/δ T-cell lymphoma (CGDTCL). Other cases not categorized into these provisional entries remain unspecified.

PRIMARY CUTANEOUS AGGRESSIVE EPIDERMOTROPIC CD8+ CYTOTOXIC T-CELL LYMPHOMA

As the name implies, PCAECTL is characterized by an aggressive clinical course. It may present as localized or disseminated eruptive papules, nodules, and tumors, some with ulceration and necrosis, or it may present as superficial, hyperkeratotic patches and plaques. There are no preexisting patches or other mycosis fungoides-like progressive skin findings. This lymphoma may disseminate to other sites, including the lung, testis, central nervous system, and mucosa, but the lymph nodes are rarely involved. Histopathologically, there is marked epidermotropism with CD8+ CD56– cytotoxic T cells. Tumor cells are small-medium or medium-large, with pleomorphic or blastic nuclei. Adnexal structures may be involved or even destroyed. The tumor cell phenotype is CD3+, CD8+, granzyme B–positive, perforin-positive, TIA-1+, CD45RA+, CD45RO–, CD2–, CD4–, CD5–, CD7±. Retention of CD7 in the absence of CD2 positivity may be a clue to diagnosis. Median survival is 32 months, with 18% survival at 5 years. Traditionally, patients have been treated with doxorubicin-based multiagent chemotherapy. More recently, patients with the diagnosis of disseminated pagetoid reticulosis (Ketron-Goodman disease) are now reclassified to either PCAETCL, CGDTCL, or tumor-stage mycosis fungoides.

PRIMARY CUTANEOUS CD4+ SMALL/MEDIUM-SIZED PLEOMORPHIC T-CELL LYMPHOMA

PCSMTCL is an indolent lymphoma, usually presenting as a solitary plaque or tumor with a predilection for the head, neck, torso, or arms. The clinical history is significant because there are no patches or plaques suggestive of preexisting mycosis fungoides and these patients have a more favorable clinical prognosis. The average age range at the time of diagnosis is 50 to 60 years, but cases ranging from 3 to 90 years of age have been documented. The diagnosis is restricted to lymphomas with a CD4+ cell phenotype, and large cells must represent less than 30% of the cell population by definition.

Histologically, this tumor is represented by sheets of small and medium-sized CD4+, CD3+, CD30–, CD8– T cells in the dermis and superficial subcutaneous fat. There is a tendency toward a perivascular or periadnexal pattern, with infiltration and sometimes destruction of the pilar units and sweat glands. Epidermotropism is absent. Typically, a significant admixture of reactive lymphohistiocytic infiltrates is present; noncaseating granulomas may also be a feature. A substantial number of reactive B lymphocytes in the infiltrate may be a diagnostic distractor; eosinophils and plasma cells are also typically seen. Clonal rearrangement of TCR-γ or TCR-β genes is nearly always detected by polymerase chain reaction (PCR) and can be useful in distinguishing this tumor from reactive T-cell infiltrates.

This is the only PCPTCL provisional classification group that has a favorable clinical prognosis, with an estimated 5-year survival rate of 60% to 80%. Surgical excision or radiation therapy is the preferred method of treatment, although cyclophosphamide may be effective in patients with more generalized skin disease.

CUTANEOUS γ/δ T-CELL LYMPHOMA

CGDTCL is composed of activated γδ cytotoxic T cells, normally a small subset of peripheral T cells with direct antigen recognition capability. These cells originate from CD4– CD8– thymic precursors in the bone marrow, with the expression of gamma and delta chains in the TCR preceding the development and expression of alpha and beta chains. The exact function of γ/δ T cells is unknown, but the cells are proposed to have roles in first-line defense against pathogens at body surfaces and the interface between the innate and the adaptive immune systems.

The two well-recognized forms of γδ TCL are hepatosplenic and primary cutaneous. In addition, there is a form characterized by mucosal presentation and it is unknown whether the mucosal type represents a variant of the same entity (e.g., mucocutaneous γ/δ T-cell lymphoma. Included in the CGDTCL group are cases previously categorized as subcutaneous panniculitis-like lymphoma with γ/δ phenotype.

This lymphoma typically presents as disseminated plaques or ulcerated, necrotic nodules and tumors, with a predilection for the extremities. The median age is 42 years with a female predominance.1 Those tumors with deeper involvement of the subcutaneous fat may mimic panniculitis, such as lupus erythematosus profundus. Involvement of mucosa or other extranodal sites is common, but lymph nodes, spleen, and bone marrow are typically spared. All cases of CGDTCL are reported to have a poor prognosis.

Histologic findings include epidermotropism, dermal aggregates, a panniculitis-like pattern, or diffuse involvement of the epidermis, dermis, and subcutaneous fat. The T cells are characteristically CD2+, CD3+, with variable expression of CD56+ and CD7+, and strong expression of cytotoxic proteins. They typically lack CD4 and CD8. Clonal rearrangement of the TCR-γ gene is found in approximately 70% of cases. The neoplastic cells are generally medium to large with coarsely clumped chromatin, but blastic cells are infrequent. Apoptosis, necrosis, angioinvasion, and angiodestruction are commonly present. Diagnosis must be made with the use of TCR-γ antibodies on frozen tissue, however, absence of βF1, the formalin-resistant epitope of the a/β TCR, may infer the diagnosis.

Median survival is 15 months, with an overall survival of approximately 10% at 5 years. There is a trend for decreased survival in those with deeper involvement. Leukopenia may portend a poorer prognosis owing to an underlying hemophagocytic syndrome in patients with a panniculitis-like pattern. Most cases are resistant to multiagent chemotherapy.

PRIMARY CUTANEOUS PERIPHERAL T-CELL LYMPHOMA, UNSPECIFIED

Excluding the aforementioned provisional entries, the remaining cases of PCPTCL, unspecified, usually display large neoplastic cells representing greater than 30% of the cell population and have been referred to as "cutaneous medium/large pleomorphic T-cell lymphoma, not otherwise specified (NOS)," by some authors. This category has diverse clinical and histologic presentations. In general, CD30 staining is negative or scattered; rare cases may show co-expression of CD56. The prognosis for all lymphomas termed *not otherwise specified* is generally poor, with a 5-year survival rate of less than 20% despite multiagent chemotherapy.

The aggressive clinical behavior of these tumors may be explained by the gene expression patterns. Comparative genomic hybridization of primary cutaneous lymphomas, NOS, has shown gains of large regions on chromosome 7, 8, and 17 and losses on chromosome 9. The most frequently affected minimal common region (MCR) with chromosomal gain was 7q36, which encodes the antiapoptotic *FASTK* gene that is also overexpressed in mycosis fungoides. The MCR gain on chromosome 8 is associated with the *MYC* oncogene that is amplified in patients with Sézary syndrome and aggressive B-cell lymphomas. The region of loss on chromosome 9 contains the *CDKN2A* tumor suppressor gene. In comparative analysis of gene expression, peripheral T-cell lymphoma PTL, NOS, was characterized by high expression of the *PRKCQ* gene required for T-cell activation and diminished expression of FAS and caspase 10 relative to cutaneous anaplastic large cell lymphoma.

Within the unspecified category, multiple variants with unique clinical and histologic behavior have been described. Currently, more studies are needed to further define these entities. There are multiple reports of a CD8+ primary cutaneous T-cell lymphoma, most commonly occurring on the ears, which has demonstrated indolent behavior. These tumors fairly uniformly express CD8, CD3, CD5, and CD45RA but lack CD4, CD7, CD56, CD30, and cytotoxic proteins and are successfully treated with radiotherapy without recurrence. Debate exists whether these cases are CD8+ variants of PCSMTCL or a unique entity.

There is a report of two cases of peripheral T-cell lymphoma (PTCL)-NOS, follicular variant, occurring as a primary cutaneous tumor similar to the nodal variant. This presentation must also be further distinguished from CD4+ small/medium-sized pleomorphic T-cell lymphoma.

A FOXP3+, CTLA-4+ primary cutaneous T-cell lymphoma has been reported, supporting the existence of lymphoproliferative malignancies of regulatory T cells. This is in contrast to other PCPTCLs in which only the reactive infiltrating T reg cells showed FOXP3 positivity. This tumor presented similarly to mycosis fungoides but showed pleomorphic medium-large cells with marked epidermotropism and behaved aggressively. Conventional treatments for mycosis fungoides failed and the patient was eventually treated with multiagent chemotherapy, which did induce remission.

In addition, three cases of primary cutaneous T-cell lymphoma localized to the lower leg have been described. Histopathologically, these were distinct from subcutaneous panniculitis-like T-cell lymphoma and localized pagetoid reticulosis, which also show a predilection for the lower extremity, and behaved aggressively. Each consisted of dense infiltrates of atypical mature helper T cells that were CD3+/CD4+, CD8–/CD30–. Although these cases would histopathologically be classified under tumor stage mycosis fungoides (two cases) and PCPTCL, NOS (one case), the clinical presentation and behavior were distinct, and the authors proposed these cases may represent a unique entity.

Multiple reports of CD20+ primary cutaneous T-cell lymphomas exist as well. It is unknown whether CD20+ positivity in these tumors represents aberrant expression, malignant transformation of a small population of T cells that normally express CD20, or a marker of T-cell activation.

Whereas the three provisional categories given to PCPTCLs, unspecified, in the 2005 WHO/EORTC classification have offered significant guidance for clinical and molecular characterization of this group of tumors, further molecular analysis and long-term follow-up will help facilitate further appropriate categorization.

SUGGESTED READINGS

Aguilera P, Mascaró JM, Martinez A, Esteve J, Puig S, Campo E, et al. Cutaneous γ/δ T-cell lymphoma: a histopathologic mimicker of lupus erythematosus profundus (lupus panniculitis). *J Am Acad Dermatol.* 2007;56:643–647.

Baum C, Link B, Neppalli V, Swick B, Liu V. Reappraisal of the provisional entity primary cutaneous CD4+ small/medium pleomorphic T-cell lymphoma: a series of 10 adult and pediatric patients and review of the literature. *J Am Acad Dermatol.* 2011;65:739–748.

Betraminelli H, Leinweber B, Kerl H, Cerroni L. Primary cutaneous CD4+ small/medium-sized pleomorphic T-cell lymphoma: a cutaneous nodular proliferation of pleomorphic T lymphocytes of undetermined significance? A study of 136 cases. *Am J Dermatopathol.* 2009;31: 317–322.

Burg G, Kempf W, Cozzio A, Feit J, Willemze R, Jaffe E, et al. WHO/EORTC classification of cutaneous lymphomas 2005: histologic and molecular aspects. *J Cutan Pathol.* 2005;32:647–674.

Ghobrial I, Weenig R, Pittlekow M, Qu G, Kurtin PJ, Ristow K, et al. Clinical outcome of patients with subcutaneous panniculitis-like T-cell lymphoma. *Leuk Lymphoma.* 2005;46:703–770.

Gormley R, Hess S, Anand D, Junkins-Hopkins J, Rook AH, Kim EJ. Primary cutaneous aggressive epidermotropic CD8+ T-cell lymphoma. *J Am Acad Dermatol.* 2010;62: 300–307.

Grogg K, Jung S, Erickson L, McClure R, Dogan A. Primary cutaneous CD4-positive small/medium-sized pleomorphic T-cell lymphoma: a clonal T-cell lymphoproliferative disorder with indolent behavior. *Mod Pathol.* 2008;21:708–715.

Le Tourneau A, Audouin J, Molina T, Qubaja M, Gaulard P, Leroy JP, et al. Primary cutaneous follicular variant of peripheral T-cell lymphoma NOS. A report of two cases. *Histopathology.* 2010;56:548–555.

Marzano A, Vezzoli P, Fanoni D, Venegoni L, Berti E. Primary cutaneous T-cell lymphoma expressing

FOXP3: a case report supporting the existence of malignancies of regulatory T cells. *J Am Acad Dermatol.* 2009;61:348–355.

Oshima H, Matsuzaki Y, Takeuchi S, Nakano H, Sawamura D. CD20+ primary cutaneous T-cell lymphoma presenting as a solitary extensive plaque. *Br J Dermatol.* 2009;160:881–898.

Petrella T, Maubec E, Cornillet-Lefebvre P, Willemze R, Pluot M, Durlach A, et al. Indolent CD8-positive lymphoid proliferation of the ear: a distinct primary cutaneous T-cell lymphoma? *Am J Surg Pathol.* 2007; 31:1887–1892.

Poligone B, Wilson L, Subtil A, Heald P. Primary cutaneous T-cell lymphoma localized to the lower leg. *Arch Dermatol.* 2009;145:677-682.

Ryan AJA, Robson A, Hayes BD, Sheahan K, Collins P. Primary cutaneous peripheral T-cell lymphoma, unspecified with an indolent clinical course: a distinct peripheral T-cell lymphoma? *Clin Exp Dermatol.* 2010;35:892–896.

Tripodo C, Iannitto E, Florena A, Pucillo CE, Piccaluga PP, Franco V, et al. Gamma-delta T-cell lymphomas. *Nat Rev Clin Oncol.* 2009;6:707–717.

Van Kester M, Tensen C, Vermeer M, Dijkman R, Mulder AA, Szuhai K, et al. Cutaneous anaplastic large cell lymphoma and peripheral T-cell lymphoma NOS show distinct chromosomal alterations and differential expression of chemokine receptors and apoptosis regulators. *J Invest Dermatol.* 2010;130:563–575.

Weaver J, Mahindra AK, Pohlman B, Jin T, Hsi E. Non-mycosis fungoides cutaneous T-cell lymphoma: reclassification according to the WHO-EORTC classification. *J Cutan Pathol.* 2010;37:516–524.

Willemze R, Jaffe ES, Burg G, Cerroni L, Berti E, Swerdlow SH, et al. WHO-EORTC classification for cutaneous lymphomas. *Blood.* 2005;105:3768–3785.

CUTANEOUS B-CELL LYMPHOMAS

Maria Angelica Selim, MD, and Mai P. Hoang, MD

The term *cutaneous B-cell lymphomas (CBCLs)* alludes to a diverse group of B-cell lymphomas that presents in the skin without evidence of extracutaneous disease at the time of diagnosis. Therefore, in each patient with a diagnosis of B-cell lymphoma in the skin, detailed physical examination, complete blood count with differential and comprehensive blood chemistry including lactate dehydrogenase (LDH), bone marrow cytology, and histology (in intermediate to aggressive lymphomas like diffuse large B-cell lymphoma, leg type), and appropriate imaging studies such as positron emission tomography/computed tomography (PET/CT) are required to rule out secondary cutaneous disease by a nodal lymphoma. Primary CBCLs have a different clinical behavior and prognosis than their nodal counterparts; it is of paramount importance to differentiate and classify them separately and recognize the necessity of different therapeutic approaches to avoid unnecessarily aggressive treatment.

Primary CBCL incidence varies widely among continents, with several European studies reporting that 20% to 25% of all primary cutaneous lymphomas are CBCLs in contrast to 3.2 to 7.7% published by three institutions in the United States. This difference may represent true regional divergences (disparities) of factors yet to be known.

B-cell lymphocytes are not normally present in the skin. B cells can accumulate in response to different types of antigenic stimuli originating a reactive B-cell response also known as *pseudolymphoma* or *cutaneous lymphoid hyperplasia*. As potential stimuli, we can find drugs, arthropod bites (e.g., *Borrelia burgdorferi*), acupuncture, and tattoo pigments among others. A body of evidence supports the concept that cutaneous lymphoid hyperplasia and cutaneous low-grade lymphomas form part of a spectrum of cutaneous B-cell lymphoproliferative disorders with a stepwise progression from hyperplasia to a neoplasm. This may partially explain the difficulty in separating cutaneous lymphoid hyperplasia from low-grade B-cell lymphomas. These two entities not only share some similarities in clinical and histologic presentation but also present clonal immunoglobulin gene rearrangements as defined by immunohistochemical and molecular techniques. There is an intense search of genetic alteration that may explain the mechanisms in the development of these lymphomas and can be used as diagnostic tool. However, specific cytogenetic abnormalities as seen in nodal B-cell lymphomas have still not been identified for CBCLs.

Until the 1980s, any lymphoma beside mycosis fungoides was interpreted as a manifestation of a systemic lymphoma. Among dermatologists and dermatopathologists, there is the belief that CBCLs are specific entities of extranodal lymphomas with distinct clinical presentation and different behavior of their nodal counterparts. In 2008, the new World Health Organization (WHO) classification of tumors of hematopoietic and lymphoid tissues acknowledged this concept by including cutaneous follicle center lymphomas and cutaneous diffuse large B-cell lymphomas, leg type, as separate entities in the classification. Conversely, cutaneous marginal zone B-cell lymphomas have been included within the group of extranodal marginal zone lymphomas of mucosal-associated lymphoid tissue (MALT). The other classification that has been used for CBCLs is the one proposed by the European Organization for Research and Treatment of Cancer (EORTC) and the WHO that categorizes these lymphomas into three main groups: cutaneous marginal zone B-cell lymphomas, cutaneous follicle center lymphomas, and cutaneous diffuse large B-cell lymphomas, leg type. The terminology used by these classifications is quite comparable (Table 13-1), reducing the confusion and potential misinterpretation among specialists taking care of these patients. This is also important to pave the way in the categorization of these patients to accrue clinicopathologic information and unify criteria for therapeutic trials.

The TNM (tumor-node-metastasis) staging system used for mycosis fungoides and Sézary's syndrome did not adapt to the biology of CBCLs.

TABLE 13-1   Comparison of the World Health Organization/European Organization for Research and Treatment of Cancer Classification of 2005 and World Health Organization Classification of 2008 for Cutaneous B-Cell Lymphomas

WHO/EORTC Classification 2005	WHO Classification 2008
Primary cutaneous marginal zone B-cell lymphoma	Extranodal marginal zone lymphoma of mucosa-associated lymphoid tissue (MALT lymphoma)
Primary cutaneous follicle center lymphoma	Primary cutaneous follicle center lymphoma
Primary cutaneous diffuse large B-cell lymphoma, leg type	Primary cutaneous diffuse large B-cell lymphoma, leg type
Primary cutaneous diffuse large B-cell lymphoma	Intravascular large B-cell lymphoma
• Intravascular large B-cell lymphoma	

EORTC, European Organization for Research and Treatment of Cancer; MALT, mucosa-associated lymphoid tissue; WHO, World Health Organization.

In 2007, the International Society of Cutaneous Lymphomas (ISCL) and the EORTC Task Force Group for cutaneous lymphomas proposed a T system (Table 13-2). Additional studies are needed to determine whether this T classification has prognostic or therapeutic implications.

PRIMARY CUTANEOUS FOLLICLE CENTER LYMPHOMA

Cutaneous follicle center lymphoma consists of the neoplastic proliferation of germinal center cells confined to the skin. In the WHO/EORTC classification, this category includes cases with follicular growth pattern as well as those with diffuse growth pattern or mixed.

Clinical Features

Primary cutaneous follicle center lymphomas (PCFCLs) commonly affect adults of both genders, although rare cases in childhood have been reported. The median age is 59 years. Clinically, it presents with solitary or grouped erythematous papules, plaques, and tumors on the scalp or forehead, trunk, and rarely, on the leg. *Crosti's lymphoma* or *reticulohistiocytoma of the dorsum* refers to erythematous plaques and nodules of the back surrounded by erythematous macules and papules that expand centrifugally around

the central tumors. Although there is no specific clinical presentation that predicts the histologic growth pattern (follicular vs. diffuse); Crosti's lymphoma corresponds mainly to the diffuse presentation. If untreated, the tumors grow in size but spread to extracutaneous sites is uncommon. Sporadic cases associated with infections by human herpesvirus-8 (HHV-8), hepatitis C, or *B. burgdorferi*, have been identified; however, these do not appear to be significant etiologic factors in these lymphomas. Regardless of the number of lesions, follicular or diffuse growth pattern, or the number of blast cells, PCFCLs have an excellent prognosis, with a 5-year survival greater than 95%. Only tumors present in the leg have a bad prognosis as seen in cutaneous diffuse large B-cell lymphoma, leg type.

Histologic Features and Immunophenotype

PCFCLs are tumors located in dermis with extension to the subcutaneous tissue (Figure 13-1). As in most of the CBCLs, the epidermis is spared. They consist of proliferations of small, medium, and large cleaved cells (centrocytes) admixed with variable number of large cells with features of centroblasts. Small reactive T cells are also seen. These proliferations may acquire a diffuse growth pattern or follicular pattern of growth (Figure 13-2). The neoplastic follicles need to be differentiated from reactive normal follicles.

TABLE 13-2 **International Society for Cutaneous Lymphoma/European Organization for Research and Treatment of Cancer Proposal on T Classification of Cutaneous Lymphomas Other than Mycosis Fungoides and Sézary Syndrome**

Solitary	T1	Small	T1a	One solitary lesion ≤ 5 cm in diameter
		Large	T1b	One solitary lesion > 5 cm in diameter
Multiple	T2	Small	T2a	All-encompassing in < 15 cm in diameter
		Medium	T2b	All-encompassing in >15 cm and ≤ 30 cm in diameter
		Large	T2c	All-encompassing in > 30 cm in diameter
Generalized	T3		T3a	Two noncontiguous body regions
			T3b	≥ Three body regions
	N0			No clinical or pathologic lymph node involvement
	N1			Involvement of one peripheral lymph node draining current or prior lesion
	N2			Involvement of two or more peripheral lymph nodes or involvement of any lymph node that does not drain current or prior skin lesion
	N3			Involvement of central lymph nodes
	M0			No evidence of extracutaneous non—lymph node disease
	M1			Evidence of extracutaneous non–lymph node disease

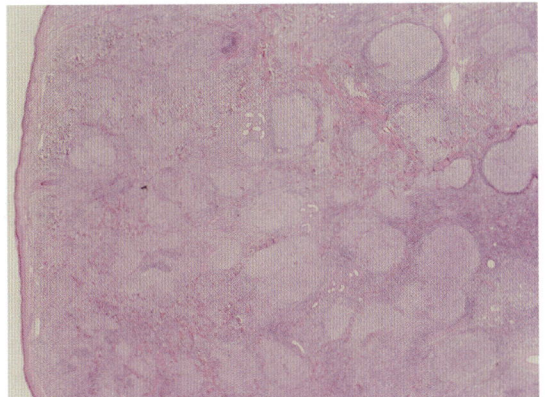

Figure 13-1 PCFCLs are tumors located in dermis with extension to the subcutaneous tissue.

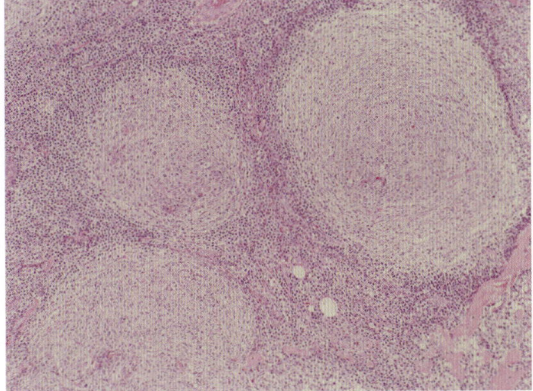

Figure 13-2 PCFCLs with follicular pattern of growth.

The histologic features seen in neoplastic follicles are the reduction of the mantle zone, the rarity or absence of tingible body macrophages, and monomorphism due to the absence of dark and light areas (Figure 13-3). When diffuse and follicular pattern coexist, the neoplastic follicles are localized to the periphery of the tumor. A rare variant formed by spindle cells have been reported and named *spindle cell B-cell lymphoma*. Although in the past, these cases were classified as large B-cell

lymphomas, it is now demonstrated that the spindle cells are centrocytes that show germinal center B-cell origin, and therefore, they are part of the spectrum of PCFCLs.

The neoplastic follicle center cells are typically CD20+, CD79a+, bcl-6+, CD10+, and bcl2– (Figures 13-4a and 13-4b). CD10 is frequently lost in diffuse forms of this lymphoma. Beside bcl-6 and CD10 as germinal center signature differentiation markers, paired box gene (PAX) 5 and

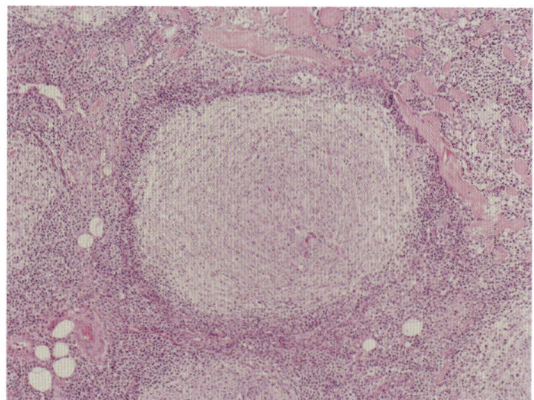

Figure 13-3 The histologic features seen in neoplastic follicles are the reduction of the mantle zone, the rarity or absence of tingible body macrophages and monomorphism due to the absence of dark and light areas.

interferon regulatory factor-8 (IRF-8) can also be used. When in doubt whether the follicles are reactive or neoplastic in nature, Ki-67 can be used.

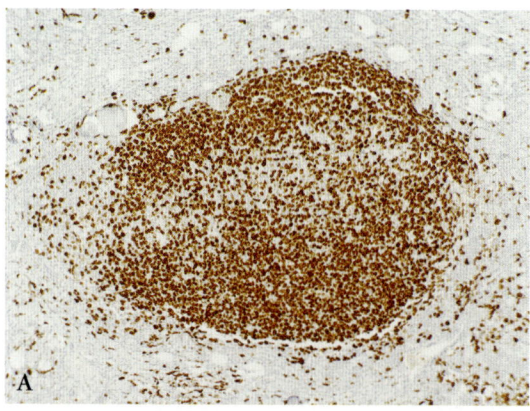

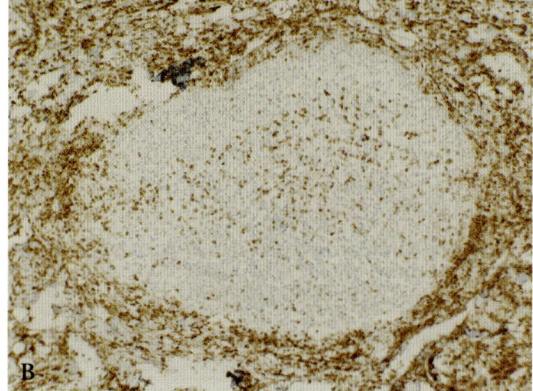

Figures 13-4a and 13-13-4b The neoplastic follicle center cells are typically CD20+, CD79a+, Bcl-6+ (Figure 4a), CD10+, and Bcl2- (Figure 4b).

In reactive follicles, approximately 90% of the cells react to this marker whereas neoplastic follicles have a positivity of less than 50%. Bcl-2 is a classic diagnostic marker for nodal follicular center lymphoma. Although bcl-2 is absent in the majority of PCFCLs, in the 10% to 25% of the cases identified, it is virtually diagnostic and incompatible with a reactive disease. For practical purposes, the detection of bcl-2 by rearrangements and or protein expression should raise the concern of nodal follicular lymphoma with secondary cutaneous involvement. PCFCL involving the leg with a diffuse growth pattern has a large component of large cells and can mimic cutaneous diffuse large B-cell lymphoma, leg type. The presence of large cleaved lymphocytes in PCFCLs and the absence of reactivity to bcl-2, MUM-1, and forkhead box protein (FOX-P1) can differentiate this lymphoma from the cutaneous diffuse large B-cell lymphoma, leg type. Of note, classically, the neoplastic follicle center cells are typically positive for the B-cell marker CD20. However, recurrent lymphoma after treatment with anti-CD20 monoclonal antibody (rituximab) can cause loss this marker; therefore, other B-cell markers like CD79a should be considered in this clinical scenario.

Genetic Features

PCFCLs show a monoclonal rearrangement of the immunoglobulin heavy chain (JH) gene by polymerase chain reaction (PCR) in the majority of cases. This clone can be identified in different follicles of the lymphoma as well as interfollicular areas. It is well accepted that PCFCLs are morphologically identical to nodal counterparts but differ on the genetic pathway. The classic translocation (t14;18) seen in the systemic counterpart of this lymphoma is only rarely seen in PCFCLs.

Therapy

Radiotherapy is the preferred treatment for solitary or few lesions of PCFCLs. Solitary lesions can also be surgically excised with postradiation treatment of the surgical field and surrounded skin. Interferon-alpha (systemically or intralesional) has been used in these patients, sometimes associated with other treatment. A novel treatment with anti-CD20 monoclonal antibodies (rituximab) has been proposed as local treatment with intralesional injections or systemically. Controlled multicenter studies are necessary to investigate rituximab's effectiveness. Anthracycline-based chemotherapy is considered only in patients with very extensive cutaneous disease or in those developing extracutaneous dissemination.

PRIMARY CUTANEOUS MARGINAL ZONE B-CELL LYMPHOMA (PCMZL)

The tumor cells are small B cells that are composed of marginal (centrocyte-like) cells, lymphoplasmacytoid cells, and plasma cells. Primary cutaneous marginal zone B-cell lymphomas (PCMZLs) include cases previously reported as primary cutaneous immunocytoma and primary cutaneous plasmacytoma.

Clinical Features

PCMZLs can present as solitary or multiple erythematous papules to small nodules on the trunk or extremities of young adults with a male predominance. The median age is 39 years. Complete staging studies are necessary to exclude cutaneous involvement by other types of extranodal marginal zone lymphoma of MALT. It appears that detection of specific cells in bone marrow does not affect prognosis in PCMZLs; therefore, its role has been questioned in these patients. Although staging is essential to distinguish PCMZL from secondary cutaneous involvement by a systemic marginal zone lymphoma (MZL), PCMZL may be seen in younger patients and favors the trunk and extremities whereas secondary cutaneous involvement is seen in older patients and frequently affects the head and neck. Association with *B. burgdorferi* in a subset of European cases from endemic and non-endemic areas, tattoo pigment, recurrent herpes simplex virus type-1 infection on the lower lip over 15 years, and influenza vaccination has been reported. It has been proved that different samples of cutaneous marginal cell lymphoma recognize similar antigens, supporting the hypothesis of an antigen-driven lymphoma parallel to what occurs in MALT lymphoma of the stomach. Conversely, the presence of PCMZL in a patient treated with fluoxetine therapy raises the possibility that an inhibitory effect on T-suppressor lymphocytes may originate an excessive antigen-driven B-cell proliferation with PCMZL as the end result.

Although immunocytomas are now considered a variant of PCMZL, they have certain characteristics that differ from the classic PCMZL cases such as its increased frequency in older population, increased involvement of lower extremities, and its frequent association with *B. burgdorferi* infection.

Recurrence is common, but systemic involvement is rare. The recurrences, affecting nearly half of the successfully treated patients, maintain the low-grade features of the primary tumor. The prognosis of PCMZLs is excellent with 5-year survival close to 100%.

Histologic Features and Immunophenotype

PCMZL affects the dermis and, occasionally, the subcutis in a patchy, nodular, or diffuse growth pattern. As with most of the B-cell lymphomas, the epidermis is not involved (Figure 13-5). The most characteristic presentation of PCMZL in

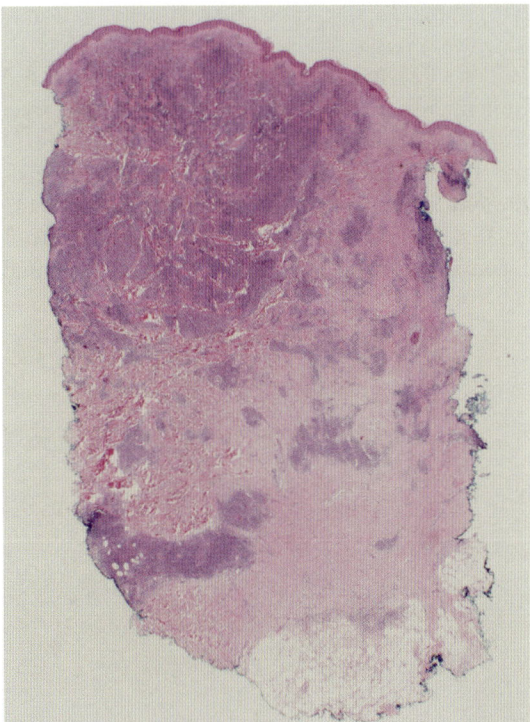

Figure 13-5 PCMZL affects the dermis and occasionally the subcutis in a patchy, nodular or diffuse growth pattern, the epidermis is not involved.

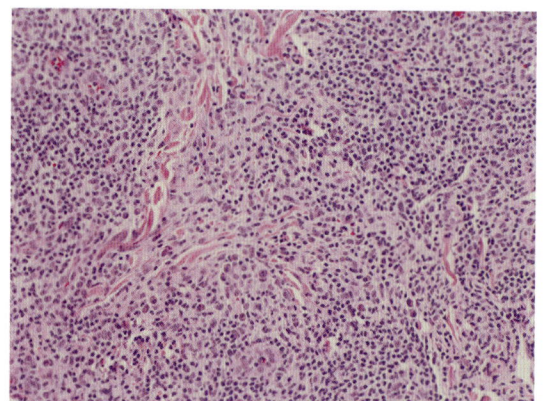

Figure 13-6 PCMZL consists of a proliferation of marginal zones cells (small to medium sized cells with indented nuclei and pale cytoplasm).

low power is the nodular growth pattern with reactive germinal centers and peri- and interfollicular proliferation of marginal zone cells (small to medium-sized cells with indented nuclei and pale cytoplasm) (Figure 13-6). Commonly, plasma cells aggregate at the periphery of the tumor (Figure 13-7). Lymphoplasmacytoid cells and small lymphocytes are not uncommon in this lymphoma. In rare cases, plasma cells predominate over marginal cells, and these cases are classified as PCMZL plasmacytic variant. PCMZL and noncutaneous MZL cannot be differentiated on histologic grounds. It should be noted that reactive B and T cells as well as histiocytes and eosinophils are represented in PCMZL, creating the challenge of differentiating this lymphoma from reactive processes. The expansion of the marginal

cell population in association with a clonal population of plasma cells in PCMZL allows differentiating between these two entities.

The marginal zone B cells are typically CD20+, CD79a+, bcl-2+ (Figures 13-8a-c), and there is monotypic light chain expression by the plasma cells. In contrast to PCFCLs, they are CD5–,

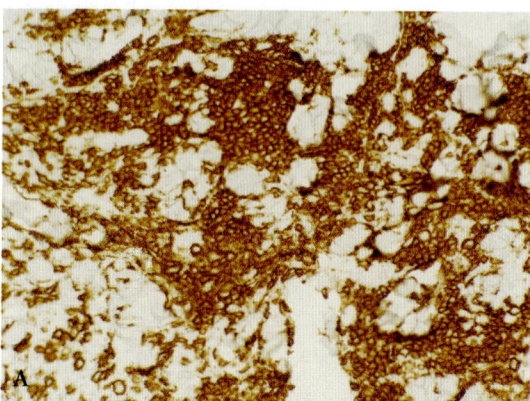

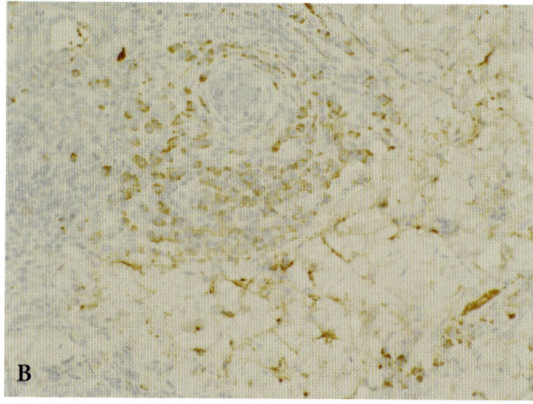

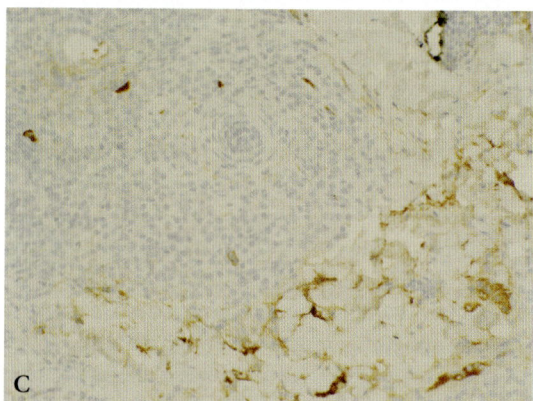

Figures 13-8 The marginal zone B cells are typically CD20+ (A), with plasma cell restriction (B:kappa and C:lambda).

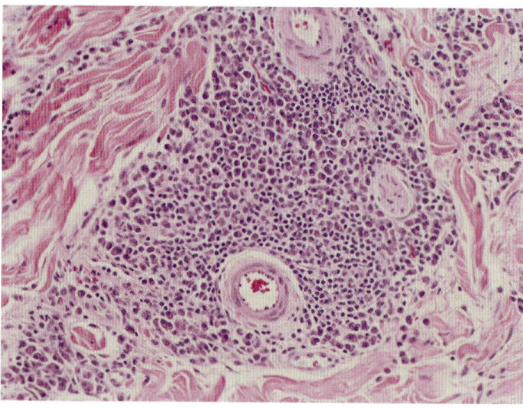

Figure 13-7 Commonly, plasma cells aggregate are noted at the periphery of PCMZLs.

CD10–, and bcl6–. In situ hybridization for the immunoglobulin light chains is a more sensitive method than immunohistochemistry detection of clonality.

Genetic Features

Approximately 50% to 60% of the cases present a monoclonal rearrangement of the immunoglobulin heavy chain (JH). A distinct interchromosomal 14;18 translocation affecting immunoglobulin H (IgH) and MALT1 has been detected in a subset of PCMZL. The latter has been also identified in other extranodal marginal cell lymphomas involving the liver, ocular, adnexal, and salivary glands, highlighting some relationship among a subgroup of PCMZLs with extracutaneous ones. Rare cases of PCMZL may show a conventional t(14;18) involving *IgH* and *bcl2*. A recently described translocation (3;14) (p14;q32) affecting IgH and FOXP1 seen in extranodal MALT has been detected in few PCMZLs. Contrary to extranodal MZLs of MALT that express IgM, PCMZLs express IgG, IgA, and IgE and lack the chemokine receptor CXCR3. The use of detection of class-switched cases to subclassify PCMZL is still under discussion. Aberrant somatic hypermutations could play a role in the pathogenesis of this disease by mutating regulatory and proto-oncogenes such as *PAX5*, *c-MYC*, and *PIM1*, among others. Inactivation of tumor-suppressor genes *CDKN2A* and *DAPK* by hypermethylation has frequently been detected in PCMZL.

Therapy

The solitary or few lesions of PCMZL are often treated with radiotherapy or excision. Many patients can be managed with "watchful waiting" strategy. For multifocal lesions, intralesional interferon-alpha or oral chlorambucil has been reported to produce complete responses in approximately 50% of patients. Treatment with rituximab (anti-CD20) has resulted in complete remissions in a subset of patients; however, this is often accompanied by recurrence. Systemic multiagent chemotherapy should be reserved for the unusual cases with extracutaneous dissemination.

PRIMARY CUTANEOUS LARGE B-CELL LYMPHOMA, LEG-TYPE

Clinical Features

Primary cutaneous large B-cell lymphoma (PCLBCL), leg-type, is included as "large B-cell lymphoma of the leg" in EORTC classification, whereas it is included as "diffuse large B-cell lymphoma" in the WHO classification. PCLBCLs characteristically present as rapidly growing tumors on one or both lower legs of elderly women. Ulceration is common. Approximately 10% to 15% of cases of PCLBCLs present with skin lesions at sites other than the leg. They often disseminate to extracutaneous sites and possess a 5-year survival of approximately 55%. Multiple skin lesions at diagnosis are an adverse risk factor.

Histologic Features

Histologic sections show a diffuse proliferation of uniform and large neoplastic cells (centroblasts and immunoblasts) in the dermis (Figure 13-9). Mitoses are frequent and Ki-67 proliferation index is high (Figure 13-10). These neoplastic B cells are typically CD20+ (Figure 13-11), CD79a+, bcl-2+, MUM-1/IRF-4+ (Figure 13-12), PAX-5+, Fox-P1+, bcl-6+, and CD10–.

Genetic Features

PCLBCLs (leg type) have the gene expression profile of activated B-cell–like diffuse large B-cell

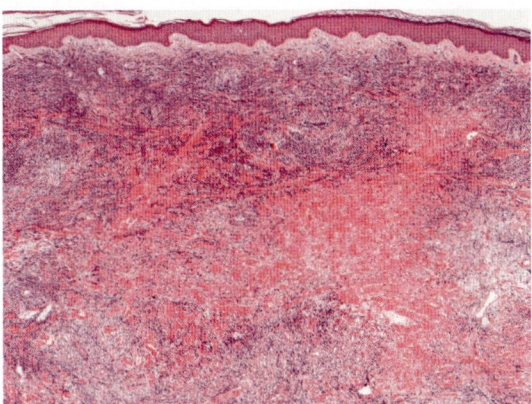

Figure 13-9 A diffuse infiltrate of atypical lymphoid cells is seen in the dermis.

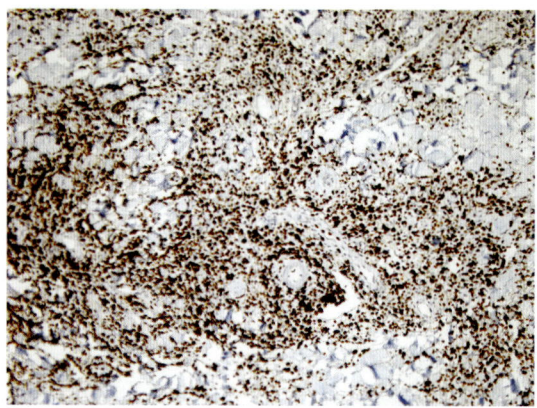

Figure 13-10 High Ki-67 proliferation index is noted.

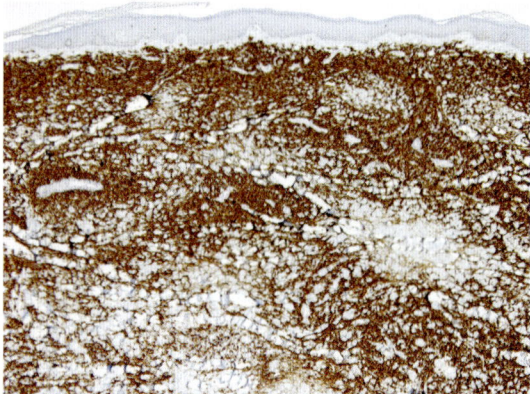

Figure 13-11 The neoplastic cells are strongly positive for CD20.

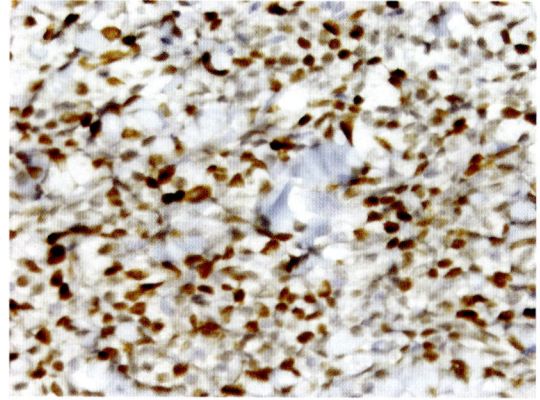

Figure 13-12 Nuclear MUM1 expression is noted.

lymphoma. Although the t(14;18) is absent, amplification of *bcl-2* gene is present in some cases. Inactivation of p15 and p16 tumor suppressor genes by promotor hypermethylation is noted in 11% and 14%, respectively. Chromosomal imbalances, including gains in 18q and 7p and loss of 6q, can be detected in up to 85%. Translocations involving *MYC*, *BCL-6*, and *IgH* genes were documented in 11 of 14 patients with PCLBCLs (leg type) but not in those with PCFCLs. Deletion of a small region on chromosome 9p21.3 was detected in 67% of PCLBCLs (leg type).

Therapy

PCLBCLs should be treated as systemic diffuse large B-cell lymphomas with combination therapy (R-CHOP [rituximab, cyclophosphamide, hydroxydaunomycin, Oncovin/vincristine, and prednisone]). The solitary lesion is often treated by radiotherapy.

OTHER PRIMARY CUTANEOUS LARGE B-CELL LYMPHOMAS

Primary Cutaneous T-Cell/Histiocyte-rich B-Cell Lymphoma

Clinical Features

This rare variant often presents as solitary lesions on the head, trunk, or extremities. Its biologic course is similar to those of PCFCL and PCMZL.

Histologic Features

It is characterized by scattered neoplastic B cells (<15% of the infiltrate) in a background of numerous reactive T cells. The neoplastic B cells are CD20+, CD30−, and often bcl6+. The reactive T cells are CD3+, CD4+, and CD8+.

Genetic Features

Molecular studies show a monoclonal rearrangement of the immunoglobulin heavy chain gene.

Therapy

Surgical excision and/or local radiotherapy is often the treatment.

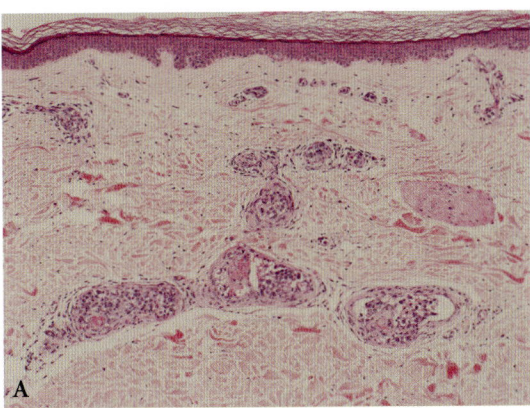 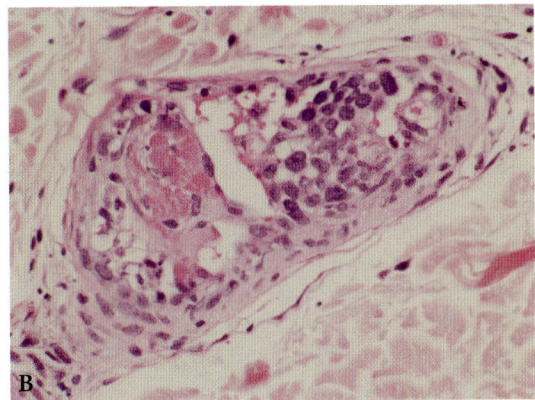

Figures 13-13 In primary cutaneous intravascular large B-cell lymphoma numerous large neoplastic B-cells are seen occluding vascular lumens in the dermis.

Primary Cutaneous Intravascular Large B-Cell Lymphoma

Clinical Features

Initially classified as a vascular neoplasm (malignant angioendotheliomatosis), it is a rare type of large B-cell lymphoma that can involve the central nervous system, lungs, and skin and is generally associated with poor prognosis. It may be a skin primary and present as violaceous patches and plaques or telangiectatic lesions on the lower legs or trunk. Patients presenting with only skin lesions have better prognosis than those with other organ involvement (3-year survival 56% vs. 22%). It has been hypothesized that absence of certain adhesion molecules (CD29, CD54) results in inability of neoplastic cells to escape the vascular wall.

Histologic Features

Numerous large neoplastic B cells are seen occluding the vascular lumen (Figure 13-13a and 13-13b). Colonization of capillaries of hemangioma by tumor cells has been reported. The tumor cells are CD19+, CD20+, CD22+, CD79a+ (Figure 13-14) and have monotypic immunoglobulin expression. Aberrant CD5 expression can be seen in a subset of tumor.

Genetic Features

Molecular studies demonstrate a monoclonal rearrangement of the immunoglobulin heavy chain gene. Fluorescence in situ hybridization (FISH) studies revealed karyotype abnormalities.

Therapy

The preferred treatment is multiagent chemotherapy even for patients with only cutaneous disease.

Plasmablastic or Anaplastic Lymphoma

Clinical Features

Plasmablastic lymphoma (PBL) is a rare subtype of diffuse large B-cell lymphoma that was first reported in human immunodeficiency virus (HIV)–infected individuals, but it can be seen in patients with transplants or receiving chemotherapy.

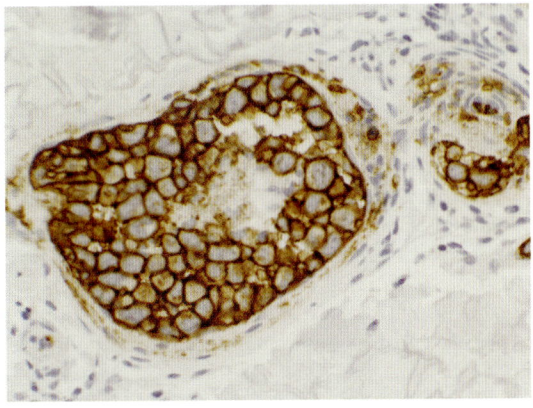

Figure 13-14 The tumor cells are CD79a positive.

It preferentially involves the oral cavity and has a poor prognosis with an average survival of 6 months. Cutaneous involvement has rarely been reported.

Histologic Features

A dense infiltrate of atypical large plasmablastic cells is typically seen in the dermis and often the subcutaneous tissue. The tumors cells are CD38+, CD138+, CD43+, CD45+ and show immunoglobulin light chain restriction. They are negative for B-cell (CD20, CD79a) and T-cell (CD3, CD4, CD5, CD8) markers, CD10, CD15, bcl-2, bcl-6, CD56, CD57, TIA-1, CD34, and myeloperoxidase.

Genetic Features

Epstein-Barr virus mRNA and HHV-8 were detected by in situ hybridization and PCR, respectively.

Therapy

Treatment often consists of polychemotherapy and in combination with antiretroviral treatment in the appropriate setting.

SUGGESTED READINGS

Bekkenk M, Vermeer MH, Geerts ML, Noordijk EM, Heule F, van Voorst Vader PC, et al. Treatment of multifocal primary cutaneous B-cell lymphoma: guidelines of the Dutch Cutaneous Lymphoma Group. *J Clin Oncol*. 1999;17:2471–2478.

Berti E, Alessi E, Caputo R, Gianotti R, Delia D, Vezzoni P. Reticulohistiocytoma of the dorsum. *J Am Acad Dermatol*. 1988;19:259–272.

Cerroni L, Arzberger E, Pütz B, Höfler G, Metze D, Sander CA, et al. Primary cutaneous follicular center cell lymphoma with follicular growth pattern. *Blood*. 2000;95:3922–3928.

Cerroni L, Signoretti S, Hofler G, Arnessi G, Pütz B, Lackinger E, et al. Primary cutaneous marginal B-cell lymphoma: a recently described entity of low-grade malignant cutaneous B-cell lymphoma. *Am J Surg Pathol*. 1997;21:1307–1315.

Cerroni L, Zöchling N, Pütz B, Kerl H. Infection by *Borrelia burgdorferi* and cutaneous B-cell lymphoma.*J Cutan Pathol*. 1997;24:457–461.

Chetty R, Hlatswayo N, Muc R, Sabaratuam R, Gutter K. Plasmablastic lymphoma in HIV+ patients:

an expanding spectrum. *Histopathology*. 2003;42:605–609.

Child FJ, Scarisbrick JJ, Calonje E, Orchard G, Russell-Jones R, Whittaker SJ. Inactivation of tumor suppressor genes p15INK4b and p16INK4a in primary cutaneous B cell lymphoma. *J Invest Dermatol*. 2002;118:941–948.

Crosti A. Mycosis fungoides and malignant cutaneous reticulo-histiocytomas [in French]. *Ann Dermatol Syphiligr (Paris)*. 1951;78:576–578.

De Leval L, Harris NL, Longtine J, Ferry JA, Duncan LM. Cutaneous B-cell lymphomas of follicular and marginal zone types: use of Bcl-6, CD10, Bcl-2, and CD21 in differential diagnosis and classification. *Am J Surg Pathol*. 2001;25:732–741.

Delecluse HJ, Anagnostopoulos I, Dallenbach F, Hummel M, Marafioti T, Schneider U, et al. Plasmablastic lymphomas of the oral cavity: a new entity associated with the human immunodeficiency virus infection. *Blood*. 1997;89:1413–1120.

Dunphy CH, Nahass GT. Primary cutaneous T-cell-rich B-cell lymphomas with flow cytometric immunophenotypic findings: report of 3 cases and review of the literature. *Arch Pathol Lab Med*. 1999;123:1236–1240.

Fink-Puches R, Zenahlik P, Bäck B, Smolle J, Kerl H, Cerroni L. Primary cutaneous lymphomas: applicability of current classification schemes (European Organization for Research and Treatment of Cancer, World Health Organization) based on clinicopathologic features observed in a large group of patients. *Blood*. 2002;99:800–805.

Gatter KC, Warnke RA. Diffuse large B-cell lymphoma. In: Jaffe ES, Harris NL, Stein H, Vardiman JW, eds. *World Health Organization Classification of Tumors: Tumors of Haematopoietic and Lymphoid Tissues*. Lyon, France: IARC Press, 2001:171–4.

Goodlad JR, Davidson MM, Hollowood K, Ling C, MacKenzie C, Christie I, et al. Primary cutaneous B-cell lymphoma and *Borrelia burgdorferi* infection in patients from the Highlands of Scotland. *Am J Surg Pathol*. 2000;24:1279–1285.

Khalidi HS, Brynes RK, Browne P, Koo CH, Buttifora H, madeiros LJ. Intravascular large B-cell lymphoma: the CD5 antigen is expressed by a subset of cases. *Mod Pathol*. 1998;11:983–938.

Lawnicki LC, Weisenburger DD, Aoun P, Chan WC, Wickert RS, Greiner TC. The t(14;18) and bcl-2 expression are present in a subset of primary cutaneous follicular lymphoma: association with lower grade. *Am J Clin Pathol*. 2002;118:765–772.

Li S, Griffin CA, Mann RB, Borowitz MJ. Primary cutaneous T-cell rich B-cell lymphoma: clinically distinct from its nodal counterpart? *Mod Pathol*. 2001;14:10–13.

Mao X, Lillington D, Child FJ, Russell-Jones R, Young B, Whittaker SJ. Comparative genomic hybridization analysis of primary cutaneous B-cell lymphomas: identification of common genomic alterations in disease pathogenesis. *Genes Chromosomes Cancer.* 2002;35:144–155.

Perniciaro C, Winkelmann RK, Daoud MS, Su WP. Malignant angioendotheliomatosis is an angiotropic intravascular lymphoma: immunohistochemical, ultrastructural and molecular genetic studies. *Am J Dermatopathol.* 1995;17:242–248.

Ponzoni M, Arrigoni G, Gould VE, Del Curto B, Maggioni M, Scapinello A, et al. Lack of CD29 (beta1 integrin) and CD54 (ICAM-1) adhesion molecules in intravascular lymphomatosis. *Hum Pathol.* 2000; 31:220–226.

Rijlaarsdam JU, Toonstra J, Meijer OW, Noordijk EM, Willemze R. Treatment of primary cutaneous B-cell lymphomas of follicular center cell origin: a clinical follow-up study of 55 patients treated with radiotherapy or polytherapy. *J Clin Oncol.* 1996;14:549–555.

Rijlaarsdam JU, van der Putte SCJ, Berti E, Kerl H, Rieger R, Toonstra J, et al. Cutaneous immunocytomas: a clinicopathologic study of 26 cases. *Histopathology.* 1993;23:119–125.

Sander CA, Kaudewitz P, Kutzner H, Simon M, Schirren CG, Siotos N, et al. T-cell rich B-cell lymphoma presenting in the skin: a clinicopathologic analysis of six cases. *J Cutan Pathol.* 1996;23:101–108.

Sangueza OP, Yadav S, White CR Jr, Braziel RM. Evolution of B-cell lymphoma from pseudolymphoma. *Am J Dermatopathol.* 1992;14:408–413.

Sheibani K, Battifora H, Winberg CD, Burke JS, Ben-Ezra J, Willinger GM, et al. Further evidence that "malignant angioendotheliomatosis" is an angiotropic large-cell lymphoma. *N Engl J Med.* 1986;314:943–948.

Torne R, Su WPD, Smolle J, Kerl H. Clinicopathologic study of cutaneous plasmacytoma. *Int J Dermatol.* 1990;29:562–566.

Trent JT, Romanelli P, Kerdel FA. Topical targretin and intralesional interferon alfa for cutaneous lymphoma of the scalp. *Arch Dermatol.* 2002;138: 1421–1423.

Vermeer MH, Geelen FAMJ, van Haselen CW, van Voorst Vader PC, Geerts ML, van Vloten WA, et al. Primary cutaneous large B-cell lymphomas of the legs: a distinct type of cutaneous B-cell lymphoma with an intermediate prognosis. *Arch Dermatol.* 1996;132:1304–1308.

Viguier M, Rivet J, Agbalika F, Kerviler E, Brice P, Dubertret L, et al. B-cell lymphomas involving the skin associated with hepatitis C virus infection. *Int J Dermatol.* 2002;41:577–582.

Willemze R, Kerl H, Sterry W, Berti E, Cerroni L, Chimenti S, et al. EORTC classification for primary cutaneous lymphoma: a proposal from the Cutaneous Lymphoma Study Group of the European Organization for Research and Treatment of Cancer. *Blood.* 1997;90:354–371.

SKIN CONDITIONS CONSIDERED TO BE PRECURSORS TO CUTANEOUS LYMPHOMA

John Alan Zic, MD

INTRODUCTION

As discussed in previous chapters, the diagnosis of the primary cutaneous lymphomas can be challenging for many reasons. First, the cutaneous lymphomas are great imitators. The cutaneous T-cell lymphoma (CTCL) variants may resemble eczematous dermatitis, psoriasis, tinea corporis, pigmented purpura, hand dermatitis, contact dermatitis, arthropod bites, acne vulgaris, acne rosacea, erythema nodosum, and other skin disorders. The cutaneous B-cell lymphoma (CBCL) variants may resemble acne vulgaris, eczematous dermatitis, pigmented purpura, Kaposi's sarcoma, and rarely, cherry angiomas. For these reasons, the cutaneous lymphomas have been labeled as the "great imitators of the 21st century." Therefore, it is important for physicians to keep the cutaneous lymphomas on their radar screens.

Second, the cutaneous lymphomas may be difficult to diagnose because it may take months to years to diagnose from the onset of symptoms. Although the clinician may fail to consider the diagnosis early on, oftentimes the cutaneous lymphoma itself has not evolved enough to be strongly considered by the pathologist. For example, mycosis fungoides (MF) may begin with nonspecific patches in sun-protected areas that may resemble eczematous dermatitis for years both clinically and pathologically before a diagnosis can be made.

This chapter focuses on those skin conditions that are considered to be precursors to the primary cutaneous lymphomas. Precursor skin conditions include those well-defined skin diseases that carry an increased risk for the development of one of cutaneous lymphoma variants in the future. Outside of the cutaneous lymphomas, actinic keratoses are an excellent example of a precursor skin condition that has an increased risk of developing into a malignancy, squamous cell carcinoma. The second hit hypothesis helps to explain why some actinic keratoses go on to develop into squamous cell carcinomas after further ultraviolet (UV)-induced DNA damage. Unfortunately, there is no similar credible theory to help explain why some skin diseases carry an increased risk for the development of one of the cutaneous lymphoma variants.

Those skin conditions that are considered to be precursors to the CTCLs include chronic eczematous or psoriasiform dermatitis with an atypical lymphocytic infiltrate, parapsoriasis, poikiloderma vasculare atrophicans (PVA), lymphomatoid papulosis (LyP), follicular mucinosis (FM), and atypical lymphocytic lobular panniculitis (ALLP). The skin condition that may be considered to be a precursor to CBCL is cutaneous lymphoid hyperplasia (CLH; Table 14-1).

PRECURSORS TO CUTANEOUS T-CELL LYMPHOMA

Chronic Dermatitis with an Atypical Lymphocytic Infiltrate

Chronic dermatitis may be loosely defined as an eruption *resembling* eczema or psoriasis that has been present for more than 6 months. "Resemble" is the key descriptor. In an adult, chronic eczematous dermatitis is a diagnosis of exclusion characterized by ill-defined pink scaly patches. Before a clinician labels an eruption as chronic eczematous dermatitis he or she needs to rule out an allergic contact dermatitis, drug hypersensitivity eruption, and other skin conditions including MF. In a child, characteristic ill-defined scaly pink patches on the flexural extremities associated with atopy strongly suggests a diagnosis of atopic eczema. With the exception of nummular eczema, it is the opinion of this author that adults rarely develop the skin disease eczema, but rather develop eczema-like cutaneous reactions in which the etiology needs to be explored.

TABLE 14-1   Skin Conditions Considered to Be Precursors to Cutaneous Lymphoma

Precursor Skin Disease	Estimated Rate of Progression to Cutaneous Lymphoma	Cutaneous Lymphoma Variant(s)
Chronic dermatitis with an atypical lymphocytic infiltrate	≤25% if associated with a clonal T-cell population	Mycosis fungoides
Erythroderma with an atypical lymphocytic infiltrate	Unknown	Sézary's syndrome
Large plaque parapsoriasis	10–35%	Mycosis fungoides
Poikiloderma vasculare atrophicans	Unknown	Mycosis fungoides
Lymphomatoid papulosis	10–20%, ≤60% at referral centers	Mycosis fungoides, primary cutaneous anaplastic large cell lymphoma
Follicular mucinosis	10–20%	Mycosis fungoides, folliculotropic mycosis fungoides
Atypical lymphocytic lobular panniculitis	Unknown	Subcutaneous panniculitis-like T-cell lymphoma
Lupus profundus	Unknown	Subcutaneous panniculitis-like T-cell lymphoma
Cutaneous lymphoid hyperplasia	4%	Primary cutaneous B-cell lymphoma variants

The clinical presentation of chronic psoriasiform dermatitis is characterized by an eruption of ill-defined and well-defined indurated patches and plaques. Unlike psoriasis vulgaris, chronic psoriasiform dermatitis rarely shows pitting of the nail plates or arthritic changes. The etiology of chronic psoriasiform dermatitis must be investigated. As in chronic eczematous dermatitis, the skin conditions of allergic contact dermatitis, drug hypersensitivity eruption, nummular eczema, and others including MF need to be ruled out.

Often, a skin biopsy report from a patient with chronic eczematous or psoriasiform dermatitis will be descriptive in nature, but it may suggest a possible etiology. This should not deter a physician from performing skin biopsies yearly on patients with chronic dermatitis. Over time, perhaps years, the etiology may become clearer. If the pathologist sees an increased number of lymphocytes in the dermis and epidermis with cytologic abnormalities, the label of "atypical lymphocytic infiltrate" will be applied to the description. This should

alert the clinician that the chronic dermatitis may be a precursor to MF.

Molecular genetic studies may be helpful to clarify the potential risk of evolution to MF. T-cell receptor gene rearrangement (TCRR) studies can identify the presence of a clonal population of T cells in the skin sample. The term *clonal dermatitis* has been used to describe a form of chronic dermatitis that harbors a dominant T-cell clone but lacks histologic features diagnostic for CTCL. It is estimated that approximately 25% of clonal dermatitis cases progress to overt CTCL within 5e years. Others have coined the term *cutaneous T-cell lymphoid dyscrasia* to describe a variety of distinct skin conditions of ambiguous origin that precede the diagnosis of CTCL and are associated with a T-cell clone. Performing TCRR on skin biopsies from two different sites may be even more helpful in securing a diagnosis of MF. One small study found the presence of the same T-cell clone in two different sites to be a very promising technique with high specificity (95.7%) in distinguishing MF from inflammatory dermatoses.

If the chronic eczematous or psoriasiform dermatitis with atypical lymphocytic infiltrate progresses over months to years to involve more than 50% of body surface area (BSA) with large regions of erythema, then an evolving Sézary syndrome (SS) should be explored. As discussed in Chapter 7, patients with SS have erythroderma over 80% of their BSA with significant blood involvement with malignant T cells. Therefore, in addition to skin biopsies, patients with possible evolving SS require complete blood counts with differential and flow cytometry of peripheral blood to assess for abnormal populations of T cells. Also, TCRR studies on peripheral blood may be helpful (Table 14-2).

In summary, patients with chronic eczematous or psoriasiform dermatitis with atypical lymphocytic infiltrate should be followed closely over time for evolution to MF and SS. The risk of progression increases with the presence of clonal T cells in the skin specimen, especially when the same T-cell clone is discovered in two different skin sites. Table 14-2 provides guidelines to help clinicians decide when further testing is indicated in patients with precursor skin conditions.

Parapsoriasis

When Brocq first used the term "parapsoriasis" in 1902, he was referring to a group of diseases

TABLE 14-2 Clinical Features Heralding Progression to Cutaneous Lymphoma from the Precursor Skin Conditions

Precursor Skin Condition	Clinical Features Heralding Progression	Recommended Next Steps in Management
Chronic dermatitis with an atypical lymphocytic infiltrate	1. Dermatitis now refractory to topical therapy requiring systemic therapy 2. Development of thicker plaques from patch morphology	1. Multiple skin biopsies of oldest and thickest skin lesions off of topical or systemic steroids for 3–4 wk 2. Consider immunostains for T-cells and TCRR studies
Erythroderma with an atypical lymphocytic infiltrate	1. Development of more widespread exfoliative erythroderma 2. Development of ectropion 3. Development of peripheral adenopathy	1. Multiple skin biopsies of oldest and thickest skin lesions off of topical or systemic steroids for 3–4 wk 2. Consider immunostains for T-cells and TCRR studies 3. Peripheral blood for flow cytometry and TCRR studies 4. CT scans of chest, abdomen, pelvis and possible lymph node biopsy (not FNA)
Large plaque parapsoriasis	1. Development of fixed, not waxing and waning, patches 2. Development of plaques 3. Development of new patches of varied colors	1. Multiple skin biopsies of oldest and thickest skin lesions off of topical or systemic steroids for 3–4 wk 2. Consider immunostains for T-cells and TCRR studies
Poikiloderma vasculare atrophicans	1. Development of new patches of varied color 2. Development of plaques	1. Multiple skin biopsies of oldest and thickest skin lesions off of topical or systemic steroids for 3–4 wk 2. Consider immunostains for T-cells and TCRR studies

(continued)

TABLE 14-2 Clinical Features Heralding Progression to Cutaneous Lymphoma from the Precursor Skin Conditions (continued)

Precursor Skin Condition	Clinical Features Heralding Progression	Recommended Next Steps in Management
Lymphomatoid papulosis	1. Development of larger nodules > 1 cm without regression (PCALCL) 2. Development of patches and/or plaques in sun-protected areas (MF)	1. Multiple skin biopsies of oldest and thickest skin lesions off of topical or systemic steroids for 3–4 wk 2. Consider immunostains for T-cells and TCRR studies
Follicular mucinosis	1. Development of thick plaques on hair-bearing areas (FMF) 2. Development of patches and/or plaques in sun-protected areas (MF)	1. Multiple skin biopsies of oldest and thickest skin lesions off of topical or systemic steroids for 3–4 wk 2. Consider immunostains for T-cells and TCRR studies
Atypical lymphocytic lobular panniculitis and lupus profundus	1. Indurated plaques and/or subcutaneous nodules no longer responsive to present systemic therapy 2. Development of deeper subcutaneous nodules in a patient with only prior plaques	1. Multiple deep skin biopsies or incisional biopsies of oldest and thickest skin lesions off of topical or systemic steroids for 3–4 wk 2. Consider immunostains for T-cells and TCRR studies 3. Peripheral blood for CBC with differential and platelets, flow cytometry and TCRR studies 4. Consider CT scans of chest, abdomen, pelvis
Cutaneous lymphoid hyperplasia	1. Development of new papulonodules distant to original site or new larger lesions	1. Multiple skin biopsies of oldest and thickest skin lesions off of topical or systemic steroids for 3–4 wk 2. Consider immunostains for T- and B-cells and IgHGR studies

CBC, complete blood count; CT, computed tomography; FMF, folliculotropic mycosis fungoides; FNA, fine-needle aspiration; IgHGR, immunoglobulin heavy chain gene rearrangement; MF, mycosis fungoides; PCALCL, primary cutaneous anaplastic large T-cell lymphoma; TCRR, T-cell receptor gene rearrangement.

that included what is now recognized as large and small plaque parapsoriasis (SPP) as well as pityriasis lichenoides. The latter entity is now considered distinct from large and SPP. Nonetheless, confusion still surrounds the terminology concerning the variants of parapsoriasis.

SPP, also referred to as *digitate dermatosis* or *chronic superficial dermatitis,* presents with asymptomatic, pink or yellowish-brownish, macules and/or patches, less than 5 cm in diameter. The flanks, proximal extremities, and buttocks are often involved. Digitate or finger-shaped patches may be seen on the flanks along cleavage lines. SPP is considered a benign entity with little, if any, potential to evolve into MF, although this has been challenged by some authors.

Large plaque parapsoriasis (LPP) presents with waxing and waning mildly pruritic to asymptomatic patches usually greater than 5 cm in diameter in sun-protected areas (Figures 14-1 and 14-2). The clinical findings of LPP and early MF can be indistinguishable. However, the patches of

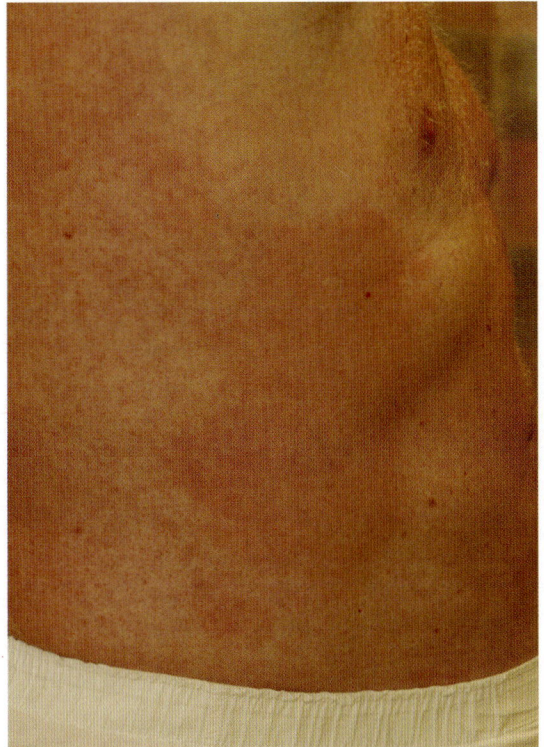

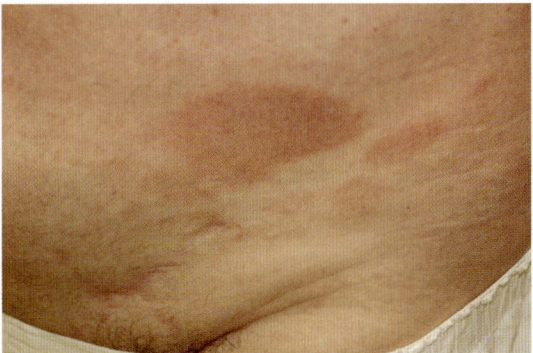

Figure 14-2 Left lower abdomen showing ill-defined pink patches in the same patient as Figure 14-1 with large plaque parapsoriasis. Note clinical similarities to early stage mycosis fungoides.

MF tend to be fixed whereas the patches of LPP tend to wane in the summer and flare in the winter. Histologically, LPP often shows a non-specific or bandlike mononuclear infiltrate with epidermal hyperplasia, vacuolization in the basal cell layer, capillary dilatation, and an absence of atypical lymphocytes or Pautrier microabscesses (Table 14-3).

Because of the difficulty in distinguishing LPP and MF, some experts have referred to LPP

Figure 14-1 Right flank showing ill-defined large pink patches in a patient with large plaque parapsoriasis.

TABLE 14-3   Differentiating Large Plaque Parapsoriasis from Early Mycosis Fungoides

	Large Plaque Parapsoriasis	Early Mycosis Fungoides
Clinical Features		
Patches usually >5 cm	Common	Common
Thin plaques*	Not present	Occasional
Sun-protected distribution	Very common	Very common
Waxing in winter, waning in summer	Common	Uncommon
Fixed skin lesions, no waxing and waning	Uncommon	Common
Variation in color	Uncommon	Common
Histologic Features		
Bandlike infiltrate of lymphocytes	Common	Common
Epidermotropism	Rare	Common
Pautrier microabscesses	Not present	Uncommon, but specific
Basal layer vacuolization	Common	Uncommon
Atypical lymphocytes	Not present	Present

*The term *plaque* in large plaque psoriasis refers to the European definition for large flat patches, not the English definition of a flat-topped elevated solid skin lesion.

as "a latent form of mycosis fungoides" or "an early stage of mycosis fungoides." Although LPP is considered a benign condition, progression to MF has been documented in 10% to 35%. Further support for LPP to be a precursor of MF lies in the finding of clonal populations of T cells using TCRR in approximately 50% of cases.

In summary, LPP is the most well-recognized precursor condition to CTCL, specifically MF. Therefore, patients with LPP should be followed for the development of progression from waxing and waning patches to more fixed patches and thicker plaques that may herald the development of MF (see Table 14-2).

Poikiloderma Vasculare Atrophicans

PVA is considered by most experts to be a rare variant of MF. And, like LPP, some clinicians believe that PVA may potentially precede or coexist with MF whereas others believe that PVA represented an early form of CTCL. The macules and patches of PVA usually involve sun-protected sites, most commonly the buttocks, breasts, and flexural areas; however, many patients may have diffuse involvement. More importantly, the patches of PVA show the poikilodermatous features of hypopigmentation, hyperpigmentation, atrophy, and telangiectasias. Histologically, PVA demonstrates chronic, ill-defined inflammatory changes in the dermis, dilated capillaries, and a thin epidermis. Frequently, normal-appearing lymphoid cells form a bandlike pattern in the superficial dermis with only rare cells in the epidermis that may support the view that not all cases of PVA are a rare variant of MF. However, more often, the poikilodermatous variant of MF and PVA may be indistinguishable and patients presenting with large poikilodermatous patches should be followed closely for the development of MF (see Table 14-2).

Lymphomatoid Papulosis

Prior to the 2005 World Health Organization (WHO) reclassification of the cutaneous lymphomas, LyP was classified as a benign CD30+ lymphoproliferative disorder of the skin. The benign nature of LyP is supported by the

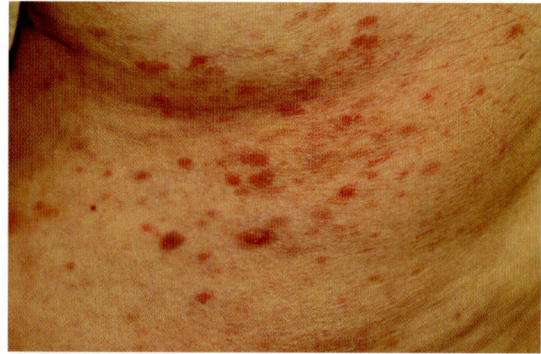

Figure 14-3 Left flank showing a cluster of thin and crusted papules in a patient with lymphomatoid papulosis.

spontaneous remission of the target skin lesions, papules, and the lack of spread to extracutaneous organs. Since the 2005 WHO classification, LyP has been designated a distinct variant of the CTCLs. Together with primary cutaneous anaplastic T-cell lymphoma (PCALCL), LyP is subclassified as one of the malignant CD30+ lymphoproliferative disorders of the skin. The malignant nature of LyP is supported by the finding of abnormal T cells in the skin infiltrate coupled with the presence of a clonal population of T cells in over 50% of cases.

Patients with LyP present with red papules appearing in crops. The crops may contain several to over 100 papules, which may cause considerable pruritus (Figure 14-3). Over the next 4 to 8 weeks, the papules ulcerate until spontaneous resolution leaves hyperpigmented macules.

LyP is a skin condition considered to be a precursor to cutaneous lymphoma because of the potential for MF and PCALCL to develop in patients with LyP. Several reports have documented the same T-cell clone in LyP and the subsequent MF. In some cases, LyP develops after the diagnosis of MF. Commonly reported rates of progression to lymphoma are 10% to 20%, although higher rates of 40% to 60% have recently been reported in cancer referral centers.

In summary, LyP should be considered in any patient with recurrent crops of papules that show spontaneous resolution over 4 to 8 weeks. Once the diagnosis is established, patients with LyP should be followed for the development of MF, PCALCL, and other lymphomas.

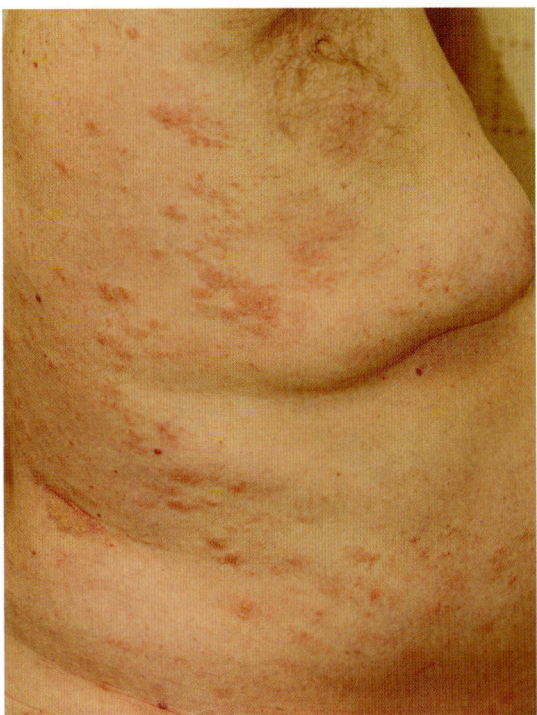

Figure 14-4 Right flank showing thin pink oval plaques in a patient with follicular mucinosis.

Follicular Mucinosis

FM is a benign skin disorder characterized by patches of alopecia studded with follicular papules and/or edematous boggy plaques devoid of hair (Figure 14-4). It is sometimes referred to as *alopecia mucinosa*. Histologically, the dermis shows disrupted hair follicles infiltrated with mucin and normal-appearing lymphocytes. Idiopathic or primary follicular mucinosis (PFM) has a benign self-limiting course and is seen primarily in children and young adults. In older adults, however, some patients with FM will go on to develop classic MF and, more frequently, folliculotropic mucosis fungoides (FMF). This form of FM is termed *MF-associated FM* or lymphoma-associated follicular mucinosis (LAFM). Unlike classic MF, the malignant T cells in FMF infiltrate the hair follicle epithelium more so than the epidermis. For reasons that are not entirely clear, patients with FMF have a worse prognosis than patients with classic MF.

The potential for adult patients with FM to develop MF or one if its variants is well recognized.

Some estimate that between 10% to 20% of adults with FM may go on to develop MF or one of its variants. Unfortunately, the presence of a clonal population of T cells does not appear to predict which patients will progress. Because of considerable overlap between PFM and MF-associated FM, no single clinical or laboratory finding can be used to distinguish them. Hopefully, the use of multiple clinical, histologic, immunopathologic, and molecular genetic criteria will be useful in evaluation of these patients.

In summary, two forms of FM exist, a primary or idiopathic FM and MF-associated FM. Because reliable criteria do not exist to differentiate the two, physicians should follow patients for the development of new skin lesions and perform skin biopsies at regular intervals.

Atypical Lymphocytic Lobular Panniculitis

The WHO classification of the CTCLs recognizes two variants that show malignant infiltrates in the deep dermis and subcutaneous fat, the more indolent subcutaneous panniculitis-like T-cell lymphoma (SPTCL) and the highly aggressive γ/δ T-cell lymphoma. Because of its aggressive nature and rapid progression, γ/δ T-cell lymphoma is less likely to have a prolonged premalignant phase.

ALLP is a recently described entity that is considered a clonal T-cell dyscrasia characterized by waxing and waning indurated deep plaques (Figure 14-5). A morphologic and biologic continuum with SPTCL has been suggested, although, in

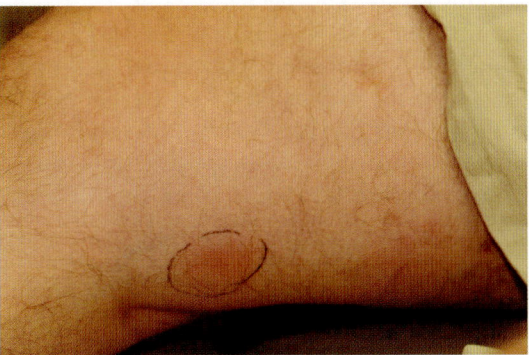

Figure 14-5 Right medial thigh showing a 4-cm subcutaneous indurated deep pink plaque outlined in pen in a patient with atypical lymphoid lobular panniculitis.

one study, several patients followed for years did not go on to develop SPTCL. Therefore, ALLP may not be a true precursor to cutaneous lymphoma as compared with those previously discussed. However, more long-term follow-up of patients with ALLP is needed.

It is not uncommon for patients with SPTCL to have a history of nonspecific waxing and waning tender subcutaneous nodules prior to the development of more fixed subcutaneous nodules diagnostic of SPTCL. In many cases, SPTCL is preceded by an inflammatory phase with features of a lobular lymphocytic panniculitis resembling lupus profundus clinically and histologically. Some investigators have suggested that lupus profundus, ALLP, and SPTCL represent a spectrum of histologic, immunophenotypic, and molecular abnormalities that range from those that are clearly benign to those that are clearly neoplastic.

In summary, patients with ALLP or lupus profundus need to be counseled about the potential for progression to SPTCL and clinicians should stay vigilant for the development of more fixed subcutaneous nodules heralding SPTCL.

PRECURSORS TO CUTANEOUS B-CELL LYMPHOMA

Cutaneous Lymphoid Hyperplasia/ Cutaneous B-Cell Pseudolymphoma

CLH is the preferred term to describe benign growths of the skin characterized by dense deep infiltrates of normal-appearing lymphocytes on pathologic examination. Others use the terms "cutaneous pseudolymphoma" or "lymphocytoma cutis" (now archaic) to describe the same condition. Although most cases of CLH show mixed T- and B-cell infiltrates, uncommon cases may show T-cell predominance.

CLH may resemble the primary CBCLs clinically but do not meet the histologic, immunophenotypic and molecular genetic criteria. Clinically, CLH often presents with a solitary nodule or grouped papulonodules. A history of an arthropod bite at the site is not uncommon. Other reported triggers include a wide variety of foreign antigens, including arthropod stings and

infestations, *Borrelia burgdorferi*, tattoos, vaccinations, trauma, injection of foreign substances, pierced ear jewelry, and drugs.

The vast majority of CLHs do not progress to malignancy, and physicians and their patients should not be unduly alarmed by this diagnosis. However, while the natural history of most CLH remains indolent, clinicians should not assume that all cases of CLH will remain benign. Only a small minority of CLH cases (~ 4%), including those with clonal B-cell rearrangements, in several series have progressed to cutaneous B-cell lymphoma. It is important to recognize that the potential exists for certain lesions of CLH to progress to CBCL. Whether these progressive cases represent benign lesions that become malignant or whether a malignant process was present from inception, but undetectable early on, is not known.

CONCLUSIONS

The precursor skin conditions described in this chapter require clinical vigilance and a low threshold to consider performing additional skin biopsies. Patient expectations must align with the actual risk of developing a cutaneous lymphoma so that the physician can be alerted when a change develops. In few other areas of medicine is the correlation of clinical and pathologic findings more important than in the diagnosis of the cutaneous lymphomas.

SUGGESTED READINGS

Chronic Dermatitis with an Atypical Lymphocytic Infiltrate

Guitart J, Magro C. Cutaneous T-cell lymphoid dyscrasia: a unifying term for idiopathic chronic dermatoses with persistent T-cell clones. *Arch Dermatol.* 2007;143:921–932.2.

Ponti R, Quaglino P, Novelli M, Fierro MT, Comessatti A, Peroni A, et al. T-cell receptor? gene rearrangement by multiplex polymerase chain reaction/heteroduplex analysis in patients with cutaneous T-cell lymphoma (mycosis fungoides/Sézary syndrome) and benign inflammatory disease: correlation with clinical, histological and immunophenotypical findings. *Br J Dermatol.* 2005;153:565–573.

Thurber SE, Zhang B, Kim YH, Schrijver I, Zehnder J, Kohler S. T-cell clonality analysis in biopsy specimens from two different skin sites shows high specificity in the diagnosis of patients with suggested mycosis fungoides. *J Am Acad Dermatol.* 2007;57: 782–790.

Wood GS. Analysis of clonality in cutaneous T cell lymphoma and associated diseases. *Ann N Y Acad Sci.* 2001;941:26–30.

Large Plaque Parapsoriasis

Benmaman O, Sanchez JL. Comparative clinicopathological study on pityriasis lichenoides chronica and small plaque parapsoriasis. *Am J Dermatopathol.* 1988;10:189–196.

Bordignon M, Fortina AB, Pigozzi B, Alaibac M. γδ d T cells as potential contributors to the progression of parapsoriasis to mycosis fungoides. *Mol Med Rep.* 2008;1:485–488.

Brocq L. Les parapsoriases. *Ann Dermatol Venereol.* 1902;3:433–468.

Kikuchi A, Naka W, Harada T, Sakuraoka K, Harada R, Nishikawa T. Parapsoriasis en plaques: its potential for progression to malignant lymphoma. *J Am Acad Dermatol.* 1993;29:419–422.

Lazar A, Caro W, Roenigk HH Jr, Pinski KS. Parapsoriasis and mycosis fungoides: the Northwestern University experience, 1970 to 1985. *J Am Acad Dermatol.* 1989;21:919–923.

Staib G, Sterry W. Use of polymerase chain reaction in the detection of clones in lymphoproliferative diseases of the skin. *Recent Results Cancer Res.* 1995;139:239–247.

Väkevä L, Sarna S, Vaalasti A, Pukkala E, Kariniemi AL, Ranki A. A retrospective study of the probability of the evolution of parapsoriasis en plaques into mycosis fungoides. *Acta Derm Venereol.* 2005;85: 318–3.

Poikiloderma Vasculare Atrophicans

Burg G, Dummer R, Nestle FO, Doebbeling U, Haeffner A. Cutaneous lymphomas consist of a spectrum of nosologically different entities including mycosis fungoides and small plaque parapsoriasis. *Arch Dermatol.* 1996;132:567–572.

Dougherty J. Poikiloderma atrophicans vasculare. *Arch Dermatol.* 1971;103:550–552.

Kreuter A, Hoffmamm K, Altmeyer P. A case of poikiloderma vasculare atrophicans, a rare variant of cutaneous T-cell lymphoma, responding to extracorporeal photopheresis. *J Am Acad Dermatol.* 2005;52:706–708.

Nakai K, Yoneda K, Moriue T, Miyamoto I, Fukita N, Yokoi I, et al. Narrow-band ultraviolet B decreases serum interleukin-2 receptor levels in patients with poikiloderma vasculare atrophicans. *J Eur Acad Dermatol Venereol.* 2009;23:835–862.

Lymphomatoid Papulosis

Kunishige JH, McDonald H, Alvarez G, Johnson M, Prieto V, Duvic M. Lymphomatoid papulosis and associated lymphomas: a retrospective case series of 84 patients. *Clin Exp Dermatol.* 2009;34:576–581.

Liu HL, Hoppe RT, Kohler S, Harvell JD, Reddy S, Kim YH. CD30+ cutaneous lymphoproliferative disorders: the Stanford experience in lymphomatoid papulosis and primary cutaneous anaplastic large cell lymphoma. *J Am Acad Dermatol.* 2003;49:1049–1058.

Willemze R, Jaffe ES, Burg G, Cerroni L, Berti E, Swerdlow SH, et al. WHO-EORTC classification for cutaneous lymphomas. *Blood.* 2005;105:3768–3785.

Willemze R, Meijer CJ. Primary cutaneous CD30-positive lymphoproliferative disorders. *Hematol Oncol Clin North Am.* 2003;17:1319–1332.

Follicular Mucinosis

Agar NS, Wedgeworth E, Crichton S, Mitchell TJ, Cox M, Ferreira S, et al. Survival outcomes and prognostic factors in mycosis fungoides/Sézary syndrome: validation of the Revised International Society for Cutaneous Lymphomas/European Organization for Research and Treatment of Cancer Staging Proposal. *J Clin Oncol.* 2010;28:4730–4739.

Brown HA, Gibson LE, Pujol RM, Lust JA, Pittelkow MR. Primary follicular mucinosis: long-term follow-up of patients younger than 40 years with and without clonal T-cell receptor gene rearrangement. *J Am Acad Dermatol.* 2002;47:856.

Rongioletti F, De Lucchi S, Meyes D, Mora M, Rebora A, Zupo S, et al. Follicular mucinosis: a clinicopathologic, histochemical, immunohistochemical and molecular study comparing the primary benign form and the mycosis fungoides associated follicular mucinosis. *J Cutan Pathol.* 2010;37:15–19.

Atypical Lymphocytic Lobular Panniculitis

Guitart J. Subcutaneous lymphoma and related conditions. *Dermatol Ther.* 2010;23:350–355.

Magro CM, Schaefer JT, Morrison C, Porcu P. Atypical lymphocytic lobular panniculitis: a clonal subcutaneous T-cell dyscrasia. *J Cutan Pathol.* 2008;35:947–954.

Lupus Profundus

Magro CM, Crowson AN, Kovatich J, Burns F. Lupus profundus, indeterminate lymphocytic lobular panniculitis and subcutaneous T-cell lymphoma: a spectrum of subcuticular T-cell lymphoid dyscrasia. *J Cutan Pathol.* 2001;28:235–247.

Cutaneous Lymphoid Hyperplasia

Bergman R, Khamaysi K, Khamaysi Z, Arie YB. A study of histologic and immunophenotypical staining patterns in cutaneous lymphoid hyperplasia. *J Am Acad Dermatol.* 2011;65:112–124.

Gilliam AC, Wood GS. Cutaneous lymphoid hyperplasias. *Semin Cutan Med Surg.* 2000;119:133–141.

Kulow BF, Cualing H, Steele P, VanHorn J, Breneman JC, Mutasim DF, et al. Progression of cutaneous B-cell pseudolymphoma to cutaneous B-cell lymphoma. *J Cutan Med Surg.* 2002;6:519–528.

Nihal M, Mikkola D, Horvath N, Gilliam AC, Stevens SR, Spiro TP, et al. Cutaneous lymphoid hyperplasia: a lymphoproliferative continuum with lymphomatous potential. *Hum Pathol.* 2003;34:617–622.

CLINICAL MIMICS OF CUTANEOUS LYMPHOMA

Derek Thomas Bernstein, BS, Maura Jane Holcomb, MD,
and Ted Rosen, MD

INTRODUCTION

Numerous benign and malignant conditions present with clinical manifestations suggestive of primary cutaneous lymphoma. Correctly recognizing such mimics is essential because they tend to have better prognoses and require considerably different therapeutic approaches than their malignant counterparts. Unfortunately, despite many recent technologic advances, a uniformly reliable and straightforward set of diagnostic criteria remains elusive for many of these clinical mimics. This is partly related to the facts that lymphoid infiltrates lie on a wide spectrum, ranging from clearly benign to overtly malignant, and that there is significant overlap in cell types identifiable in various infiltrates. In general, polyclonal lymphoid infiltrates often represent the most benign lesions, whereas monoclonal infiltrates may or may not be neoplastic, and wildly anaplastic infiltrates represent the most overtly malignant lesions. As a result, differentiation between cutaneous lymphoma and its various clinical mimics relies upon the integration of historical information, clinical morphology, routine histopathologic findings, and immunohistochemical and molecular studies (when and where available). Table 15-1 outlines some important parameters in the consideration of cutaneous lymphoma versus pseudolymphomatous states.

Pseudolymphomas (cutaneous lymphocytic hyperplasia) are often categorized as B-cell–rich, T-cell–rich, mixed lymphocyte–rich, lymphocyte-poor, or neutrophil-rich. Common B-cell–rich pseudolymphomas mimic cutaneous follicular

TABLE 15-1   Criteria Differentiating Pseudolymphoma and Lymphoma

	Benign	Malignant
Clinical criteria	Solitary or localized, smaller lesions	Multiple or disseminated, larger lesions
	Slower growth	More rapid growth
	Spontaneous resolution or improvement with elimination of any etiologic factor or offending agent	Treatment requires more aggressive therapy; success of therapy variable in some states
Histologic criteria	Small, mature lymphocytes with surrounding reactive cells	Large, atypical lymphocytes
	Prominent papillary dermal involvement	Prominent deep dermal involvement
	Lack of bcl-2 staining	Presence of bcl-2 staining
	Presence of pan-T-cell markers (CD2, CD3, CD5, CD7)	Lack of pan-T-cell markers (CD2, CD3, CD5, CD7)
	Presence of pan-B-cell markers (CD19, CD20, CD22, CD79a)	Lack of pan-B-cell markers (CD19, CD20, CD22, CD79a)
	T-cell receptor gene polyclonality	T-cell receptor gene monoclonality and rearrangement
	Mixed lambda and kappa light chain antibody production	Single lambda or kappa light chain antibody production

B-cell lymphoma, cutaneous marginal zone B-cell lymphoma, or diffuse large B-cell lymphoma. Common T-cell–rich pseudolymphomas mimic mycosis fungoides (MF), Sézary's syndrome (SS), or less commonly, one of the other types of cutaneous T-cell lymphomas. Mixed lymphocyte-rich and lymphocyte-poor pseudolymphomas may present similar to any of the recognized primary cutaneous lymphomas. Neutrophil-rich pseudolymphomas may also mimic a host of true cutaneous lymphoma types. In addition, several common and uncommon benign and malignant dermatoses occasionally may be misdiagnosed as primary cutaneous lymphomas and several specific morphologic patterns of skin disease can closely simulate primary cutaneous lymphoma. We discuss each of these categories separately.

B-CELL–RICH PSEUDOLYMPHOMAS (TABLE 15-2)

Borrelia Lymphocytoma Cutis

Borrelia lymphocytoma cutis occurs in approximately 1% of patients who develop Lyme disease in endemic regions of Europe. It is caused by strains of the spirochete *Borrelia burgdorferi*, which is transmitted by *Ixodes ricinus* tick bites. This disease is very rarely encountered in the United States because the endemic strains are different from those encountered in Europe. Lesions present as erythematous or violaceous nodules and plaques with a predilection for the nose, earlobe, nipple, and scrotum, reflective of the spirochete's preference for areas of lower body temperature. These lesions may ulcerate or appear concurrently with erythema chronicum migrans and acrodermatitis chronica atrophicans, two additional cutaneous manifestations of Lyme disease. Because many infections with *Borrelia* are asymptomatic, the pseudolymphoma may be the first indication of infection. Treatment with anti-*Borrelia* antibiotics (such as doxycycline) results in regression of the cutaneous lesions. Lack of response to a course of antibiotics should prompt the clinician to reconsider the diagnosis of lymphoma.

Herpes

Herpes viruses commonly present as painful, vesicular dermatoses. Diagnosis is made primarily by classic clinical findings, with or without isolation and identification in viral culture. Atypical cutaneous manifestations may be seen, particularly in immunocompromised patients as well as those with underlying hematologic malignancies. A prototype of this phenomenon is vegetative herpes simplex. These cases in particular may mimic primary cutaneous lymphoma. Therefore, biopsy

TABLE 15-2   B-Cell–rich Infiltrates Mimicking Follicular, Marginal Zone, and Diffuse Large B-Cell Lymphomas

B-Cell–rich Pseudolymphoma	Differentiating Features
Borrelia lymphocytoma cutis	Association with erythema chronicum migrans and acrodermatitis chronica atrophicans
	History of tick bite in endemic regions of Europe
	Response of lesion to antibiotics
HSV-associated pseudolymphoma	Lesions present in herpetic clusters
	Response of lesions to acyclovir analogues
VZV-associated pseudolymphoma	Dermatomal distribution of painful lesions
	Response of lesions to acyclovir analogues
Vaccine-associated lymphocytoma cutis	Temporal association with vaccination
	Subsequent pseudolymphoma formation at additional injection sites
	Detection of aluminum deposits by Morin's technique or ion microscopy

HSV, herpes simplex virus; VZV, varicella-zoster virus.

showing a polymorphous reactive pattern or typical viral changes, coupled with clinical response to acyclovir or one of its analogues, may aid in elucidating the proper diagnosis. *Post-zoster scar lymphocytoma cutis,* also known as *zoster folliculitis,* may present as juicy red papules with a tendency to progress to ulceration that may mimic any of the primary B-cell lymphomas. Differentiation techniques enumerated previously may be helpful. Temporal association is also important for differentiation in these cases.

Reactions to Vaccines

Relatively common reactions to vaccines include erythema, edema, pain, and deep induration at the injection site. Rarely, erythematous, mildly pruritic and firm nodules and plaques may present a few weeks to several months following vaccination; these may persist for months to years and closely simulate primary cutaneous lymphoma. These pseudolymphomas have been primarily associated with tetanus, hepatitis B, and varicella-zoster virus vaccination, all of which contain aluminum hydroxide as an adjuvant. A history of recent vaccination strongly points toward pseudolymphoma, although differentiation from lymphoma may be difficult when the temporal association is les clear. Histologically, pseudolymphoma may be best diagnosed in this scenario by the detection of aluminum deposits by Morin's technique or ion microscopy. The literature suggests that patients developing pseudolymphoma from vaccination tend to manifest the same reaction in alternative injection sites. Treatment options include topical and local steroids, surgical excision, and radiotherapy. Long-term follow-up is important because of the evidence reporting rare vaccine-associated true lymphoma.

T-CELL–RICH PSEUDOLYMPHOMAS (TABLE 15-3)

Nodular Scabies

Nodular scabies is marked by an atypical lymphomatoid immune response that accompanies acute infection and may persist for months after proper treatment is administered. It typically manifests

TABLE 15-3   T-Cell–rich Infiltrates Mimicking Mycosis Fungoides and Sézary's Syndrome

T-Cell–rich Pseudolymphoma	Differentiating Features
Nodular scabies	Demonstration of causative ectoparasite Prominent eosinophils within infiltrate
Actinic reticuloid	Striking photodistribution Lack of Pautrier's microabscesses on biopsy
Anticonvulsant-induced pseudolymphoma	Temporal association with anticonvulsant therapy Resolution with drug removal
Lichenoid pigmented purpuric dermatitis	Irritant exposure Hemosiderin deposition
Pseudolymphomatous folliculitis	Hyperplastic hair follicles and lack of Pautrier's microabscesses on biopsy
Small plaque (premycotic) parapsoriasis	Lack of Pautrier's microabscesses on biopsy
HIV-associated pseudolymphoma	Resolution with HAART Reactive, predominantly CD8+ T-cell infiltrate in patient with HIV infection; low CD4 count
Tattoo-induced cutaneous lymphoid hyperplasia	Reactive infiltrate limited to distribution of single tattoo ink color

HAART, highly active antiretroviral therapy; HIV, human immunodeficiency virus.

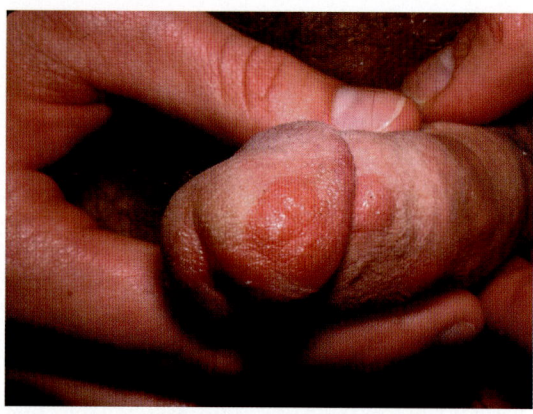

Figure 15-1 The location of nodular scabies suggests the correct diagnosis.

as multiple erythematous nodules with associated pruritus. The condition can be differentiated from lymphoma by contemporary or previous unequivocal demonstration of the etiologic mite, typical distribution of lesions (e.g., head of the penis; Figure 15-1), and/or by the appearance of numerous eosinophils within a biopsy specimen. Assuming that treatment for scabies has already been given, management of persistent nodular lesions is best accomplished with topical calcineurin inhibitors such as pimecrolimus and tacrolimus.

Actinic Reticuloid

Actinic reticuloid is a specific histologic variant of chronic actinic dermatitis, a photodermatosis presenting initially as pruritic, erythematous scaly papules or plaques on sun-exposed areas. With progression, the lesion may involve large portions of the skin surface and include crusting, edema, lichenification, or purpura. This heterogeneous appearance closely mimics many cases of classic MF. Variable degrees of photosensitivity to a broad action spectrum (including ultraviolet A [UVA] and ultraviolet B [UVB]) for years, or even for life, is typical. Phototesting is diagnostic. Actinic reticuloid is primarily treated with desensitization via incremental exposure to PUVA (psoralen + UVA) therapy, with or without adjunctive topical or systemic corticosteroid therapy. Steroids alone have been shown to be beneficial, but rapid recurrence occurs after corticosteroid cessation.

Hypersensitivity Reactions to Anticonvulsants

Cutaneous eruptions occur in 2% to 4% of patients taking anticonvulsants. Cutaneous hypersensitivity reactions to this class of drugs may include life-threatening conditions such as toxic epidermal necrolysis and Stevens-Johnson syndrome, as well as more benign eruptions such as pseudolymphoma formation. Typical causative agents include carbamazepine, phenytoin, phenobarbital, and valproic acid. Anticonvulsant-induced pseudolymphoma mimics MF, presenting as reddish-brown plaques or as a morbilliform maculopapular rash sparing the palms and soles. Less commonly, systemic signs of fever, lymphadenopathy, hepatosplenomegaly, and facial edema may be suggestive of SS. Pseudolymphoma may appear within weeks or, alternatively, after years of anticonvulsant use. Following discontinuation of the offending drug, resolution typically begins within 1 to 2 weeks and is the diagnostic gold standard. Systemic or topical steroids and antihistamines may provide partial regression and a degree of symptomatic relief, but they generally will not induce complete resolution. Of note, substitution of one anticonvulsant for another may lead to recurrence of the original pseudolymphoma.

Lichenoid Pigmented Purpuric Dermatitis

Lichenoid pigmented purpuric dermatitis clinically manifests similar to purpuric variants of MF, presenting initially as nonblanching, pruritic, petechial patches with variable degrees of scaling, vesiculation, and lichenification. As the lesion progresses, hemosiderin accumulation caused by extravasation of red blood cells causes the lesion to appear brown. Although most cases are idiopathic, some have been related to irritant chemicals, clothing, and drugs. It is best differentiated from neoplastic processes by histologic examination showing perivascular lymphocytic infiltration around dilated or ruptured venules in the papillary dermis with prominent erythrocyte extravasation. Lichenoid pigmented purpuric dermatitis may be a longstanding disease with a widespread and relapsing course. It has been shown to progress to MF in some instances, so long-term clinical and histologic follow-up is essential. Irritant removal is important when identified. Because of the potential for malignant transformation, aggressive treatment with PUVA or topical mechlorethamine is prudent. Topical or intralesional steroids, oral pentoxifylline, topical calcineurin inhibitors, oral methotrexate and cyclosporine, and knee-high compression hose to reduce venous stasis are other potential treatment options, but these have been ineffective in refractory cases.

Folliculitis

Pseudolymphomatous folliculitis primarily presents as a solitary red nodule or plaque on the face, scalp, or trunk with mild tenderness and/or pruritus; less common cases of multiple nodules have been reported. Typically, there is no preceding history of bacterial folliculitis. It can be differentiated from follicular MF, marginal zone lymphoma, and anaplastic large cell lymphoma based on characteristic histology. Enlarged, hyperplastic hair follicles with or without destruction and a reactive infiltrate is suggestive of pseudolymphoma versus lymphoma. Pseudolymphomatous folliculitis may exhibit regression after biopsy. Intralesional triamcinolone acetonide and oral cyclosporine are therapeutic. Topical corticosteroids, oral antihistamines, topical tacrolimus, narrow-band UVB radiation and interferon-gamma have all proved generally ineffective.

Small Plaque Parapsoriasis

Plaque-type parapsoriasis is the most common cutaneous manifestation preceding histologically typical MF, thus the term *premycotic parapsoriasis.* Currently, the World Health Organization considers "large plaque" parapsoriasis to be premalignant, whereas "small plaque" parapsoriasis (also known as "digitate dermatosis" in some countries) is considered to be a benign disease because it almost never evolves into MF. However, clinicians may have some difficulty distinguishing "small" from "large" plaque parapsoriasis. Clinically, small plaque parapsoriasis presents as single or multiple 3 to 6 × 0.5 to 2-cm erythematous patches, often ovoid in shape (resembling the ends of fingers) with fine scaling (Figure 15-2). Differentiation from MF is typically histologic. Therapy for small

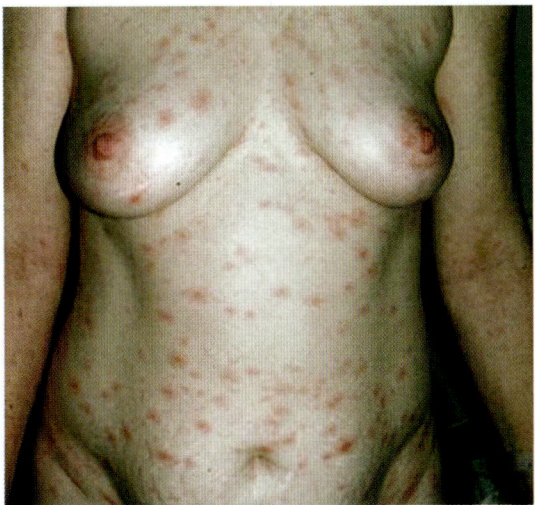

Figure 15-2 Small plaque parapsoriasis mimics premycotic parapsoriasis.

plaque parapsoriasis includes topical steroids as well as phototherapy (broad- or narrow-band UVB or PUVA).

Human Immunodeficiency Virus–related Pseudolymphoma

Human immunodeficiency virus (HIV) infection is associated with an increased risk of aggressive B-cell lymphoma as well as less common T-cell–dominant lymphomas. These are defined by a CD4+ infiltrate and tend to occur in patients with relatively intact immune systems, lower viral loads, and higher CD4 counts. Conversely, HIV-related pseudolymphomas are primarily CD8+ infiltrates that become more prevalent with greater immune dysfunction. They present as erythematous, scaly plaques that can coalesce and crust as they develop on the limbs, face, and trunk. Hyperkeratosis of the palms and soles may develop as well as vitiligo-like hypopigmentation. HIV-related pseudolymphomas may also present as an erythroderma, thereby mimicking SS. Differentiation of this benign condition is defined by a clinical response to highly active antiretroviral therapy (HAART) therapy or steroids, the two mainstays of treatment. Of note, polyclonality in HIV-related lymphoid lesions is not a good indicator of benign clinical course because many polyclonal lymphocyte proliferations have been documented to ultimately behave in a malignant fashion.

Reactions to Tattoos

Tattoos may elicit an early lichenoid or granulomatous response, which may occasionally progress to persistent cutaneous lymphoid hyperplasia (CLH). Lesions present as pruritic solitary or multiple nodules located within a single color, most often red. Histologic examination shows a reactive infiltrate in the dermis with epidermal spongiosis, differentiating this entity from cutaneous lymphoma. Onset typically occurs months to years after the tattoo is placed. Although spontaneous resolution has been documented, complete excision and CO_2 laser ablation may be required. Corticosteroid therapy has a poor response rate. Long-term follow up is essential because relapse may occur and rare evolution to primary cutaneous lymphoma has been documented.

MIXED CELL TYPE, LYMPHOCYTE-RICH PSEUDOLYMPHOMA (SEE TABLE 15-4)

Gold-associated Contact Dermatitis

Gold-associated contact dermatitis has only recently been recognized as a significant problem. Direct inoculation via ear piercing and acupuncture with gold-tipped needles, however, is well known for its ability to cause pseudolymphomatoid reactions. Mildly tender or pruritic violaceous, firm nodules or papules lacking eczematous changes develop at the puncture site, reminiscent of MF. Diagnosis is based upon a history of piercing, patch test positivity to gold, and visualization of birefringent multinucleated giant cells

TABLE 15-4   Mixed Lymphocyte-rich Infiltrates Mimicking Primary Cutaneous Lymphoma

Mixed Lymphocyte-rich Pseudolymphoma	Cutaneous Lymphoma	Differentiating Features
Gold trauma–associated pseudolymphoma	Classic mycosis fungoides	Clinical history of piercing/acupuncture Positive patch test for gold Reactive infiltrate on biopsy
Lymphomatoid contact dermatitis	Classic mycosis fungoides	Positive patch test for allergen Resolution with allergen removal Infiltrate may have prominent B cell component
Lymphomatoid drug reactions	Classic mycosis fungoides Granulomatous mycosis fungoides Pleomorphic T-cell lymphoma Marginal zone lymphoma Angiocentric lymphoma	Resolution with cessation of drug Reactive infiltrate on biopsy
APACHE/papular angiolymphoid hyperplasia	Classic mycosis fungoides	Infiltrate lacking epidermotropism and interface dermatitis, with prominent, thick-walled vessels on biopsy
Syphilis Cutaneous leishmaniasis	Nodular mycosis fungoides Marginal zone lymphoma	Positive dark-field microscopy Positive VDRL or RPR serology Response to penicillin
Lupus erythematosus	Mycosis fungoides Marginal aone lymphoma	Biopsy demonstrating leishmania PCR demonstrating leishmania Response of lesions to antimonial or oral azole therapy

Mixed Lymphocyte-rich Pseudolymphoma	Cutaneous Lymphoma	Differentiating Features
	Various (see Table 15-6)	Autoantibody detection
		Positive phototesting
Lymphomatoid keratosis		Characteristic histologic features on biopsy
	Unilesional mycosis fungoides	Mixed T and B cells on biopsy

APACHE, acral pseudolymphomatous angiokeratoma; PCR, polymerase chain reaction; RPR, rapid plasma reagin; VDRL, Venereal Disease Research Laboratory.

indicating gold phagocytosis on biopsy. Resolution of lesions has been documented following shave biopsy as well as following intralesional steroid injection. Avoidance of gold is recommended to prevent recurrence.

Lymphomatoid Contact Dermatitis

Lymphomatoid contact dermatitis has two different primary presentations, a localized form characterized by solitary or multiple nodules or plaques in the region of direct contact with the offending agent and an eczematous and lichenified type that progresses to erythroderma. Multiple agents have been implicated in this type of pseudolymphoma since its first description in 1976 including polidocanol, paraphenylenediamine, ethylenediamine, benzydamine hydrochloride, phosphorus sesquisulfide, para-tertiary butylphenol formaldehyde resin, nickel, gold, cobalt naphthenate, and zinc. Despite potential for either B- or T-cell–rich infiltrates, differentiation from MF is the primary diagnostic challenge. History demonstrating temporal relationship between the agent and the skin lesion, resolution after withdrawal of the sensitizing agent, and reactive mixed cell–type histologic infiltrate all suggest pseudolymphoma. Excision has also been curative. Topical and oral corticosteroid therapy has shown variable efficacy. Long-term follow-up is essential in lesions that do not resolve because true malignant transformation may occur.

Lymphomatoid Drug Reactions

Lymphomatoid drug reactions provide a potential diagnostic challenge because the skin eruption may occur within weeks to years of drug administration, thereby obscuring the temporal relation. The pathogenesis of such lesions is believed to be based upon immune dysregulation, as evidenced by the majority of such reactions occurring in immunocompromised patients. Lesions are typically erythematous papules or plaques, with or without pruritus, frequently seen on the face and proximal upper extremities. A list of the common causes of lymphomatoid drug reactions can be found in Table 15-5. Treatment involves withdrawal of the offending agent and supportive care. Regression may occur over a period of weeks to months.

TABLE 15-5 Medications Causing Lymphomatoid Reactions

Amphetamines
Antibiotics (fluoroquinolones, cephalosporins, penicillins, tetracyclines, sulfonamides)
Anticoagulants
Antimuscarinics
Antivirals (ganciclovir in particular)
Diuretics (furosemide in particular)
Immunosuppressants (including anakinra, thalidomide, infliximab, adalimumab, etanercept)
Laxatives (senna)
ACE inhibitors
Histamine antagonists (H1 and H2 blockers)
Calcium channel vlockers
Antidepressants (fluoxetine in particular)
Lipid-lowering agents
Benzodiazepines

ACE, angiotensin-converting enzyme.

Acral Pseudolymphomatous Angiokeratoma

Acral pseudolymphomatous angiokeratoma (APACHE), originally thought to be a vascular malformation seen in children, is currently classified as a pseudolymphoma occurring at any age based on the increased number of adult cases. The typical presentation consists of solitary or multiple, asymptomatic, erythematous to violaceous angiomatous papules with hyperkeratotic collars located in acral regions. Differentiation from classic MF is made histologically. Prominent thick-walled blood vessels are characteristic in APACHE. Clinically, this entity is chronic and benign, with lesions often lasting for more than 10 years. Corticosteroid therapy, removal by curettage, and liquid nitrogen cryosurgery have all been complicated by recurrence. Excision when feasible, owing to size and location, is curative.

Syphilis

Syphilis is a multistage, sexually transmitted infectious disease notable for a wide range of clinical presentations ("the great imitator"). Syphilis is caused by the spirochete *Treponema pallidum*. An atypical nodular presentation often, but not exclusively, associated with HIV infection may mimic lymphoma. This type of syphilis presents as multiple smooth, red, firm, mobile, and nontender dome-shaped nodules or large erythematous plaques that can be suggestive of nodular MF or cutaneous marginal zone B-cell lymphoma (Figure 15-3). Perioral, perirectal,

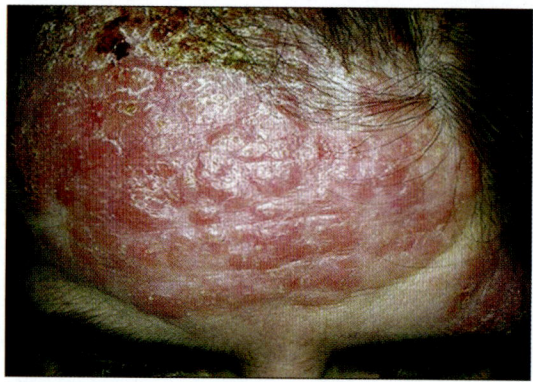

Figure 15-3 Atypical secondary syphilis may mimic lymphoma.

or genital involvement may suggest the proper diagnosis. Fifty percent to 80% of patients may present with generalized lymphadenopathy as well, further convoluting the clinical picture. The proper diagnosis can be made based on positive dark-field microscopy of the lesions demonstrating the spirochete or positive serologic tests for syphilis (Venereal Disease Research laboratory [VDRL] and rapid plasma regain [RPR]). Histologic examination may show a large number of plasma cells within the infiltrate, but biopsy results are not uniformly reliable in establishing this diagnosis. Treatment with benzathine penicillin resolves cutaneous lesions.

Leishmaniasis

Cutaneous leishmaniasis is a parasitic infection seen most frequently in the United States among travelers and military personnel returning from endemic tropical and subtropical countries. It presents as painless, brown, crusted nodules with a tendency to centrally ulcerate, suggestive of aggressive MF or cutaneous marginal zone B-cell lymphoma. A high clinical suspicion is essential. Diagnosis is based on a compatible travel history as well as routine histology or polymerase chain reaction (PCR) analysis providing evidence for the presence of *Leishmania* spp. Of note, histologic analysis may demonstrate significant cellular and mitotic atypia. Also, bcl-2 staining may be positive, a molecular marker typically suggestive of malignancy. Remission of cutaneous lesions can be achieved following intravenous/intramuscular administration of pentavalent antimonial medication, use of thermotherapy, or in susceptible organisms, oral azole (fluconazole, ketoconazole) therapy.

Lupus Erythematosus

Several forms of lupus erythematosus, especially deep-seated variants, may be clinically suggestive of lymphoma (Table 15-6 and Figure 15-4). Differentiation is based on the slowly progressive clinical course, histologic examination, and the presence of antinuclear antibody (ANA), anti-Ro, anti-La, and anti-dsDNA autoantibodies. The location of cutaneous lesions can be

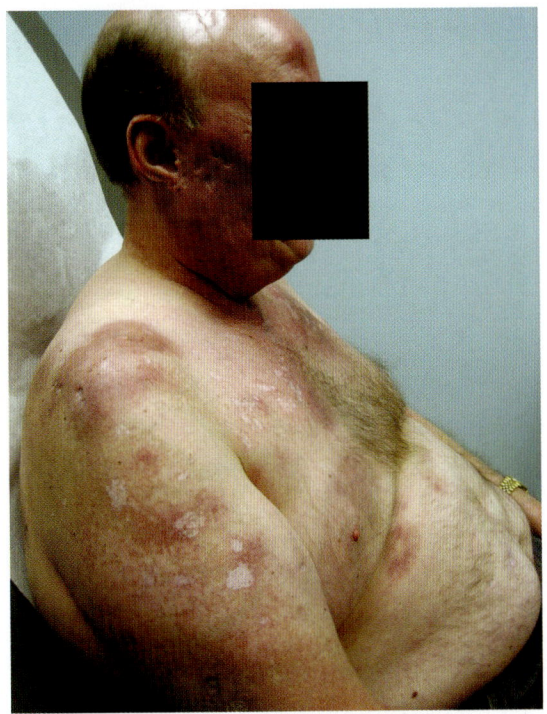

Figure 15-4 Lupus panniculitis resembles deep-seated lymphoma.

helpful in distinction from lymphoma because lupus favors cutaneous regions exposed to sunlight. Antimalarial drugs, oral corticosteroids, and various immunosuppressives (e.g., azathioprine and methotrexate) are used for treatment.

Lymphomatoid Keratosis

Lymphomatoid keratosis is an epidermotropic cutaneous lymphoid hypertrophy that presents initially as solitary tiny papule with progression to a scaly plaque most commonly on the face, but also on the upper trunk and extremities. Most cases are idiopathic, but arthropod bites, stings, tattoos, and vaccinations have all been implicated. Lymphomatoid keratosis simulates classic MF, but it can be differentiated based on the heterogeneous infiltrate, as well as the mixed presence of B and T cells. Complete excision of this solitary lesion is curative.

LYMPHOCYTE-POOR PSEUDOLYMPHOMA (TABLE 15-7)

Leprosy

Leprosy, caused by *Mycobacterium leprae* infection, remains prevalent in certain geographic areas of the world. In fact, 75% of the global disease burden is accounted for by only a few countries, most notably Brazil, India, Madagascar, Mexico, Mozambique, and Nepal. Presentation depends upon whether the disease is paucibacillary or multibacillary. Tuberculoid (paucibacillary) leprosy presents as nonpruritic, flesh-colored to red-brown coalescing papules to annular plaque. On the other end of the spectrum, lepromatous (multibacillary) leprosy presents as widespread

TABLE 15-6 Variants of Cutaneous Lupus Erythematosus That Mimic Lymphoma

Lupus Subtype	Cutaneous Lymphoma Simulated	Clinical Description of mimic
Oral lupus erythematosus	Follicular T-cell lymphoma	Irregularly cobblestoned and polypoid plaque on buccal mucosa, hard and soft palate, tongue, larynx, or epiglottis
Lupus tumidus	Mycosis fungoides	Large, indurated, erythematous, scaly, nonscarring, light-sensitive plaque in sun-exposed regions, especially face and upper arms
Lupus panniculitis	Panniculitis-like T-cell lymphoma Intravascular large B-cell lymphoma	Moderate to large-sized erythematous deep subcutaneous nodules, often with associated systemic symptoms

TABLE 15-7   Lymphocyte-poor Diseases Mimicking Primary Cutaneous Lymphoma

Lymphocyte-poor Pseudolymphoma	Cutaneous Lymphoma Mimicked	Differentiating Features of Mimic
Leprosy	Granulomatous mycosis fungoides Granulomatous slack skin Primary cutaneous B-cell lymphoma	Skin split smear positivity for *Mycobacterium leprae*
Disseminated coccidioidomycosis	Classic mycosis fungoides	*Coccidioides immitis* spherules on GMS stain Fungal culture reveals organism Positive fungal serology
Cutaneous tuberculosis	Classic mycosis fungoides	Detection of organism on AFB stain Recovery of organism on culture Positive PPD test Response to antituberculous therapy
Exfoliative dermatitis	Sézary's syndrome	Clinical history Reactive infiltrate on biopsy CD4+/CD27− cells
Psoriasis	Primary cutaneous B-cell lymphoma Primary cutaneous T-cell lymphoma	Family history Ancillary findings (e.g., nail changes) Typical histology for psoriasis
Sarcoidosis	Classic, granulomatous and hypopigmented mycosis fungoides Pleomorphic T-cell lymphoma	Noncaseating granulomas with paucity of lymphocytes on biopsy Hilar adenopathy Hypercalcemia Elevated ACE level
Granuloma annulare	Marginal zone lymphoma Classic and granulomatous mycosis fungoides Hodgkin's lymphoma (skin) Follicular lymphomas	Lesions are consistent color Dermal mucin within palisading granulomas and paucity of lymphocytes without epidermotropism
Venous stasis ulcer	Diffuse large B-cell lymphoma, leg type	Varicose veins and edema present Hemosiderin-induced dyschromia

ACE, angiotensin-converting enzyme; AFB, acid-fast bacillus; GMS, Gomori methenamine silver; PPD, purified protein derivative.

erythematous nodules or plaques or diffuse cutaneous infiltration (Figure 15-5). Loss of cutaneous sensation with hyper- or hypopigmented, inelastic, sagging or atrophic skin may be seen in advanced leprosy. Classic and granulomatous MF, granulomatous slack skin, and primary cutaneous B-cell lymphoma may be clinically simulated. Diagnosis of leprosy depends upon history of residence in endemic areas, compatible clinical features (such as loss of sensation, loss of eyebrows, thickened earlobes), and detection of *M. leprae* on biopsy or skin split smear. Treatment typically consists of dapsone and rifampin or clofazimine; however, other antibiotics such as clarithromycin, ofloxacin, levofloxacin, and minocycline may be used. Treatment duration in paucibacillary leprosy is 6 months versus 12 months in multibacillary forms.

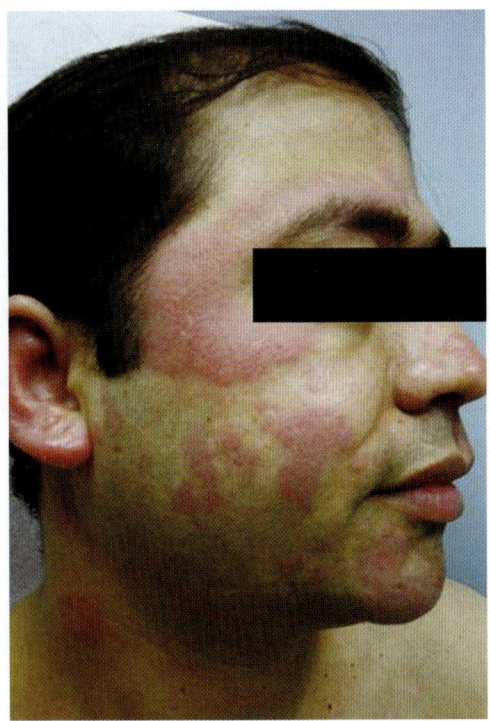

Figure 15-5 Multibacillary Hansen's disease mimics lymphoma.

Coccidioidomycosis

Disseminated coccidioidomycosis is a fungal infection endemic to the southwestern United States, typically acquired by inhalation of arthroconidia. Most cases are asymptomatic or present as mild flulike illnesses. In 0.5% to 1.5% of cases, dissemination can occur approximately 6 months after onset of pulmonary symptoms, particularly in African Americans, the elderly, pregnant women, and patients with deficient cellular immunity. Cutaneous manifestations of this disease include numerous papules, particularly on the face or extremities, slowly evolving into violaceous, exudative plaques suggestive of classic plaque stage MF. Differentiation from lymphoma can be made via positive fungal cultures or skin biopsy showing granulomatous inflammation with *Coccidioides immitis* spherules. In addition, positive specific enzyme immunoassay for immunoglobulin M (IgM) and IgG seropositivity with complement fixation (CF) titers are highly diagnostic. Treatment includes amphotericin B followed by an oral azole.

Tuberculosis

Tuberculosis is again becoming an increasingly serious problem in the United States and other developed countries, largely owing to its association with HIV co-infection. Cutaneous manifestations may be acquired after hematogenous spread of airborne-acquired exogenous disease or, much less commonly, through direct inoculation secondary to trauma. Cutaneous lesions account for less than 1% of all reported cases of tuberculosis and may be classified into one of several subtypes. Most typically, lesions present as painless red, brown, or violaceous papules or plaques, with or without ulceration. Differentiation of characteristic cutaneous tuberculosis from lymphoma is particularly difficult owing to the low sensitivity of diagnostic techniques, such as direct demonstration of the etiologic organism by Ziehl-Neelsen staining, recovery of the organism via acid-fast bacillus (AFB) culture, and application of tissue PCR. Histologic examination demonstrating a typical necrotic granulomatous infiltrate is suggestive, particularly when coupled with clinical history and positive tuberculin skin test. Response of cutaneous lesions to treatment is also suggestive of the diagnosis. Therapy is identical to systemic tuberculosis and consists of a multidrug regimen (isoniazid, rifampin, pyrazinamide, and ethambutol).

Exfoliative Dermatitis

Exfoliative dermatitis (erythroderma) is a potentially life-threatening condition defined by an extreme state of skin inflammation manifested by a generalized, pruritic erythema accompanied by variable scaling and desquamation, which covers greater than 90% of the body's surface. Fever and lymphadenopathy may also be present. Previous dermatoses are the most likely etiology. Additional causes include a variety of medicinal drugs, underlying systemic malignancies (often reticuloendothelial in origin), infections, and an idiopathic etiology. Onset is typically insidious, except in drug reactions, which tend to be acute and florid. Differentiation from SS may be difficult (Figure 15-6). Histologic examination aids in the diagnosis in approximately 50% of cases, with the remainder showing nonspecific inflammation. Furthermore, the presence of CD4+/CD27– cells

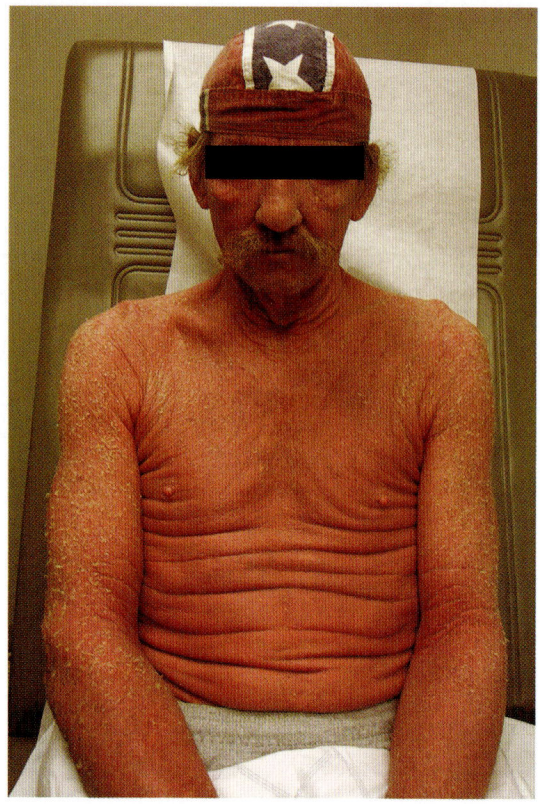

Figure 15-6 Exfoliative erythroderma mimics Sézary's syndrome.

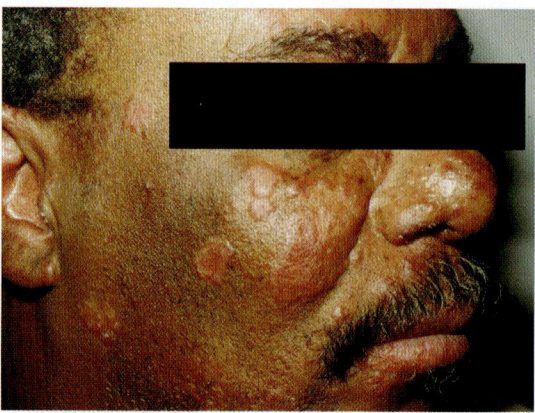

Figure 15-7 Sarcoidal plaques closely resemble cutaneous lymphoma.

is suggestive of erythroderma, whereas CD4+/CD27+ cells are typically seen in SS. Resolution of erythroderma is accomplished by treatment of the underlying condition.

Psoriasis

Psoriasis, an inflammatory skin disease due to immune dysregulation, presents as localized red to silver, dry, scaly plaques. Occasionally, differentiation from primary cutaneous lymphomas may be required and, in such cases, is based on family history of psoriasis, noncutaneous findings (e.g., nail pitting), and histologic examination.

Sarcoidosis

Sarcoidosis is characterized by noncaseating granulomatous lesions and is typically seen in lymph nodes, liver, lung, and spleen. Cutaneous involvement often presents concurrently with associated bone involvement. Cutaneous sarcoidosis may assume a wide variety of morphologic presentations. The prototypical example is lupus pernio in which indolent red-brown to violaceous, indurated papules and plaques form on the nose, cheeks, ears, lips, or forehead (Figure 15-7). The cutaneous lesions of sarcoidosis often present symmetrically, but they can also be quite heterogeneous with regard to pigmentation and coloration. This complicates the accurate differentiation of sarcoidosis from many primary cutaneous lymphomas. In addition, sarcoidosis may develop as a Koebner-type response to underlying lymphoma, further clouding the clinical picture. Whereas detection of sarcoid granulomas in other organs may be suggestive, a skin biopsy is essential for diagnosis. Findings include reactive, noncaseating granulomas with many epithelioid histiocytes and giant cells with sparse peripheral lymphocytes. Common laboratory abnormalities include hypercalcemia and an elevated angiotensin-converting enzyme level. Conventional first-line treatments include oral antimalarial agents, methotrexate, and corticosteroids. A wide range of additional therapeutic interventions are based largely on anecdotal evidence.

Granuloma Annulare

Granuloma annulare (GA) presents typically as acrally distributed, flesh-colored to red, nonscaling macules or papules before the third decade of life; atypical forms are more common in the elderly.

No clear etiology has been determined, but associations with trauma, various infections, arthropod bites, and systemic diseases (including diabetes mellitus) have been described. Differentiation from lymphoma may be challenging because the two conditions may coexist. Key studies include biopsy showing a paucity of lymphocytes, a lack of epidermotropism, and dermal mucin within palisading granulomas. In addition, lesions of GA tend to be a consistent color, whereas lymphoma demonstrates multiple reddish hues in the same lesion. GA has a chronic, indolent course and may persist for years. Localized lesions can be treated with topical or intralesional steroids or calcineurin inhibitors such as tacrolimus or pimecrolimus. Conversely, generalized GA is typically treated by PUVA or systemic vitamin A analogues. Long-term follow-up is essential because GA very rarely may evolve into lymphoma.

Venous Stasis Ulcers

A nonhealing venous stasis ulcer on the leg may mimic cutaneous diffuse large B-cell lymphoma, leg type, because both present with ulceration on the distal aspect of one leg. Venous stasis ulcers tend to present on the distal portion of the leg, immediately above the ankles. Treatment includes leg elevation, reduction of accompanying edema with pressure stockings, wet to dry or hydrocolloid dressings to the wound, and judicious débridement. Skin grafts may be indicated. The diagnosis of cutaneous diffuse large B-cell lymphoma, leg type, is suggested when additional signs of venous insufficiency (prominent varicose veins, hemosiderin-induced hyperpigmentation, and thickening/hardening of the peri-lesional skin) are absent.

NEUTROPHIL-RICH PSEUDOLYMPHOMAS (TABLE 15-8)

Bacterial Infections

The initial presentation of a variety of superficial bacterial infections may occasionally mimic cutaneous lymphoma. All of these entities are typically rich in neutrophils, as appropriate for a bacterial infection. The treatment of cellulitis, erysipelas, furuncles, and folliculitis requires oral antibiotic therapy targeted toward the most likely bacterial cause and should be modified based on antibiotic sensitivities obtained at the time of culture. For furuncles, incision and drainage is the most important therapeutic intervention. Although such infections are only rarely mistaken for cutaneous lymphoma, clinical clues suggestive of the

TABLE 15-8   Common Bacterial Infections Mimicking Cutaneous Lymphoma

Disease	Clinical Presentation	Location	Lymphoma Mimic(s)	Common Organism(s) and Treatment Options
Cellulitis	Red, hot, edematous, painful plaque with ill defined border preceded by fever, chills, and malaise	Head, extremities	Primary cutaneous T-cell lymphoma Primary cutaneous B-cell lymphoma	MSSA: dicloxacillin MRSA: doxycycline GAS-penicillin V
Erysipelas	Dark red, hot plaque with sharp borders; spreading by peripheral extension Associated painful lymphadenopathy	Legs, face	Intravascular large B-cell lymphoma	GAS-penicillin V

(continued)

TABLE 15-8   Common Bacterial Infections Mimicking Cutaneous Lymphoma (continued)

Disease	Clinical Presentation	Location	Lymphoma Mimic(s)	Common Organism(s) and Treatment Options
Furuncle	Firm tender nodules < 2 cm, that become fluctuant with abscess formation	Beard, neck, axillae, trunk, buttocks	Primary cutaneous T-cell lymphoma Primary cutaneous B-cell lymphoma	MSSA: dicloxacillin MRSA: doxycycline or trimethoprim-sulfamethoxazole
Folliculitis	Erythematous papules or pustules	Beard, neck, axillae, trunk, buttocks	Lymphomatoid papulosis	MSSA: dicloxacillin MRSA: doxycycline or trimethoprim-sulfamethoxazole *Pseudomonas aeruginosa:* ciprofloxacin

GAS, group A β-hemolytic *Streptococci;* MRSA, methicillin-resistant *Staphylococcus aureus;* MSSA, methicillin-sensitive *Staphylococcus aureus.*

latter include lack of warmth and/or pain on palpation, unresponsiveness to proper systemic antibiotics, and negative cultures.

MISCELLANEOUS BENIGN DERMATOSES ACTING AS PSEUDOLYMPHOMAS (TABLE 15-9)

Localized Pagetoid Reticulosis

The localized subtype of pagetoid reticulosis known as Woringer-Kollop disease is a diagnostic challenge given its clinical and histologic similarities to MF. It presents typically as an acrally distributed erythematous, scaling, infiltrated plaque with sharp margins. Distinguishing factors include its prominent demarcation because MF is often poorly circumscribed. Furthermore, the degree of epidermotropism in Woringer-Kollop greatly exceeds that of MF, largely owing to a high expression of alpha E beta 7. Infiltrating cells can often present with monoclonality, cellular atypia, and loss of pan-T-cell markers, which complicates the diagnosis; however, absence of CD45 expression, which is crucial for lymphocyte growth and

transformation, accounts for the benign clinical course of this disease. Spontaneous regression of the cutaneous lesion may occur, although many cases persist for years or even decades. Surgery and radiotherapy are curative in most cases. Ultrapotent topical or systemic corticosteroids may also be used.

Ecthyma Contagiosum

Ecthyma contagiosum (orf) is a zoonotic parapoxvirus infection requiring contact with infected animals, particularly sheep and goats. Therefore, lesions commonly affect farmers, butchers, and others who are routinely in contact with farm animals. Several reports suggest orf is common among Muslim populations as well, citing the sacrifice of lambs in various religious practices. Lesions progress through six stages and are large and painful. Hand involvement is most common, but facial lesions can also be seen. Detection of parapoxvirus by PCR and characteristic histologic findings (hyperkeratosis with epidermal cell vacuolization and eosinophilic intracytoplasmic inclusions) are suggestive of the proper diagnosis. In the vast majority of individuals, the disease course is self-limited with resolution in 6 to 8 weeks.

TABLE 15-9 Miscellaneous Benign Pseudolymphomas

Pseudolymphoma	Cutaneous Lymphoma	Differentiating Features
Woringer-Kollop disease	Mycosis fungoides	Sharp demarcation of lesion CD8+-heavy infiltrate with alpha E beta 7 expression and loss of CD45 and greater degree of epidermotropism than mycosis fungoides
Ecthyma contagiosum (orf)	CD30+ lymphoma lymphomatoid papulosis	Contact with infected animals Detection of parapoxvirus Characteristic hyperkeratosis and cell vacuolization with eosinophilic intracytoplasmic inclusions in superficial epidermis
Molluscum contagiosum	Mycosis fungoides CD30+ lymphoma	Molluscum contagiosum bodies on biopsy
Kimura's disease	Hodgkin's lymphoma (skin)	Reactive follicular infiltrate with central hyalinization from IgE deposition on biopsy
	Peripheral T-cell lymphoma	Eosinophilia Elevated serum IgE
Castleman's disease	Diffuse large B-cell lymphoma	"Lollipop on a stick" on biopsy Detection of lesional HHV-8
Cutis laxa	Granulomatous slack skin	Lack of malignant cells on biopsy Genetic analysis
	Primary cutaneous T-cell lymphoma	History of sun exposure with progressive intolerance
Polymorphic light eruption	Primary cutaneous B-cell lymphoma	Positive phototesting Intense itching

HHV-8, human herpesvirus-8; IgE, immunoglobulin E.

Immunocompromised hosts are at increased risk for persistent or recurring lesions. Treatment options include imiquimod, cryotherapy, and antivirals. Excision followed by split skin grafting may be required for very large or persistent lesions. In a small number of patients, amputation is performed to prevent further disease spread.

Molluscum Contagiosum

Molluscum contagiosum is a poxvirus infection presenting as well-defined, small pearly papules with a central umbilication. Following trauma to these lesions, rupture occurs, spewing forth molluscum bodies into the dermis. This leads to a florid localized CD4+ or CD30+ lymphocytosis. Clinically, this results in larger and more erythematous lesions that may suggest lymphoma. Atypical presentations leading to a lymphoma mimics are often associated with immunosuppression and facial/head involvement. Reports of molluscum contagiosum arising within lesions of MF further convolute this picture, providing a particularly difficult challenge to the clinician. The correct diagnosis requires histologic evaluation demonstrating molluscum bodies surrounded by a heterogeneous, reactive, and non-neoplastic infiltrate. Surgical excision of these lesions is curative. Use of topical immune response modifiers, such as imiquimod, is variably successful.

Kimura's disease presents as nontender, poorly circumscribed, gradually stiffening masses, occasionally associated with pigmentation and itching. It is most commonly seen in the periauricular, inguinal, epicranial, and orbital regions of young Asian men. Twelve percent to 16% of patients have associated nephrotic syndrome. Lymphadenopathy and salivary gland involvement may suggest lymphoma; however, histologic examination showing follicular hyperplasia with hyalinized central IgE deposition and a prominence of eosinophils and mast cells in the serum and lesions points toward the correct diagnosis. This is a particularly important distinction to make because Kimura's disease lacks malignant potential and may persist for decades. It appears that radiotherapy is superior to local excision or steroid treatment. Imatinib and cyclosporine also appear effective.

Castleman's Disease

Cutaneous involvement in Castleman's disease, also known as angiofollicular lymph node hyperplasia, is uncommon, but presents as nodules and plaques. The correct diagnosis may be difficult owing to this condition's association with HIV, human herpesvirus-8 (HHV-8), and hepatitis C virus (HCV) infections, all of which may be associated with cutaneous lymphoma. Ninety percent of localized cutaneous lesions exhibit a "lollipop on a stick" histologic picture, in which sclerotic blood vessels enter hyalinized lymphoid follicles. Conversely, 10% will exhibit a more variable degree of vascular proliferation with sheets of plasma cells infiltrating the mass. Surgical excision is curative for single lesions; however, no effective therapy has been discovered for generalized, multicentric disease. As a result, these patients have a median survival of 48 months after diagnosis despite the use of systemic chemotherapy, steroids, interferons, and rituximab. Long-term follow-up is particularly important in HIV-infected patients because the incidence of non-Hodgkin's lymphoma subsequent to Castleman's disease is 15 times higher than in the general population.

Cutis Laxa

Cutis laxa is rare condition marked by wrinkled, redundant, inelastic, and sagging skin. Most cases are acquired; however, congenital forms may be inherited in an autosomal dominant, recessive, or X-linked manner. Granulomatous slack skin, a subtype of cutaneous T-cell lymphoma, must be ruled out. This is accomplished via a skin biopsy showing the lack of a malignant cellular infiltrates, normal collagen fibers, and a marked deficit of elastic fibers. Surgical repair is currently the best treatment option for cutis laxa and may provide important psychological benefit to the patient. Unfortunately, benefits are variable and temporary.

Polymorphic Light Eruption

Polymorphic light eruption is the most common photodermatosis, affecting 10% to 20% of people in the Europe and the United States. Ninety percent of cases are due to exposure to the UVA spectrum of radiation. Cutaneous lesions are heterogeneous, presenting as macular, papular, papulovesicular, urticarial, multiforme, or plaquelike lesions. Distinguishing features include severe pruritus as well as the predominance of a single morphology in any given patient. Lesions may occur at any age and anywhere on the skin; however, routinely sun-exposed regions are the most common locations. It is important to distinguish this mimic from cutaneous lymphoma. The history is the most important diagnostic tool in these patients. Lesions develop typically in the spring and early summer, but not later in the season, a characteristic attributed to the development of photoresistance over time. Upon cessation of sun exposure, lesions completely resolve within days and without residual. Therefore, this is considered the primary treatment. However, prolonged, chronic PUVA and UVB therapy may induce tolerance. Topical steroids may accelerate remission and antihistamines may reduce pruritus. Topical sunscreen is largely ineffective because UVA sensitivity thresholds are often too low; however, topical sunscreen is beneficial when the disease action spectrum lies within the UVA range.

MALIGNANT DISORDERS ACTING AS PSEUDOLYMPHOMA (TABLES 15-10 AND 15-11)

Neoplastic cells from systemic malignancies, including leukemias, lymphomas, and visceral metastasis, may invade the skin producing skin lesions resembling cutaneous lymphoma. However, systemic symptoms, physical examination findings, and routine blood work, in conjunction with

TABLE 15-10   Leukemia Cutis Mimicking Primary Cutaneous Lymphoma

Systemic Leukemia	Cutaneous Lymphoma Mimic
Acute myelomonocytic or monocytic leukemia	Primary cutaneous marginal zone B-cell lymphoma
Chronic myeloid leukemia	Any primary cutaneous T-cell or B-cell lymphoma
Adult T-cell leukemia	Mycosis fungoides
	Sézary's syndrome
Acute granulocytic (myelocytic) leukemia	Primary cutaneous marginal zone B-cell lymphoma
	Lymphomatoid papulosis
Chronic lymphocytic leukemia, T-cell type	Sézary syndrome
Chronic lymphocytic leukemia, B-cell type	Primary cutaneous CD4+ small/medium-sized pleomorphic T-cell lymphoma

TABLE 15-11   Systemic B-Cell Lymphomas, Lymphoproliferative Diseases, and Monoclonal Gammopathies Simulating Primary Cutaneous Lymphoma

Systemic Lymphoid Neoplasm	Cutaneous Lymphoma Mimic	Unique features of mimic
Waldenström's macroglobulinemia	Any primary cutaneous B-cell or T-cell lymphoma	Lymphadenopathy Hepatosplenomegaly Epistaxis
Lymphomatoid granulomatosis	Subcutaneous panniculitis-like T-cell lymphoma Cutaneous γ/δ T-cell lymphoma Extranodal NK/T-cell lymphoma, nasal type	Pulmonary manifestations with constitutional symptoms
Mantle cell lymphoma	Any primary cutaneous B-cell or T-cell lymphoma	Lymphadenopathy Hepatosplenomegaly Bone marrow involved Aggressive course
Follicular lymphoma	Primary cutaneous follicle center B-cell lymphoma	Lymphadenopathy
Marginal zone B-cell lymphoma	Primary cutaneous marginal zone B-cell lymphoma	Lymphadenopathy Splenomegaly

NK, natural killer.

a skin biopsy, will readily differentiate between the two in the large majority of cases.

Metastases from Visceral Malignancies

Cutaneous metastases from visceral malignancies occur in approximately 5% of cases. Such lesions are most often red, hard, and hairless and, thus, may mimic cutaneous lymphoma (Figure 15-8). This is especially true when multiple metastatic lesions are present. Whereas metastases tend to occur in relatively close proximity to the primary cancer, the chest, abdomen and scalp are the most common locations. Breast cancer is by far the most common cutaneous metastasis, followed by lung, colorectal, renal, and ovarian cancers.

Leukemia

Leukemia has been associated with a wide variety of cutaneous manifestations, including infiltration

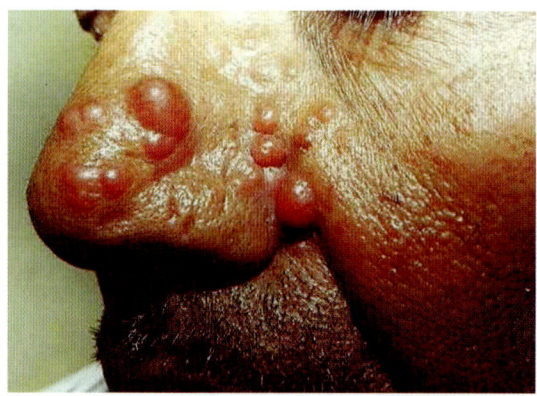

Figure 15-8 Visceral metastases mimic cutaneous lymphoma.

of neoplastic cells into the skin, referred to as *leukemia cutis* (Figure 15-9). The most common types of leukemia cutis that can mimic lymphoma and the corresponding lymphoma(s) they mimic are listed in Table 15-10. Histopathologically, leukemia cutis is characterized by a diffuse monomorphous infiltrate of leukemic cells involving the dermis and subcutaneous tissue. Leukemia cutis, which carries a grim prognosis, almost invariably occurs in patients previously diagnosed with leukemia, and most have both characteristic signs and symptoms (e.g., pallor, purpura and ecchymoses, dyspnea on exertion) and easily detected peripheral blood abnormalities.

Systemic B-Cell Lymphoma

Several of the systemic B-cell lymphomas, lymphoproliferative diseases, and monoclonal

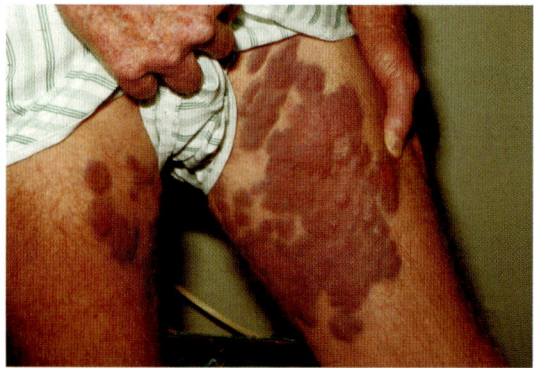

Figure 15-9 Extensive chronic granulocytic leukemia cutis mimics lymphoma.

gammopathies can involve the skin and mimic primary cutaneous lymphoma. The lymphoid neoplasms that commonly mimic cutaneous lymphoma, the corresponding lymphoma(s) mimic, and features unique to the systemic mimicker are listed in Table 15-11. A definitive diagnosis is obtained through biopsy, with the exception of follicular lymphoma and marginal zone B-cell lymphoma, in which a systemic evaluation must be done.

Angiosarcoma

Cutaneous angiosarcoma is an extremely malignant neoplasm of endothelial derivation and provides an example of a cutaneous malignancy mimicking lymphoma. This tumor commonly presents as a poorly defined, bruiselike lesion progressing to a purplish-colored, infiltrative plaque or nodule on the face or scalp of elderly patients. It mimics the clinical appearance of primary cutaneous follicle center B-cell lymphoma. Treatment of cutaneous angiosarcoma consists of wide surgical excision and palliative radiation; however, the 5-year survival rate is less than 15%.

Both B-cell and T-cell primary cutaneous lymphomas have widely variable and overlapping clinical presentations and, therefore, may mimic each other. As an example, tumor stage MF may look like primary cutaneous B-cell lymphoma and vice versa. Either of these may resemble primary cutaneous CD30+ lymphoma.

SELECTED MORPHOLOGIES WITH LYMPHOMA IN THE DIFFERENTIAL DIAGNOSIS (TABLES 15-12 AND 15-13)

Hypopigmented Patch

Hypopigmented MF is seen primarily in children and adolescents as well as dark-complected adult patients. This uncommon variant presents with hypopigmented patches. The most common dermatoses presenting in a similar manner and thereby potentially mimicking hypopigmented MF are listed in Table 15-12, including location, differentiating points, biopsy, and treatment options. Epidemiologic factors are of little

TABLE 15-12   Hypopigmented Patches Mimicking Hypopigmented Mycosis Fungoides

Disease	Location	Differentiating points	Biopsy or Scraping	Therapy
Pityriasis (tinea) versicolor	Chest, back, shoulders	More common in warm, humid weather	Budding yeast or hyphae	Oral or topical ketoconazole
Tuberculoid leprosy	Variable; localized and asymmetrical	Endemic countries	Perineural granulomatous infiltrate	Dapsone plus rifampin and clofazimine
		Decreased sensation on lesions	Paucibacillary	
Pityriasis alba	Face, arms, shoulders	Coexisting atopic dermatitis	Loss of melanin	Emollient and low-potency topical steroid
Vitiligo	Eyes, lips, digits, groin, elbows, knees	Positive family history	Absence of melanocytes	Phototherapy
		Complete loss of pigment with sharp borders and follicular macules of repigmentation		Topical calcineurin inhibitors
Hypopigmented sarcoidosis	Face, extremities	Hilar lymphadenopathy	Dermal noncaseating granulomas	Antimalarials
		Elevated ACE		Methotrexate
		Hypercalcemia		Oral steroids
				Topical steroids
Postinflammatory hypopigmentation	Variable	Caused by many inflammatory dermatoses	Variable	Benign neglect
		Any age		

ACE, angiotensin-converting enzyme.

TABLE 15-13   Subcutaneous Nodules That May Mimic Cutaneous Lymphoma

Diseases	Location	Distinguishing Features	Epidemiology
Erythema nodosum	Bilateral shins	No ulceration, spontaneously resolves in 6 wk Fever and arthralgias common Etiologies include infections, medications, and autoimmune disorders	Mostly females
Erythema induratum	Bilateral posterior lower legs	Ulceration is common Association with *Mycobacterium tuberculosis* infection	Mostly females
Inflamed epidermal cyst	Face, neck, upper trunk	History of thick white discharge from lesion; typically size < 5 cm	Young to middle-aged adults
Lupus panniculitis	Head, upper arms	Associated arthralgia/arthritis Positive ANA and anti-dsDNA	Mostly females
Superficial thrombophlebitis	Legs	Single nodule with a palpable cord, warmth, and surrounding redness	More females

ANA, antinuclear antibody.

help because most of these lymphoma simulators also tend to affect children, adolescents, and dark-skinned adult patients. Pityriasis versicolor is seen mainly in young adults as hypopigmented macules and patches on the upper body during hot or humid weather. Tuberculoid leprosy is rare outside of endemic regions and is almost always accompanied by decreased sensation on the lesions and extremities. Pityriasis alba is mostly seen on the face and upper extremities in the setting of concomitant atopic dermatitis. Lesions of vitiligo have distinct borders and are depigmented (complete loss of pigment) rather than hypopigmented. Hypopigmented sarcoidosis can be differentiated from cutaneous lymphoma by the presence of extracutaneous disease-specific manifestations.

Subcutaneous Nodule

Any disease resulting in a hard, deep, slightly movable lump may mimic those cutaneous lymphomas that involve the subcutaneous fat. Most notably, subcutaneous panniculitis-like T-cell lymphoma, cutaneous γ?δ T-cell lymphoma, and intravascular large B-cell lymphoma should be considered in the differential diagnosis of this general morphology.

Table 15-13 lists some examples of benign causes of subcutaneous nodules, along with their typical location and distinguishing features. However, there are many other potential causes of subcutaneous nodules that are beyond the scope of this text. Perhaps the most common cause of a subcutaneous nodule mimicking cutaneous lymphoma is superficial thrombophlebitis; however, the presence of a palpable cord strongly suggests the proper etiology. In the presence of subcutaneous nodules, clinical clues to a diagnosis of cutaneous lymphomas are generalized/multifocal lesions, the presence of overlying telangiectasias, or the development of hemophagocytic syndrome; which results in coagulopathies, cytopenias, and hepatosplenomegaly. By contrast, features suggesting a benign cause include head or neck distribution, localized lesions, and associated joint pain.

SUGGESTED READINGS

General Subject of Pseudolymphoma

Bergman R. Pseudolymphoma and cutaneous lymphoma: facts and controversies. *Clin Dermatol.* 2010; 28:568–574.

Gilliam A, Wood G. Cutaneous lymphoid hyperplasias. *Semin Cutan Med Surg.* 2000;19:133–141.

Minakshi N, Mikkola D, Horvath N, Gilliam A, Stevens S, Spiro T, et al. Cutaneous lymphoid hyperplasia: a lymphoproliferative continuum with lymphomatous potential. *Hum Pathol.* 2003;34:617–622.

Nashan D, Faulhaber D, Stander S, Luger TA, Stadler R. Mycosis fungoides: a dermatological masquerader. *Br J Dermatol.* 2007;156:1–10.

Ploysangam T, Breneman D, Mutasim D. Cutaneous pseudolymphomas. *J Am Acad Dermatol.* 1998;38: 877–905.

Specific Disease States

B-Cell–rich Pseudolymphoma

Albrecht S, Hofstadter S, Artsob H, Chaban O, From R, From L. Lymphadenosis benigna cutis resulting from *Borrelia* infection (*Borrelia* lymphoctyoma). *J Am Acad Dermatol.* 1991;24:621–625.

Aram G, Rohwedder A, Nazeer T, Shoss R, Fisher A, Carlson J. Varicella-zoster-virus folliculitis promoted clonal cutaneous lymphoid hyperplasia. *Am J Dermatopathol.* 2005;27:411–417.

Cerroni L, Borroni R, Massone C, Chott A, Kerl H. Cutaneous B-cell pseudolymphoma at the site of vaccination. *Am J Dermatopathol.* 2007;29:538–542.

Chong H, Brady K, Metze D, Calonje E. Persistent nodules at injection sites (aluminum granuloma)—clinicopathological study of 14 cases with a diverse range of histological reaction patterns. *Histopathology.* 2006;48:182–188.

Colli C, Leinweber B, Müllegger R, Chott A, Kerl H, Cerroni L. *Borrelia burgdorferi*–associated lymphocytoma cutis: clinicopathologic, immunophenotypic, and molecular study of 106 cases. *J Cutan Pathol.* 2004;31:232–240.

Maubec E, Pinquier L, Viguier M, Caux F, Amsler E, Aractingi S, et al. Vaccination-induced cutaneous pseudolymphoma. *J Am Acad Dermatol.* 2005;52:623–629.

Porto D, Comfere N, Myers L, Abbott J. Pseudolymphomatous reaction to varicella zoster virus vaccination: role of viral in situ hybridization. *J Cutan Pathol.* 2010;37:1098–1102.

Requena L, Kutzner H, Escalonilla P, Ortiz S, Schaller J, Rohwedder A. Cutaneous reactions at sites of herpes zoster scars: an expanded spectrum. *Brit J Dermatol.* 1998;138:161–168.

T-Cell–rich Pseudolymphoma

Bakels V, Oostveen J, Preesman A, Meijer C, Willemze R. Differentiation between actinic reticuloid and cutaneous T cell lymphoma by T cell receptor ? gene rearrangement analysis and immunophenotyping. *J Clin Pathol.* 1998;51:154–158.

Belousova I, Vanecek T, Samtsov A, Michal M, Kazakov D. A patient with clinicopathologic features of small plaque parapsoriasis presenting later with plaque-stage mycosis fungoides: report of a case and comparative retrospective study of 27 cases of "nonprogressive" small plaque parapsoriasis. *J Am Acad Dermatol.* 2008;59: 474–482.

Choi T, Doh K, Kim S, Jang M, Suh K, Kim S. Clinicopathological and genotypic aspects of anticonvulsant-induced pseudolymphoma syndrome. *Brit J Dermatol.* 2003;148:730–736.

Guitart J, Variakojis D, Kuzel T, Rosen S. Cutaneous CD8+ T cell infiltrates in advanced HIV infection. *J Am Acad Dermatol.* 1999;41:722–727.

Gül Ü, Kiliç A, Dursun A. Carbamazepine-induced pseudo mycosis fungoides. *Ann Pharmacother.* 2003; 37:1441–1443.

Hanna S, Walsh N, D'Intino Y, Langley R. Mycosis fungoides presenting as pigmented purpuric dermatitis. *Pediatr Dermatol.* 2006;23:350–354.

Hoesly F, Huerter C, Shehan J. Purpura annularis telangiectodes of Majocchi: case report and review of the literature. *Int J Dermatol.* 2009;49:1129–1133.

Kazakov D, Belousova I, Kacerovska D, Sima R, Vanecek T, Vazmitel M, et al. Hyperplasia of hair follicles and other adnexal structures in cutaneous lymphoproliferative disorders: a study of 53 cases, including so-called pseudolymphomatous folliculitis and overt lymphomas. *Am J Surg Pathol.* 2008;32:1468–1478.

Kluger N, Vermeulen C, Moguelet P, Cotten H, Koeb M, Balme B, et al. Cutaneous lymphoid hyperplasia (pseudolymphoma) in tattoos: a case series of seven patients. *J Eur Acad Derm Venereol.* 2010;24:208–213.

Lee H, Ahn S, Lee M, Choi J, Moon K, Koh J. A case of pseudolymphomatous folliculitis. *J Eur Acad Derm Venereol.* 2006;20:230–231.

Muche J, Toppe E, Sterry W, Haas N. Palpable arciform migratory erythema in an HIV patient, a CD8+ pseudolymphoma. *J Cutan Pathol.* 2004;31:379–382.

Ugajin T, Satoh T, Tokozeki H, Nishioka K. Mycosis fungoides presenting as pigmented purpuric eruption. *Eur J Dermatol.* 2005;15: 489–491.

Väkevä L, Sarna S, Vaalasti A, Pukkala E, Kariniemi A, Ranki A. A retrospective study of the probability of evolution of parapsoriasis en plaques into mycosis fungoides. *Acta Derm Venereol.* 2005;85:318–323.

Vandermaesen J, Roelandts R, Degreef H. Light on the persistent light reaction–photosensitivity dermatitis—actinic reticuloid syndrome. *J Am Acad Dermatol.* 1986;15: 685–692.

Walton S, Bottomley W, Wyatt E, Bury H. Pseudo T-cell lymphoma due to scabies in a patient with Hodgkin's disease. *Br J Dermatol.* 1991;124:277–278.

Wilkins K, Turner R, Dolev J, LeBoit P, Berger T, Maurer T. Cutaneous malignancy and human immunodeficiency virus disease. *J Am Acad Dermatol.* 2006;54: 189–206.

Mixed Cell Type Pseudolymphoma

Arai E, Shimizu M, Tsuchida T, Izaki S, Ogawa F, Hirose T. Lymphomatoid keratosis: an epidermotropic type of cutaneous lymphoid hyperplasia: clinico-pathological, immunohistochemical, and molecular biological study of 6 cases. *Arch Dermatol.* 2007;143: 53–59.

Chedraoui A, Malek J, Tamraz H, Zaynoun S, Kibbi A, Ghosn S. Acral pseudolymphomatous angiokeratoma of children in an elderly man: report of a case and review of the literature. *Int J Dermatol.* 2010;49:184–188.

Conde-Taboada A, Rosón E, Fernández-Redondo V, García-Doval I, De La Torre C, Cruces M. Lymphomatoid contact dermatitis induced by gold earrings. *Contact Dermatitis.* 2007;56:179–181.

Esparza E, Takeshita J, George E. Lymphomatoid hypersensitivity reaction to levofloxacin during autologous stem cell transplantation: a potential diagnostic pitfall in patients treated for lymphoma or leukemia. *J Cutan Pathol.* 2011;38:33–37.

Flaig M, Rupec R. Cutaneous pseudolymphoma in association with *Leishmania donovani*. *Br J Dermatol.* 2007;157:1042–1043.

Friss A, Cohen P, Bruce S, Duvic M. Chronic cutaneous lupus erythematosus mimicking mycosis fungoides. *J Am Acad Dermatol.* 1995;33: 891–895.

Hagari Y, Hagari S, Kambe N, Kawaguchi T, Nakamoto S, Mihara M. Acral pseudolymphomatous angiokeratoma of children: immunohistochemical and clonal analyses of the infiltrating cells. *J Cutan Pathol.* 2002;29:313–318.

Hodak E, David M, Rothem A, Bialowance M, Sandbank M. Nodular secondary syphilis mimicking cutaneous lymphoreticular process. *J Am Acad Dermatol.* 1987;17:914–917.

Kim K, Lee M, Choi J, Sung K, Moon K, Koh J. CD30-positive T-cell-rich pseudolymphoma induced by gold acupuncture. *Br J Dermatol* 2002;146:882–884.

Macro C, Cruz-Inigo A, Votava H, Jacobs M, Wolfe D, Crowson A. Drug-associated reversible granulomatous T cell dyscrasia: A distinct subset of the interstitial granulomatous drug reaction. *J Cutan Pathol.* 2010;37:96–111.

Martínez-Morá C, Sanz-Muñoz C, Morales-Callaghan A, Garrido-Ríos A, Torrero V, Miranda-Romero A. Lymphomatoid contact dermatitis. *Contact Dermatitis.* 2009;60:53–55.

Moon H, Park K, Hyunkyung J, Son S. A nodular syphilid presenting as a pseudolymphoma: mimicking a cutaneous marginal zone B-cell lymphoma. *Am J Dermatopathol.* 2009;31:846–848.

Park Y, Kang H, Kim H, Cho B. Lymphomatoid eosinophilic reaction to gold earrings. *Contact Dermatitis.* 1999;40:216.

Recalcati S, Vezzoli P, Girgenti V, Venegoni L, Veraldi S, Berti E. Cutaneous lymphoid hyperplasia associated with *Leishmania panamensis* infection. *Acta Derm Venereol.* 2010;90:418–419.

Tallon B, Kaddu S, Cerroni L, Kerl H, Aberer E. Pseudolymphomatous tumid lupus erythematosus of the oral mucosa. *Am J Dermatopathol.* 2010;32: 704–707.

Welsh J, Ko C, Hsu W. Lymphomatoid drug reaction secondary to methylphenidate hydrochloride. *Cutis.* 2008;81:61–64.

Lymphocyte-poor Pseudolymphoma

Akhyani M, Ghodsi Z, Toosi S, Dabbaghian H. Erythroderma: a clinical study of 97 cases. *BMC Dermatol.* 2005;5:5.

Crum N. Disseminated coccidioidomycosis with cutaneous lesions clinically mimicking mycosis fungoides. *Int J Dermatol.* 2005;44:958–960.

Diette K, Caro W, Roenigk H. Malignant lymphoma presenting with cutaneous granulomas. *J Am Acad Dermatol.* 1984;10:896–902

Fierro M, Novelli M, Quaglino P, Comessatti A, Fava P, Ortoncelli M, et al. Heterogeneity of circulating CD4+ memory T-cell subsets in erythrodermic patients: CD27 analysis can help to distinguish cutaneous T-cell lymphomas from inflammatory erythroderma. *Dermatology.* 2008;216:213–221.

Frankel A, Penrose C, Emer J. Cutaneous tuberculosis: a practical case report and review for the dermatologist. *J Clin Aesthet Dermatol.* 2009;10:19–27.

Gutte R, Kharkar V, Mahajan S, Chikhalkar S, Khopkar U. Granulomatous mycosis fungoides with hypohidrosis mimicking lepromatous leprosy. *Ind J Dermatol Venereol Leprol.* 2010;76:686–690.

Katta R. Cutaneous sarcoidosis: a dermatologic masquerader. *Am Fam Physician.* 2002;65:1581–1584.

Kawakami T, Kawanabe T, Soma Y. Granuloma annulare–like skin lesions as an initial manifestation in a Japanese patient with adult T-cell leukemia/lymphoma. *J Am Acad Dermatol.* 2009;60:848–852.

Li A, Hogan D, Sanusi I, Smoller B. Granuloma annulare and malignant neoplasms. *Am J Dermatopathol.* 2003;25:113–116.

Loehberg L, Simon M. Granulomatous slack skin clinically and histologically masquerading as borderline leprosy in its early stages. *Eur J Dermatol.* 2009; 19:88–89.

Mainguene C, Picard O, Audouin J, Le Tourneau A, Jagueux M, Diebold J. An unusual case of mycosis fungoides presenting as sarcoidosis or granulomatous mycosis fungoides. *Am J Clin Pathol.* 1993;99: 82–86.

Röglin J, Boer A. Skin manifestations of intravascular lymphoma mimic inflammatory diseases of the skin. *Br J Dermatol.* 2007;157:16–25.

Stopajnik N, Zgavec B, Luzar B, Leskovec NK. An uncommon case of chronic leg ulcers in an 80-year-old woman. *Acta Dermatolvenerol Alp Panonica Adriat.* 2010;19:17–20.

Wu H, Barusevicius A, Lessin S. Granuloma annulare with a mycosis fungoides–like distribution and palisaded granulomas of CD68-positive histiocytes. *J Am Acad Dermatol.* 2004;51:39–44.

Yeung C, Ma S, Chan H, Trandell-Smith N, Au W. Primary CD30+ cutaneous T-cell lymphoma associated with chronic burn injury in a patient with long-standing psoriasis. *Am J Dermatopathol.* 2004;26: 394–396.

Miscellaneous Benign Pseudolymphomas

Al-Salam S, Nowotny N, Sohail M, Kolodziejek J, Berger T. Ecthyma contagiosum (orf)—report of a human case from the United Arab Emirates and review of the literature. *J Cutan Pathol.* 2008;35:603–607.

Duasn S, Zoran B, Sonja V, Jelica V, Mirjana G, Ljiljana M. Pagetoid reticulosis of Woringer-Kolopp. *Dermatol Online J.* 2008;14:18.

González J, Sanz A, Martín T, Samaniego E, Martínez S, Crespo V. Cutaneous pseudolymphoma associated with molluscum contagiosum: a case report. *Int J Dermatol.* 2008;47:502–504.

Lee J, Viakhireva N, Cesca C, Lee P, Kohler S, Hoppe R, et al. Clinicopathologic features and treatment outcomes in Woringer-Kolopp disease. *J Am Acad Dermatol.* 2008;59:706–712.

Lehmann P, Schwarz T. Photodermatoses: diagnosis and treatment. *Dtsch Arztebl Int.* 2011;108:135–141.

Lobo C, Amin S, Ramsay A, Diss T, Kocjan G. Serous fluid cytology and multicentric Castleman's disease and other lymphoproliferative disorders associated with Kaposi sarcoma–associated herpes virus: a review with case reports. *Cytopathology.* Epub ahead of print 2011;June 9.

Madan R, Chen J, Trotman-Dickenson B, Jacobson F, Hunsaker A. The spectrum of Castleman's disease: mimics, radiologic pathologic correlation and role of imaging in patient management. *Eur J Radiol.* Epub ahead of print 2010;July 17.

Mohamed M, Kouwenberg D, Gardeitchik T, Kornak U, Wevers R, Morava E. Metabolic cutis laxa syndromes. *J Inherit Metab Dis.* 2011;34:907–916.

Moreno-Ramírez D, García-Escudero A, Ríos-Martín J, Herrera-Saval A, Camacho F. Cutaneous pseudolymphoma in association with molluscum contagiosum in an elderly patient. *J Cutan Pathol.* 2003;30: 473–475.

Riveros C, Gavilán, França L, Sotto M, Takahashi M. Acquired localized cutis laxa confined to the face: case report and review of the literature. *Int J Derm.* 2004;43:931–935.

Rose C, Starostik P, Bröcker E. Infection with parapoxvirus induces CD30-positive cutaneous infiltrates in humans. *J Cutan Pathol.* 1999;26:520–522.

Sun Q, Xu D, Pan S, Ding J, Zue Z, Miao C, et al. Kimura disease: review of the literature. *Intern Med J.* 2008;38:668–674.

Malignant Pseudolymphoma

Beaty MW, Toro J, Sorbara L, Stern JB, Pittaluga S, Raffeld M. Cutaneous lymphomatoid granulomatosis: correlation of clinical and biologic features. *Am J Surg Pathol.* 2001;25:1111–1120.

Bittencourt AL, Barbosa HS, Vieira MD, Farre L. Adult T-cell leukemia/lymphoma (ATL) presenting in the skin: clinical, histological and immunohistochemical features of 52 cases. *Acta Oncologica.* 2009;48:598–604.

Gerami P, Wickles SC, Querfeld C, Rosen ST, Kuzel TM, Guitart J. Cutaneous involvement with marginal zone lymphoma. *J Am Acad Dermatol.* 2010;63: 142–145.

Kim BK, Surti U, Pandya A, Cohen J, Rabkin MS, Swerdlow SH. Clinicopathologic, immunophenotypic, and molecular cytogenetic fluorescence in situ hybridization analysis of primary and secondary cutaneous follicular lymphomas. *Am J Surg Pathol.* 2005;29:69–82.

Krathen RA, Orengo IF, Rosen T. Cutaneous metastasis: a meta-analysis of data. *South Med J.* 2003;96:164–167.

Libow LF, Mawhinney JP, Bessinger GT. Cutaneous Waldenström's macroglobulinemia: report of a case and overview of the spectrum of cutaneous disease. *J Am Acad Dermatol.* 2001;45:S202–S206.

Mallett RB, Matutes E, Catovsky D, Maclennan K, Martimer PS, Holden CA. Cutaneous infiltration in T-cell prolymphocytic leukaemia. *Br J Dermatol.* 1995;132:263–266.

Requena L, Santonja C, Stuz N, Kaddu S, Weenig RH, Kutzner H. Pseudolymphomatous cutaneous angiosarcoma: a rare variant of cutaneous angiosarcoma readily mistaken for cutaneous lymphoma. *Am J Dermatopathol.* 2007;29:342–350.

Su WP, Buechner SA, Li CY. Clinicopathologic correlations in leukemia cutis. *J Am Acad Dermatol.* 1984; 11:121–128.

Selected Morphologic Variant Pseudolymphoma

Gallardo F, Pujol R. Subcutaneous panniculitis-like T-cell lymphoma and other primary cutaneous lymphomas with prominent subcutaneous tissue involvement. *Dermatol Clin.* 2008;26:529–540.

Gilchrist H, Patterson JW. Erythema nodosum and erythema induratum (nodular vasculitis): diagnosis and management. *Dermatol Ther.* 2010;23:320–327.

Hall RS, Floro JF, King LE. Hypopigmented lesions in sarcoidosis. *J Am Acad Dermatol.* 1984;11:1163–1164.

CHAPTER 16

HISTOPATHOLOGIC MIMICS OF CUTANEOUS LYMPHOMA

Antonio Subtil, MD, MBA

INTRODUCTION

The correct diagnosis of cutaneous lymphoma is a clinicopathologic process. Careful correlation of clinical and histopathologic findings is necessary for proper diagnosis and classification. In the absence of clinical information, it is frequently impossible to unequivocally classify individual cases on histomorphologic grounds alone. This often-challenging diagnostic process is further complicated by the heterogeneity and complexity of lymphoma classification schemes as well as by the wide variety and frequency of benign entities that may histologically resemble a lymphoma. These conditions are often termed *pseudolymphomas* or cutaneous reactive lymphoid hyperplasia and may simulate both T-cell and B-cell skin lymphomas. Thorough integration of all of the available data is critical to help prevent erroneous conclusions and adverse clinical consequences. Table 16-1 lists several conditions that may demonstrate histopathologic findings reminiscent of skin lymphoma. In addition to awareness

TABLE 16-1 Entities That May Histopathologically Simulate Cutaneous Lymphoma ("Pseudolymphomas")

Lymphomatoid drug eruption
Cutaneous reactive lymphoid hyperplasia in the setting of viral infection (herpes folliculitis, inflamed molluscum contagiosum, orf, milker's nodule)
Cutaneous leishmaniasis
Syphilis
Borrelia infection
Persistent nodular scabies
Persistent arthropod bite reactions
Exaggerated bite-like reactions in the setting of systemic hematologic disorders
Pseudolymphomatous tattoo reaction
Reactive lymphoid hyperplasia at sites of vaccination
Inflammatory stage of vitiligo
Early stage of lichen sclerosus et atrophicus
Inflammatory stage of morphea
Lymphomatoid lichenoid keratosis
Pigmented purpuric dermatoses
Pityriasis lichenoides
Lupus panniculitis
Pseudolymphomatous variant of cutaneous angiosarcoma
Lymphoepithelioma-like carcinoma of the skin
Merkel cell carcinoma
Acral pseudolymphomatous angiokeratoma in children (APACHE)
Pseudolymphomatous folliculitis
Cutaneous plasmacytosis
CD8+ infiltrates in the setting of advanced AIDS

AIDS, acquired immunodeficiency syndrome.

TABLE 16-2   Suggestions to Help Prevent Misdiagnosis

Be aware of potential histopathologic mimics of skin lymphoma.

Perform more than one biopsy.

Provide adequate clinical information and differential diagnosis to the pathologist (i.e., more information than "rule out skin lymphoma").

Be cognizant of proper biopsy size and technique (e.g., broad biopsy with abundant sampling of the epidermis for suspected patch/plaque stage mycosis fungoides; deeper biopsy for nodular/tumoral lesions).

The correct diagnosis of cutaneous lymphoma is a clinicopathologic process. If the histopathologic changes do not fit the clinical findings, this discrepancy should be addressed and discussed between the clinician and the pathologist.

Consider a second opinion by an expert in skin lymphomas.

Be careful not to overinterpret molecular results. Remember that certain benign skin conditions may demonstrate clonality.

If a clone is identified in an apparently benign condition, consider dual-clonality molecular analysis with comparison of clones from two anatomically distinct skin biopsy sites.

Be careful not to overinterpret a single atypical histopathologic finding. Because prominent density and/or atypical cytology may be seen in pseudolymphomas, it is important to correlate an atypical finding with other criteria to properly diagnose a lymphoma, including aberrant immunophenotype, absence of a mixed inflammatory pattern and/or monoclonality.

Close clinical follow-up and repeat biopsies over time may be necessary for certain indeterminate cases.

about these potential mimics, a few suggestions to help in preventing misdiagnosis are delineated in Table 16-2.

Several of the entities that may simulate cutaneous lymphoma are usually diagnosed by dermatopathologists. In addition, mycosis fungoides (MF), the most common type of skin lymphoma, may exhibit a wide variety of histopathologic patterns and may resemble several types of inflammatory dermatoses (Table 16-3). Therefore, a considerable knowledge of cutaneous pathology is generally necessary to properly differentiate these patterns and potential mimics. General pathologists and hematopathologists may not be very familiar with certain skin disorders such as pityriasis lichenoides, pigmented purpuric dermatosis, or inflammatory stage of vitiligo. In fact, the current Clinical Practice Guidelines for Mycosis Fungoides/Sézary Syndrome from the National Comprehensive Cancer Network require dermatopathology review of the biopsy.

Molecular studies are frequently used in the workup of lymphoid infiltrates. However, the results of molecular genetic studies should not be interpreted in isolation, and their significance must always be determined in relation to the clinical and histopathologic findings. Pitfalls do exist in the interpretation of molecular results in this setting and include both false-positives and false-negatives. It is important to not overinterpret a clonal T-cell receptor gene rearrangement because certain benign dermatoses may frequently demonstrate T-cell clones (Table 16-4). Similarly, a monoclonal immunoglobulin heavy chain (IGH) gene rearrangement by itself does not establish a diagnosis of B-cell lymphoma because it may also be detected in benign cutaneous lymphoid hyperplasia. Nihal and coworkers identified monoclonal IGH gene rearrangements in 14 out of 44 cases (32%) of cutaneous reactive lymphoid hyperplasia. Recently, dual-clonality analysis with comparison of clones from two anatomically distinct skin biopsy sites has been proposed to improve specificity. It is also important to remember that the sensitivity of molecular tests is not 100%. The possibility of a false-negative result should be considered, and a negative molecular result would not exclude the possibility of lymphoma. Several factors can cause diminished sensitivity and include poor specimen quality, fixation artifacts, and failure of primer annealing.

TABLE 16-3   Wide Variety of Histopathologic Patterns Resembling Inflammatory Dermatoses That May Be Seen in Mycosis Fungoides

- Spongiotic
- Psoriasiform
- Interface vacuolar
- Interface lichenoid
- Superficial perivascular
- Superficial and deep perivascular
- Nodular
- Diffuse
- Folliculitis
- Vasculitis
- Subepidermal vesicular
- Panniculitis
- Granulomatous
- Interstitial

Data from Shapiro PE, Pinto FJ. The histologic spectrum of mycosis fungoides/Sézary syndrome (cutaneous T-cell lymphoma). A review of 222 biopsies, including newly described patterns and the earliest pathologic changes. *Am J Surg Pathol.* 1994;18:645-667; Su LD, Kim YH, LeBoit PE, Swetter SM, Kohler S. Interstitial mycosis fungoides, a variant of mycosis fungoides resembling granuloma annulare and inflammatory morphea. *J Cutan Pathol.* 2002;29:135-141; and Kempf W, Ostheeren-Michaelis S, Paulli M, Lucioni M, Wechsler J, Audring H, et al. Granulomatous mycosis fungoides and granulomatous slack skin: a multicenter study of the Cutaneous Lymphoma Histopathology Task Force Group of the European Organization For Research and Treatment of Cancer (EORTC). *Arch Dermatol.* 2008;144:1609–1617.

TABLE 16-4   Benign Skin Conditions That May Demonstrate T-Cell Monoclonality

- Pityriasis lichenoides et varioliformis acuta
- Pityriasis lichenoides chronica
- Lichen sclerosus et atrophicus
- Lichen planus
- Pigmented purpuric dermatoses
- Lymphomatoid lichenoid keratosis

CONDITIONS THAT MAY HISTOPATHOLOGICALLY SIMULATE CUTANEOUS LYMPHOMA

Lymphomatoid Drug Eruption

Skin manifestations are one of the most common presentations of drug allergy and may range from mild to severe. Among the several clinicopathologic variants of drug reactions, some cases may be associated with denser cutaneous lymphocytic infiltrates and resemble skin lymphoma. Several medications may be associated with this type of hypersensitivity reaction, particularly anticonvulsants such as phenytoin and carbamazepine. Other potential drugs include angiotensin-converting enzyme (ACE) inhibitors, atenolol, griseofulvin, imatinib, allopurinol, cyclosporine, antihistamines, and methylphenidate. Skin lesions include generalized papules, plaques, nodules, and even erythroderma. In addition to cutaneous manifestations, some patients may also develop fever, lymphadenopathy, leukocytosis, and/or hepatosplenomegaly. Drug eruptions may show a variety of histopathologic patterns and may simulate both T-cell and B-cell skin lymphomas. Some cases may show a bandlike pattern reminiscent of MF. A B-cell–predominant pattern showing lymphoid follicles with germinal centers may also occur. CD30+ cells may be prominent in some cases and may simulate cutaneous CD30+ lymphoproliferative disorders. Eosinophils are generally present but may be absent in some cases. Whereas molecular studies generally show a polyclonal pattern, pseudoclonality may occur in a number

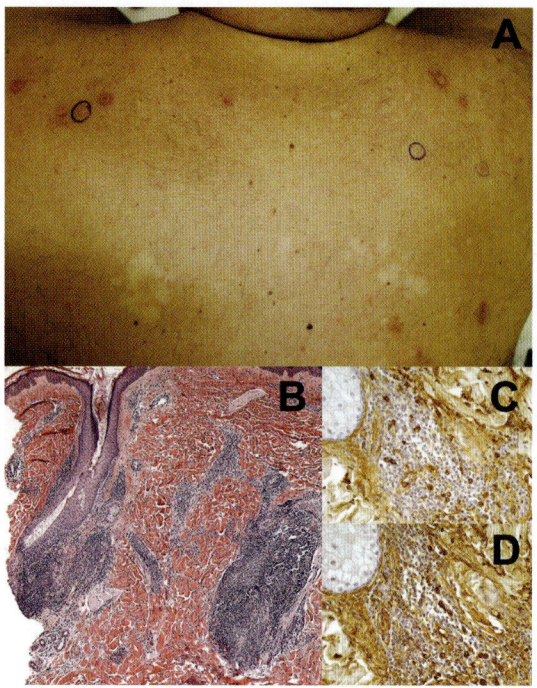

Figure 16-1 Clinical and histopathologic findings in a patient with a lymphomatoid drug eruption due to carbamazepine. **A,** Multiple pruritic papulonodules on trunk and arms, ranging in size from 3 to 10 mm. **B,** Superficial and deep periadnexal lymphocytic infiltrate reminiscent of cutaneous marginal zone B-cell lymphoma. Polytypic plasma cells with kappa (**C**) and lambda (**D**) immunoglobulin light chain immunohistochemical stains.

of cases and may cause further diagnostic difficulty. Resolution of the skin lesions in lymphomatoid drug eruptions often takes longer than other types of drug reactions and may persist for several months after cessation of the medication. Figure 16-1 shows the clinical and histopathologic findings in a patient with a lymphomatoid drug eruption due to carbamazepine.

Cutaneous Reactive Lymphoid Hyperplasia in the Setting of Viral Infection (Herpes Folliculitis, Molluscum Contagiosum, Orf, Milker's Nodule)

Several types of viral infection in the skin may be associated with florid reactive inflammatory infiltrates that may mimic skin lymphoma, including

herpes folliculitis, inflamed molluscum contagiosum, orf, milker's nodule, and inflamed warts. Histologic findings that may resemble lymphoma include dense dermal lymphoid infiltrates, angiotropism, and cytologically atypical lymphocytes. In herpetic cases, involvement of follicular units is more commonly encountered in varicella-zoster virus (VZV) compared with herpes simplex virus (HSV) infections. Most cases have a T-cell–predominant infiltrate. CD30+ cells are often prominent and may simulate cutaneous CD30+ lymphoproliferative disorders. Identification of viral cytopathic effect would facilitate a correct diagnosis; however, these changes may be present only focally, and multiple deeper sections through the tissue may be necessary. Whereas molecular studies generally show a polyclonal pattern, rare cases may show clonal T-cell receptor gene rearrangement. Figure 16-2 shows an example of herpes folliculitis with a dermal infiltrate of variable-sized lymphocytes. A hair follicle shows necrotic sebaceous glands as well as herpetic viral cytopathic effect and multinucleation.

Other Infections and Infestations

Some infectious organisms induce a florid host inflammatory response that may simulate a skin lymphoma. The density of the infiltrate in association with paucity or absence of visualizable organisms may lead to misdiagnosis. Whereas a short clinical duration would militate against a diagnosis of skin lymphoma, certain conditions such as cutaneous leishmaniasis may be associated with a persistent chronic course and cause further diagnostic confusion. Other infectious diseases to be considered include secondary syphilis and *Borrelia burgdorferi* infection. Infestation with *Sarcoptes scabiei* would not be confused with lymphoma in the vast majority of cases; however, some patients may develop reddish-brown nodules that may persist for several months despite treatment. Persistent nodular scabies likely represents a delayed hypersensitivity reaction, such as may occasionally occur with arthropod bites, including ticks. CD30+ cells may be prominent in some of these cases and may simulate lymphomatoid papulosis. Identification of the organisms as well as correlation with the clinical history and appropriate serologic studies

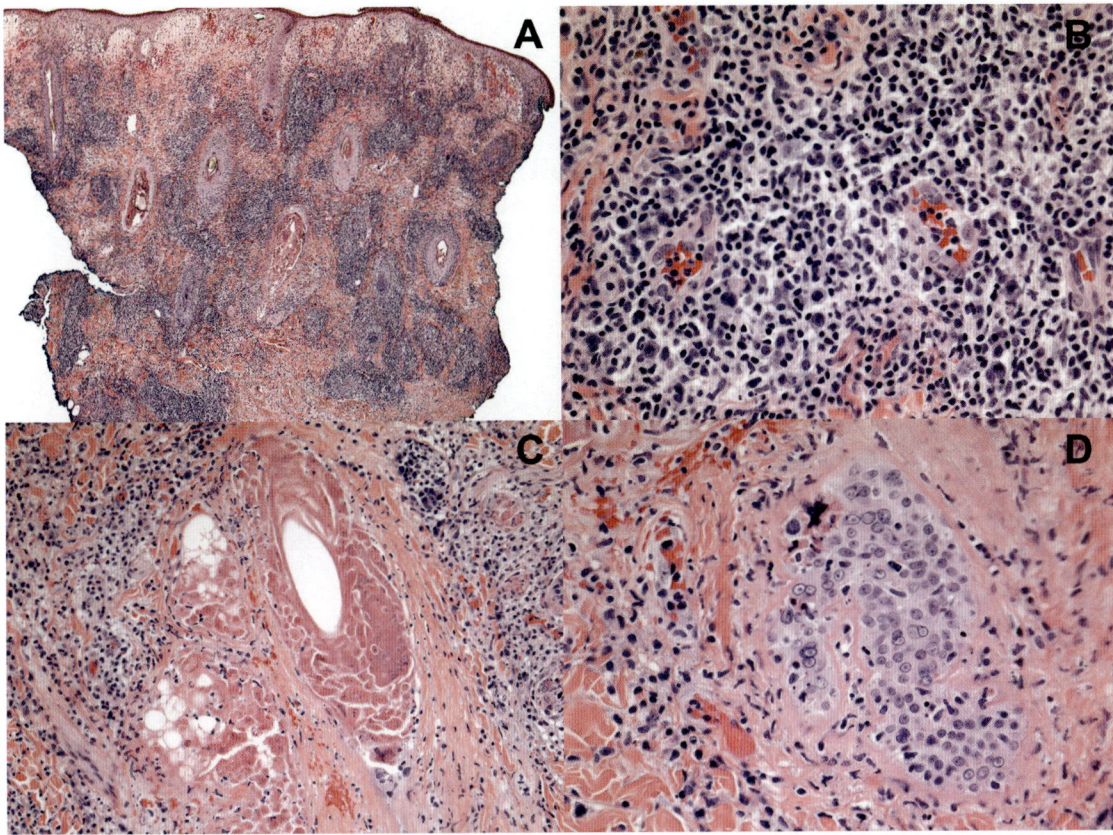

Figure 16-2 Herpes folliculitis. **A,** Moderately dense, superficial and deep dermal lymphocytic infiltrate. **B,** The infiltrate is composed of variable-sized lymphocytes, some of which exhibit atypical features. **C,** Hair follicle with necrosis of sebaceous gland lobules and acantholysis of the epithelium. **D,** Characteristic herpetic viral cytopathic effect with intranuclear inclusion and multinucleation.

are generally helpful. Figure 16-3 shows a case of cutaneous leishmaniasis in association with a dense lymphoid infiltrate.

Exaggerated Bite-like Reactions

Exaggerated arthropod bite-like reactions may occur in patients with hematologic malignant neoplasms, including chronic lymphocytic leukemia and mantle cell lymphoma. Although some of these reactions may represent hypersensitivity to mosquito bites, some patients do not recall being bitten, and it is conceivable that other factors may also be involved, such as immunodeficiency or hypersensitivity to the underlying malignancy. Skin lesions may precede the hematologic disorder or may appear months to years after the diagnosis. The inflammatory infiltrate may be

prominent but is generally associated with many eosinophils.

Tattoo Reactions

A wide range of complications may occasionally occur secondary to a tattoo and include pseudoepitheliomatous hyperplasia, granulomatous inflammation, lichenoid reaction, eczematous/spongiotic dermatitis, and various infections. Red pigment appears to be more often implicated in producing tattoo reactions. A pseudolymphomatous pattern is an uncommon type of reaction and generates a florid dermal inflammatory response. Although the density of the infiltrate may cause concern for a lymphoma, the microscopic identification of tattoo pigment, the mixed inflammatory pattern, as well as the clinical picture of

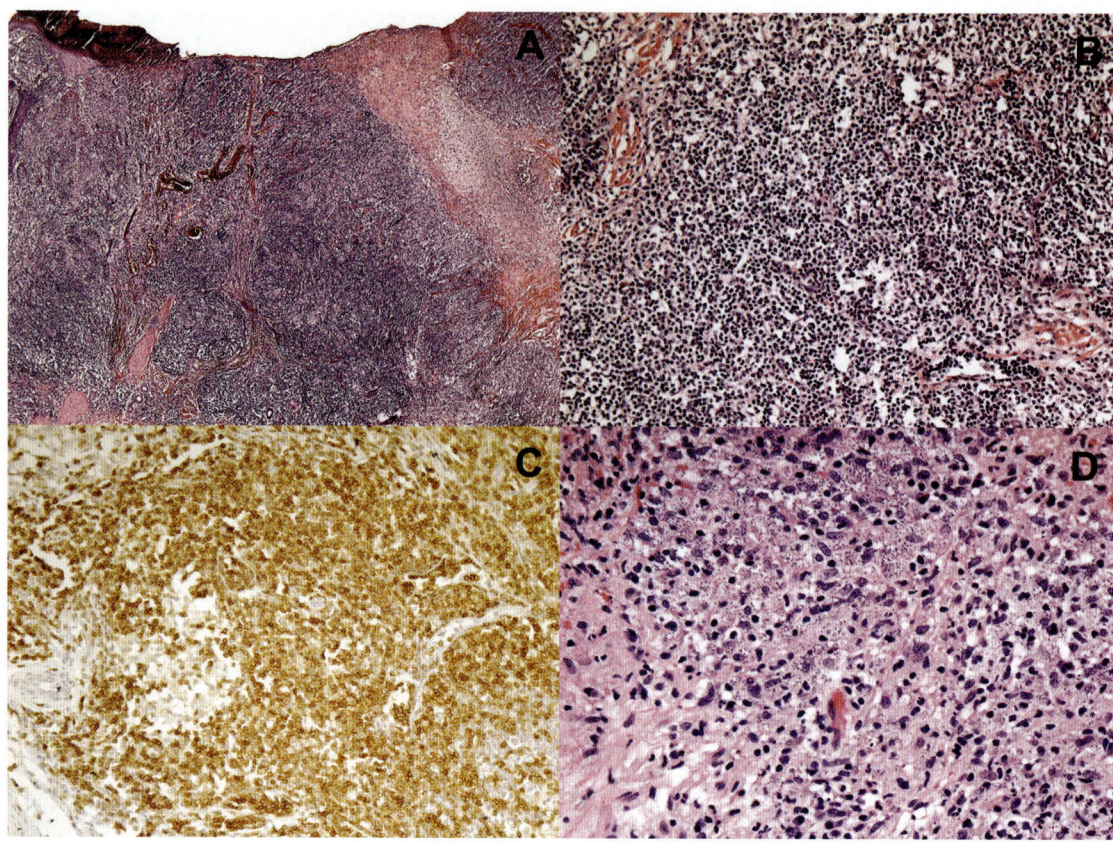

Figure 16-3 Cutaneous leishmaniasis. **A,** Dense nodular and diffuse, superficial and deep dermal infiltrate with overlying ulceration. **B,** The infiltrate is composed of lymphocytes, plasma cells, and histiocytes. **C,** The majority of the lymphocytes are CD3+ T-cells. **D,** Parasitized histiocytes with abundant intracytoplasmic *Leishmania* organisms.

lesions restricted to the tattoo can facilitate the correct diagnosis. Figure 16-4 illustrates an example of a pseudolymphomatous tattoo reaction.

Reactive Lymphoid Hyperplasia at Sites of Vaccination

Pseudolymphoma may occur as a rare complication of vaccination. The lesions may be nodular or plaquelike and may persist for several months. Dense lymphoid infiltrates often show a prominent follicular pattern and may resemble a low-grade B-cell lymphoma. In addition to the clinical history, helpful findings in this differential would include the presence of polyclonal plasma cells, eosinophils, and reactive features in the germinal centers (e.g., preserved mantle zones, tingible body macrophages, polarization).

Early Inflammatory Stage of Certain Benign Dermatoses

Sclerotic dermatoses, such as lichen sclerosus et atrophicus and morphea, may be associated with florid inflammation in their early stages. Early lichen sclerosus may show a fairly dense, bandlike infiltrate of small lymphocytes in the upper dermis with extension of lymphocytes into the lower portion of the epidermis (basilar exocytosis) and may resemble patch/plaque stage MF. Although homogenized collagen may not be present in early lesions of lichen sclerosus, loss of upper dermal elastic fibers and basement membrane thickening may be seen. Molecular studies may not be helpful in this setting because T-cell clonality may be identified in lichen sclerosus (see Table 16-4). Another benign dermatosis that may be associated with a bandlike inflammatory infiltrate with exocytosis

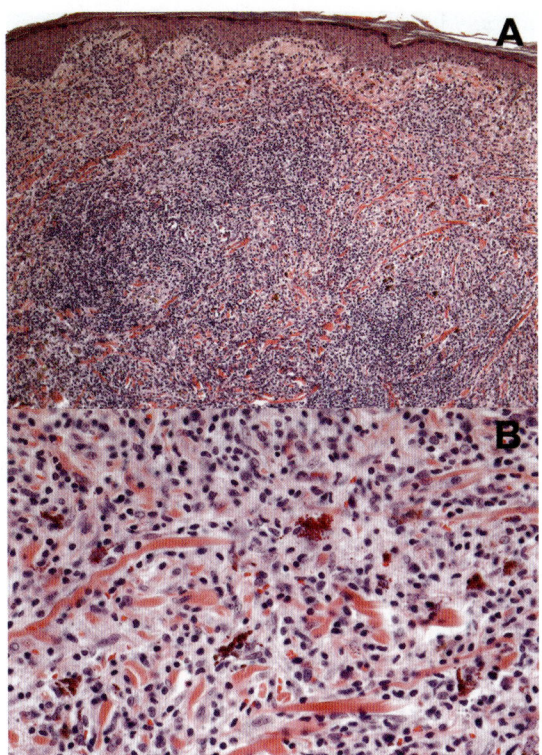

Figure 16-4 Pseudolymphomatous tattoo reaction. **A,** Dense diffuse and nodular, superficial and deep dermal lymphohistiocytic infiltrate with patchy exocytosis of lymphocytes within the epidermis. **B,** Dermal histiocytes with red tattoo pigment.

in its early stages is vitiligo. The predominance of CD8+ lymphocytes and loss of pigmentation may cause diagnostic confusion with the hypopigmented variant of MF. Careful clinicopathologic correlation and close follow-up may be necessary for a proper diagnosis.

Lymphomatoid Lichenoid Keratosis

Lichenoid keratosis or lichen planus–like keratosis (LPLK) may occasionally demonstrate a denser than usual bandlike lymphocytic inflammatory infiltrate and may mimic MF (so-called MF-LK). Exocytosis of lymphocytes in the epidermis may be prominent. Remnants of a solar lentigo or early seborrheic keratosis may be observed at the periphery of the lesion. The ratio of CD4+ and CD8+ cells is generally within normal limits, and there are often admixed B cells. Molecular studies may not be helpful because T-cell clonality may

be identified in lymphomatoid lichenoid keratosis. Clinical correlation is very important in this setting; despite the worrisome histologic findings, the clinical appearance is benign (i.e., small solitary keratotic lesion).

Pigmented Purpuric Dermatosis

There are several variants of pigmented purpuric dermatosis: progressive pigmentary dermatosis (Schamberg's disease), purpura annularis telangiectodes of Majocchi, pigmented purpuric lichenoid dermatosis of Gougerot and Blum, and lichen aureus. Pigmented purpuric dermatoses may show several histologic features reminiscent of MF, including basilar exocytosis of lymphocytes, a bandlike lymphocytic infiltrate, as well as psoriasiform lichenoid, psoriasiform spongiotic lichenoid, and atrophic lichenoid patterns. Papillary dermal edema occurs frequently in pigmented purpuric dermatosis but is not a common finding in MF; in contrast, the presence of significant cytologic atypia and exocytosis into the upper spinous layer would favor MF. Molecular studies may not be helpful in this setting because T-cell clonality may be identified in pigmented purpuric dermatosis. In addition to being a simulant, there may be a potential precursor relationship between persistent pigmented purpuric dermatosis and some cases of MF. There are documented examples of cutaneous eruptions very closely resembling pigmented purpuric dermatosis (both clinically and histologically) that, on follow-up, later developed diagnostic features of MF. Therefore, careful clinicopathologic correlation and close follow-up may be necessary for a proper diagnosis.

Pityriasis Lichenoides

Pityriasis lichenoides shows a spectrum of clinical changes and demonstrates acute (pityriasis lichenoides et varioliformis acuta [PLEVA]) and chronic (pityriasis lichenoides chronica [PLC]) forms. Pityriasis lichenoides may show some histologic features reminiscent of MF, including exocytosis of lymphocytes in the upper layers of the epidermis and a bandlike upper dermal lymphocytic infiltrate. However, cytologic atypia is generally not seen. Clinical correlation is usually helpful. Molecular studies may not be useful in this setting because T-cell clonality may be identified in pityriasis lichenoides. The correct nosology of aggressive cases of febrile ulceronecrotic PLEVA/Mucha-Haberman disease is unclear. Some of these atypical cases may potentially be related to cytotoxic cutaneous lymphomas.

Lupus Panniculitis

Lupus panniculitis is a variant of lupus erythematosus with prominent involvement of the subcutaneous tissue in the form of a lymphoplasmacytic lobular panniculitis. The density of the lymphoid infiltrate may cause concern for a lymphoma. Features favoring lupus panniculitis include changes of lupus erythematosus in the overlying skin, low proliferation rate, paucity of adipocyte rimming, hyaline fat necrosis, lack of a γ/δ immunophenotype, and presence of a significant component of B cells, plasma cells, and lymphoid follicles with germinal centers. Whereas lupus panniculitis and subcutaneous panniculitis-like T-cell lymphoma can be differentiated in the majority of cases, there are rare cases with variably overlapping clinicopathologic features, and it is conceivable that some patients may have both diseases. Close follow-up and repeat sampling may be necessary for a correct diagnosis.

Obscuring Inflammation in Nonlymphoid Neoplasms

A variety of nonlymphoid neoplasms may be associated with a dense inflammatory response that partially obscures the primary lesion. The hypercellularity of the infiltrate may simulate a lymphoma. Because this phenomenon may occur in malignant tumors, misdiagnosis could lead to erroneous therapeutic decisions. Examples include vascular neoplasms, such as the pseudolymphomatous variant of cutaneous angiosarcoma; epithelial neoplasms, such as lymphoepithelioma-like carcinoma; and neuroendocrine neoplasms, such as inflamed or dyscohesive variants of Merkel cell carcinoma. Acral pseudolymphomatous angiokeratoma in children (APACHE) appears to represent a clinicopathologic variant of pseudolymphoma rather than a vascular neoplasm. CD56 is a sensitive marker for natural killer (NK) cells but is not specific because it also

marks Merkel cell carcinoma. Strong CD56 positivity in crushed or inflamed biopsies of Merkel cell carcinoma may lead to an erroneous impression of NK-cell lymphoma. Because of the broad differential diagnoses in this setting, an extensive panel of immunohistochemical markers may be necessary to demonstrate the mixed pattern of the inflammatory infiltrate as well as to highlight the obscured neoplasm.

Pseudolymphomatous Folliculitis

Pseudolymphomatous folliculitis is a clinicopathologic variant of pseudolymphoma and generally presents with a small solitary lesion on the face. Because hair follicles may be irregularly deformed with their epithelium blurred by lymphocytic infiltrates, the histologic findings may resemble those of folliculotropic MF. Clinical correlation is useful in this setting; despite the potentially worrisome histologic findings, the clinical appearance is benign (i.e., small solitary lesion). The vast majority of cases does not exhibit B- or T-cell clonality and does not recur after excision.

Cutaneous Plasmacytosis

Cutaneous plasmacytosis is a rare entity and is most commonly seen in Asiatic countries. Some cases subsequently develop the systemic form of the disorder with lymphadenopathy and polyclonal hypergammaglobulinemia. The presence of abundant plasma cells in the skin may raise the possibility of the plasmacytic variant of cutaneous marginal zone B-cell lymphoma. However, the plasma cells show a polyclonal pattern with immunoglobulin light chain stains.

CD8+ Infiltrates in the Setting of Advanced Acquired Immunodeficiency Syndrome

Cutaneous and systemic infiltrates of polyclonal CD8+ T-cells may rarely occur in patients with advanced acquired immunodeficiency syndrome (AIDS) with profound CD4 lymphopenia. The cutaneous eruption is characterized by a dense infiltrate of lymphocytes histopathologically resembling MF but composed of CD8+ cells. Exocytosis of lymphocytes may be significant.

T-cell clonality is not identified. Regression with human immunodeficiency virus (HIV) antiviral therapy has been reported.

SUGGESTED READINGS

Arai E, Okubo H, Tsuchida T, Kitamura K, Katayama I. Pseudolymphomatous folliculitis: a clinicopathologic study of 15 cases of cutaneous pseudolymphoma with follicular invasion. *Am J Surg Pathol.* 1999;23:1313–1319.

Asakura K, Kizaki M, Ikeda Y. Exaggerated cutaneous response to mosquito bites in a patient with chronic lymphocytic leukemia. *Int J Hematol.* 2004;80:59–61.

Barnhill RL, Braverman IM. Progression of pigmented purpura-like eruptions to mycosis fungoides: report of three cases. *J Am Acad Dermatol.* 1988;19:25–31.

Barzilai A, Shpiro D, Goldberg I, Yacob-Hirsch Y, Diaz-Cascajo C, Meytes D, et al. Insect bite–like reaction in patients with hematologic malignant neoplasms. *Arch Dermatol.* 1999;135:1503–1507.

Citarella L, Massone C, Kerl H, Cerroni L. Lichen sclerosus with histopathologic features simulating early mycosis fungoides. *Am J Dermatopathol.* 2003;25:463–465.

Fung MA, LeBoit PE. Light microscopic criteria for the diagnosis of early vulvar lichen sclerosus: a comparison with lichen planus. *Am J Surg Pathol.* 1998;22:473–478.

Guitart J, Variakojis D, Kuzel T, Rosen S. Cutaneous CD8 T cell infiltrates in advanced HIV infection. *J Am Acad Dermatol.* 1999;41:722–727.

Hwong H, Jones D, Prieto VG, Schulz C, Duvic M. Persistent atypical lymphocytic hyperplasia following tick bite in a child: report of a case and review of the literature. *Pediatr Dermatol.* 2001;18:481–484.

Kiyohara T, Kumakiri M, Kawasaki T, Takeuchi A, Kuwahara H, Ueda T. Linear acral pseudolymphomatous angiokeratoma of children (APACHE): further evidence that APACHE is a cutaneous pseudolymphoma. *J Am Acad Dermatol.* 2003;48(2 Suppl):S15–S17.

Leonard DGB, ed. *Diagnostic Molecular Pathology.* Philadelphia: Elsevier Science; 2003:113–127.

Magro CM, Crowson AN, Byrd JC, Soleymani AD, Shendrik I. Atypical lymphocytic lobular panniculitis. *J Cutan Pathol.* 2004;31:300–306.

Magro CM, Crowson AN. Drug-induced immune dysregulation as a cause of atypical cutaneous lymphoid infiltrates: a hypothesis. *Hum Pathol.* 1996;27:125–132.

McComb ME, Telang GH, Vonderheid EC. Secondary syphilis presenting as pseudolymphoma of the skin. *J Am Acad Dermatol.* 2003;49(2 Suppl Case Reports):S174–S176.

McNiff JM, Glusac EJ, Lazova RZ, Carroll CB. Morphea limited to the superficial reticular dermis: an underrecognized histologic phenomenon. *Am J Dermatopathol.* 1999;21:315–319.

Moreno-Ramírez D, García-Escudero A, Ríos-Martín JJ, Herrera-Saval A, Camacho F. Cutaneous pseudolymphoma in association with molluscum contagiosum in an elderly patient. *J Cutan Pathol.* 2003;30:473–475.

Mori T, Okamoto S, Kuramochi S, Ikeda Y. An adult patient with hypersensitivity to mosquito bites developing mantle cell lymphoma. *Int J Hematol.* 2000;71:259–262.

Nathan DL, Belsito DV. Carbamazepine-induced pseudolymphoma with CD-30 positive cells. *J Am Acad Dermatol.* 1998;38:806–809.

Nihal M, Mikkola D, Horvath N, Gilliam AC, Stevens SR, Spiro TP, et al. Cutaneous lymphoid hyperplasia: a lymphoproliferative continuum with lymphomatous potential. *Hum Pathol.* 2003;34:617–622.

Petit T, Cribier B, Bagot M, Wechsler J. Inflammatory vitiligo-like macules that simulate hypopigmented mycosis fungoides. *Eur J Dermatol.* 2003;13:410–412.

Rijlaarsdam JU, Bruynzeel DP, Vos W, Meijer CJ, Willemze R. Immunohistochemical studies of lymphadenosis benigna cutis occurring in a tattoo. *Am J Dermatopathol.* 1988;10:518–523.

Rijlaarsdam U, Scheffer E, Meijer CJ, Kruyswijk MR, Willemze R. Mycosis fungoides–like lesions associated with phenytoin and carbamazepine therapy. *J Am Acad Dermatol.* 1991;24:216–220.

Rijlaarsdam U, Willemze R. Cutaneous pseudo-T-cell lymphomas. *Semin Diagn Pathol.* 1991;8:102–108.

Rose C, Starostik P, Bröcker EB. Infection with parapoxvirus induces CD30-positive cutaneous infiltrates in humans. *J Cutan Pathol.* 1999;26:520–522.

Santucci M, Pimpinelli N, Massi D, Kadin ME, Meijer CJ, Müller-Hermelink HK, et al. Cytotoxic/natural killer cell cutaneous lymphomas. Report of EORTC Cutaneous Lymphoma Task Force Workshop. *Cancer.* 2003;97:610–627.

Schartz NE, De La Blanchardiére A, Alaoui S, Morel P, Sigaux F, Vignon-Pennamen MD, et al. Regression of CD8+ pseudolymphoma after HIV antiviral triple therapy. *J Am Acad Dermatol.* 2003;49:139–141.

Shapiro PE, Pinto FJ. The histologic spectrum of mycosis fungoides/Sézary syndrome (cutaneous T-cell lymphoma). A review of 222 biopsies, including newly described patterns and the earliest pathologic changes. *Am J Surg Pathol.* 1994;18:645–667.

Su LD, Kim YH, LeBoit PE, Swetter SM, Kohler S. Interstitial mycosis fungoides, a variant of mycosis fungoides resembling granuloma annulare and inflammatory morphea. *J Cutan Pathol.* 2002;29: 135–141.

Tomasini D, Zampatti C, Palmedo G, Bonfacini V, Sangalli G, Kutzner H. Cytotoxic mycosis fungoides evolving from pityriasis lichenoides chronica in a seventeen-year-old girl. Report of a case. *Dermatology.* 2002;205:176–179.

Toro JR, Sander CA, LeBoit PE. Persistent pigmented purpuric dermatitis and mycosis fungoides: simulant, precursor, or both? A study by light microscopy and molecular methods. *Am J Dermatopathol.* 1997;19: 108–118.

Zhang P, Chiriboga L, Jacobson M, Marsh E, Hennessey P, Schinella R, et al. Mycosis fungoides–like T-cell cutaneous lymphoid infiltrates in patients with HIV infection. *Am J Dermatopathol.* 1995;17: 29–35.

SYSTEMIC INVOLVEMENT AND EVALUATION OF CUTANEOUS T-CELL LYMPHOMA

Francine M. Foss, MD

INTRODUCTION

Cutaneous T-cell lymphomas (CTCLs) are a clinically and histopathologically diverse group of malignancies that present with involvement of the skin. The most common types are mycosis fungoides (MF) and the Sézary syndrome (SS). MF typically is a more indolent form of the disease in its earlier stages, although patients may develop progression to more extensive involvement, including visceral disease or large cell transformation. SS consists of erythrodermatous skin involvement with the presence of circulating neoplastic leukemia (Sézary) cells and frequent nodal involvement. In a retrospective review of 148 uniformly staged patients who were evaluated at the National Cancer Institute (NCI) with imaging studies, bone marrow and liver biopsies, and lymph node biopsies (blind inguinal node if there were no palpable nodes), the incidence of visceral involvement at diagnosis was 15%, with 7 patients having bone marrow alone, 11 having liver involvement alone, and 4 having both bone marrow and liver involvement.

STAGING AND PROGNOSIS OF MYCOSIS FUNGOIDES/ SÉZARY'S SYNDROME

Staging systems for MF have been developed based on clinical features of skin involvement as well as infiltration of lymph nodes and viscera. The most commonly used staging system for MF/SS is based on a tumor-node-metastasis-blood (TNMB) classification (Table 17-1). Skin involvement is defined based on the type of lesions and extent. T1 and T2 disease are patches or plaques involving less than and greater than 10% of the skin surface, respectively. T3 disease is the presence of at least one cutaneous tumor. T4 disease is erythroderma, which may be flat and patchlike or may be diffusely infiltrating and associated with a leathery skin appearance or thickening and fissuring of the skin, particularly on the palms or soles of the feet. Staging studies have been recommended by the International Society for Cutaneous Lymphomas (ISCL). For all patients with T1 or limited T2 disease, imaging tests may be limited to chest x-ray and ultrasound of nodal

TABLE 17-1 Clinical Staging of Mycosis Fungoides/Sézary's Syndrome by Tumor-Node-Metastasis-Blood

TNMB Stages	Description of TNMB
Skin	
T_1	Limited patches, papules and/or plaques† covering < 10% of the skin surface. May further stratify into T_{1a} (patch only) vs. T_{1b} (plaque ± patch).
T_2	Patches, papules or plaques covering ≥ 10% of the skin surface. May further stratify into T_{2a} (patch only) vs. T_{2b} (plaque ± patch).
T_3	One or more tumors (≥1 cm diameter).
T_4	Confluence of erythema covering ≥ 80% body surface area.

(continued)

TABLE 17-1   Clinical Staging of Mycosis Fungoides/Sézary's Syndrome by Tumor-Node-Metastasis-Blood *(continued)*

TNMB Stages	Description of TNMB
Node	
N_0	No clinically abnormal peripheral lymph nodes; biopsy not required.
N_1	Clinically abnormal peripheral lymph nodes; histopathology Dutch Gr 1 or NCI LN_{0-2}
N_{1a}	Clone negative.
N_{1b}	Clone positive.
N_2	Clinically abnormal peripheral lymph nodes; histopathology Dutch Gr 2 or NCI LN_3
N_{2a}	Clone negative.
N_{2b}	Clone positive.
N_3	Clinically abnormal peripheral lymph nodes; histopathology Dutch Gr 3-4 or NCI LN_4; clone positive or negative.
N_x	Clinically abnormal peripheral lymph nodes, no histologic confirmation.
Visceral	
M_0	No visceral organ involvement.
M_1	Visceral involvement (must have pathology confirmation and organ involved should be specified).
Blood	
B_0	Absence of significant blood involvement: =5% of peripheral blood lymphocytes are atypical (Sézary) cells
B_{0a}	Clone negative.
B_{0b}	Clone positive.
B_1	Low blood tumor burden: >5% of peripheral blood lymphocytes are atypical (Sézary) cells but does not meet the criteria of B_2
B_{1a}	Clone negative.
B_{1b}	Clone positive.
B_2	High blood tumor burden: ≥1000/uL Sézary cells with positive clone. One of the following can be substituted for Sézary cells: CD4/CD8 ≥ 10, CD4+CD7– cells ≥ 40% or CD4+CD26– cells ≥ 30%.

NCI, National Cancer Institute; TNMB, tumor-node-metastasis-blood.

Stage	T	N	M	B
IA	1	0	0	0,1
IB	2	0	0	0,1
II	1-2	1,2	0	0,1
IIB	3	0-2	0	0,1
III	4	0-2	0	0,1
IIIA	4	0-2	0	0
IIIB	4	0-2	0	1
IVA_1	1-4	0-2	0	2
IVA_2	1-4	3	0	0-2
IVB	1-4	0-3	1	0-2

groups. For all other patients, imaging in the form of computed tomography (CT) scans of the chest, abdomen, and pelvis or positron emission tomography (PET) scans are recommended to detect nodal or visceral involvement.

Lymph Nodes

Lymph node involvement has been classified based on whether the nodes are palpable and on the degree of infiltration with malignant cells. Physical examination is a poor method for determining the size of peripheral lymph nodes. In general, a node greater than 1.5 cm in diameter is considered suspicious. Nodes are characterized based on the degree of involvement. The dermatopathic node demonstrates small (LN2) or large (LN3) clusters of atypical T cells with preserved nodal architecture and often with expansion of the parafollicular zones. LN4 nodes are effaced by tumor cells. There are two current staging systems for nodal involvement in CTCL. The NCI/Veterans Affairs (VA) system defines nodal classification based on the number of atypical lymphocytes, be they small (6-10 μm) or large (≥11 μm) in size, to differentiate between LN categories, whereas the Dutch system differentiates based on size of the atypical lymphocytes (>7.5 μm) to determine involvement.[5] The Dutch grade 1 node corresponds to LN0-2, Dutch grade 2 corresponds to LN3, and Dutch grade 3 (partially effaced) or grade 4 (fully effaced) corresponds to an LN4 node.

Rearrangements of the T-cell receptor (TCR) are found in half of patients with LN3 nodes and rarely in those with LN2 histology. Clonal rearrangements were found in 13% of LN2, 83% of LN3 nodes, and all LN4 nodes by Southern blotting. The prognosis of patients with clonal rearrangements was inferior irrespective of the LN stage. In a comparison of Southern blot and polymerase chain reaction (PCR) determination of clonality by TCR rearrangement in both palpable and nonpalpable lymph nodes in patients with MF/SS, only Southern blot was predictive of a poor prognosis in a multivariate analysis that included skin stage, presence or absence of lymphadenopathy, and histologic lymph node score.

Because a fine-needle aspirate is not adequate to demonstrate nodal architecture, the ISCL recommendation is that an excisional biopsy is required to accurately classify a node using the LN1-4 grading system. Lymph node biopsy is recommended if a node is palpable (>1.5 cm in diameter) or has intense fluorodeoxyglucose (FDG) uptake on PET scan. Enlarged nodes draining involved skin areas are generally preferred over nonpalpable internal nodes. Flow cytometry and studies for TCR rearrangement should be performed on node biopsies. The presence of nodal involvement as LN3 or 4 will upstage a patient to stage IVA.

Blood Involvement

Blood involvement in MF has not been included in the staging system until the most recent revisions to the staging and classification of MF/SS in 2007. According to the new criteria, three levels of blood involvement were established. B_0 is defined as the absence of clinically significant blood involvement. B_2 has been defined as leukemic involvement with Sézary cells accounting for 5% or greater of total lymphocytes, and B_1 comprises patients with less than 5% atypical circulating cells that do not fulfill B_2 criteria. The criteria for B_2 includes at least one of the following plus molecular genetic evidence of clonality of the TCR: absolute Sézary count ≥ 1.0 K/μL, CD4/CD8 ratio ≥ 10, CD4+ CD7– cells ≥ 40%, or CD4+ CD26– cells ≥ 30% of lymphocytes.

Flow cytometry has become the standard to define blood involvement in MF/SS. Loss of antigen expression, such as CD7, dim expression of CD3, or loss of CD26 are findings associated with Sézary cells, but these may not be specific. The expression of CD7 on CD4+ cells may diminish with age or with chronic inflammatory dermatoses. It has been shown, furthermore, that clonal Sézary cells may be CD4+ CD7+ or CD4+ CD7–. CD26 is a glycosylated transmembrane protein that has enzymatic activity (dipeptidyl peptidase IV) and is expressed normally on appropximately 85% of CD3+ CD4+ lymphocytes. Loss of CD26 has been shown to be a sensitive marker for Sézary cells compared with normal T cells (96% sensitivity, 98% specificity).

Visceral Disease Assessment

Visceral involvement has been documented in a number of retrospective studies to be an adverse prognostic factor in MF/SS. Visceral disease is uncommon except in patients with blood or advanced nodal disease and is defined as involvement in at least one organ outside of skin, nodes, or blood. Splenomegaly and liver involvement have been reported and may be focal or disseminated. Liver disease should be confirmed by a liver biopsy. In one series of 43 patients in whom all had liver biopsies as part of staging, 7 patients (16%) had liver involvement, and most of these patients had SS or erythroderma.

Bone marrow involvement in CTCL has been found primarily in patients with advanced disease. The type of marrow involvement has been defined as either cytologically atypical lymphoid aggregates or infiltrative disease and has been associated with inferior survival. In one prospective study done at the NCI, 90 consecutive patients underwent bone marrow biopsies as part of a staging evaluation. Thirty-seven patients had positive findings (35 had lymphoid aggregates, 11 of which were cytologically atypical, and 2 had diffuse involvement). Whereas most of the patients with infiltrative or cytologically atypical aggregates had advanced lymph node or blood involvement, 28% had early skin stage. In other retrospective studies, bone marrow involvement was associated primarily with blood involvement and advanced lymph node disease. All of these studies have primarily relied on histopathologic assessment of the bone marrow.

The ISCL has recently recommended a bone marrow biopsy for patients with B_2 blood involvement or in patients with unexplained hematologic abnormalities. If bone marrow studies are done, flow cytometry for immunophenotypic analysis to detect malignant populations of cells as well as TCR gene rearrangements are recommended, although the prognostic significance of the latter has not been fully demonstrated.

Overall outcome in MF/SS is correlated with clinical stage, and retrospective studies have identified skin involvement as well as visceral disease as the most important prognostic factors. Patients with limited patch/plaque disease covering less than 10% of their skin surface have a prognosis indistinguishable from that of age-, sex-, and race-matched controls. The 10-year disease-specific survival for patients with more extensive skin involvement with patches or plaques is 83%, whereas those with tumors or histologically

documented lymph node involvement had survivals of 42% or 20%, respectively. Patients with effaced lymph nodes or the presence of large cell transformation had a uniformly poor prognosis. A review by Willemze and coworkers and the European Organization for Research and Treatment of Cancer (EORTC) reported outcomes for subtypes of CTCL. Patients with a folliculotropic subtype had a worse outcome than other subtypes of MF, and SS patients had a significantly inferior 5-year disease-free survival (Table 17-2)

SYSTEMIC THERAPY FOR ADVANCED MYCOSIS FUNGOIDES/SÉZARY'S SYNDROME

Patients with advanced MF or SS are often treated with topical and local modalities, such as ultraviolet light–based therapies, topical nitrogen mustard, retinoids, or electron beam irradiation to the skin. Because most patients with advanced disease develop progression and will eventually succumb to their disease, systemic therapies are often employed early in the course of therapy. The National Comprehensive Cancer Network (NCCN) guidelines recommend that patients with tumor stage disease (T3), erythroderma with blood involvement (B1 or B2), or visceral involvement be treated with systemic therapies. In addition, patients with extensive patch or plaque stage disease (T2) with blood involvement (B1 or B2) should also receive systemic therapy along with skin directed treatment. Systemic therapies in category A include biologic agents as well as denileukin diftitox and methotrexate. Categories B and C includes single-agent chemotherapy drugs, nucleoside analogues, and newer agents, such as pralatrexate and romidepsin. Therapeutic options for MF/SS are summarized in Table 17-3.

Biologic Therapies

Interferons

Interferon-alpha (IFN-α) has been demonstrated in a number of studies to be a highly active agent in CTCL, with response rates ranging from 40% to 80%. Doses have ranged from 1 to 18 MU administered subcutaneously on a number of schedules,

TABLE 17-2 **Outcomes for Cutaneous T-Cell Lymphoma Subtypes According to World Health Organization Classification**

WHO-EORTC Classification	N	Frequency (%)	Disease-specific 5-Year Survival (%)
Indolent Clinical Behavior			
MF	800	44	88
Folliculotropic MF	86	4	80
Pagetoid reticulosis	14	<1	100
Granulomatous slack skin	4	<1	100
Primary cutaneous anaplastic large cell lymphoma	146	8	95
Lymphomatoid papulosis	236	12	100
Aggressive Clinical Behavior			
Sézary's syndrome	52	3	24
Primary cutaneous NK/T-cell lymphoma, nasal-type	7	<1	NR
Primary cutaneous aggressive CD8+ T-cell lymphoma	14	<1	18
Primary cutaneous gamma delta T-cell lymphoma	13	<1	NR
Primary cutaneous peripheral T-cell lymphoma, unspecified	47	2	16

EORTC, European Organization for Research and Treatment of cancer; MF, mycosis fungoides; NK, natural killer; NR not reported, WHO, World Health organization.

Adapted from Willemze R, Jaffe ES, Burg G, Cerroni L, Berti E, Swerdlow SH, et al. WHO-EORTC classification for cutaneous lymphomas. *Blood*. 2005;105:3768–3785.

the most common being three times a week. IFN-γ has also demonstrated activity but is not as widely used. Constitutional symptoms and bone marrow suppression have limited aggressive and long-term use of IFNs for many patients. Early studies with high-dose interleukin-2 (IL-2) have demonstrated activity in relapsed CTCL but with significant toxicity. In a study of intermediate-dose IL-2, 11 patients (median age, 60 yr) with advanced or refractory CTCL underwent 8-week cycles of daily subcutaneous injections of 11 MIU, 4 days/wk for 6 weeks, followed by 2 weeks off therapy. This dose was well tolerated, and there were 4 partial responses, 3 of which were sustained. IL-12 has also demonstrated activity in early and advanced MF. A phase II study demonstrated responses in 43% of the patients, with response durations ranging from 3 to 45 weeks. The drug has not been subsequently evaluated further in clinical trials.

Photopheresis (Extracorporeal Photochemotherapy)

Extracorporeal photochemotherapy (ECP), or photopheresis, involves a leukapheresis to isolate mononuclear cells that are exposed ex vivo to ultraviolet A (UVA) in the presence of methoxypsoralen and then reinfused back into the patient. Methoxypsoralen incorporates into DNA and, in the presence of ultraviolet light, induces strand breaks and subsequently apoptosis. The mechanism of action of ECP is believed to be related to the induction of apoptosis in clonal Sézary T cells, leading to uptake and processing of tumor antigens by immature dendritic cells generated from the effects of the ECP process on circulating monocytoid precursors. The process of ECP has been shown to induce a cell-mediated anti-tumor response. Clinical improvement with ECP has been demonstrated in both patients with SS

TABLE 17-3   Therapies for Advanced Mycosis Fungoides/ Sézary's Syndrome

Single Agents—Biologic Therapies

Denileukin diftitox (Ontak, Eisai)

Extracorporeal photopheresis

HDACi: Romidepsin (Istodax, Celgene/ Gloucester)

Vorinostat (Zolinza, Merck)

Interferons	IFN-α
	IFN-γ
Retinoids	Acitretin (Soriatane, Stiefel)
	All-trans-retinoic acid
	Bexarotene (Targretin, Eisai)
	Isotretinoin

Combinations

Bexarotene + denileukin diftitox

Photopheresis + IFN

Photopheresis + retinoid

Photopheresis + retinoid + IFN

Retinoid + IFN

Single Agents—Cytotoxic Therapies

Methotrexate

Bortezomib (Velcade, Millennium)

Chlorambucil (Leukeran, GlaxoSmithKline)

Cyclophosphamide

Etoposide

Gemcitabine

Liposomal doxorubicin

Pentostatin

Temozolomide

Pralatrexate

Combination Chemotherapy

EPOCH

GND

Hyper-CVAD

ICE

EPOCH, etoposide, prednisone, vincristine, cyclophosphamide, doxorubicin; GND, gemcitabine (Gemzar, Lilly), vinorelbine, liposomal doxorubicin (Doxil, Ortho Biotech); HDACi, histone deacetylase inhibitor; hyper-CVAD, cyclophosphamide, vincristine, doxorubicin, dexamethasone; ICE, etoposide, methylprednisolone, ifosfamide; IFN, interferon.

and patients with tumor and plaque stage CTCL. The immunomodulatory effects of ECP have been augmented by the use of cytokines and retinoids. The NCCN guidelines include combinations of ECP with bexarotene or other retinoids or with IFN.

ECP is initially administered on a once-a-month schedule, with therapy continued until maximal clearing is established. An additional 6 months of therapy may be administered to consolidate the clinical response. After the patient's disease has stabilized, the interval between ECP treatments is gradually prolonged by 1 week per cycle every three cycles. After the interval between treatments has reached 8 weeks for three cycles, therapy can be discontinued.

Bexarotene (Retinoid Therapy)

Retinoid analogues have been categorized based on their binding patterns with respect to the major classes of retinoid receptors RAR and RXR. Bexarotene is an oral RXR-selective retinoid with activity both topically and orally. In a clinical trial of heavily pretreated refractory CTCL, oral monotherapy with bexarotene had a response rate of 54% in early stage and 45% in advanced stage CTCL patients. The median response duration was 299 days with continuous dosing at a dose of 300 mg/m²/day, and responses occurred in all groups of patients (57% at stage IIB, 32% at stage III, 44% at stage IVA, and 40% at stage IVB) including those with large cell transformation. Pruritus decreased significantly in the treated patients and led to overall improvement in quality-of-life indices.

The major toxicities of bexarotene included elevations in serum lipids and cholesterol and suppression of thyroid function. Elevations in the lipids occurred rapidly, within 2 to 4 weeks, requiring the use of lipid-lowering agents in the majority of patients. Patients taking bexarotene also developed a dose-dependent central hypothyroidism with low thyroid-stimulating hormone and free thyroxine levels within weeks of starting the medication. Bexarotene has been widely used as a first systemic oral therapy for patients with both early and advanced MF/SS. Therapy is often initiated at a low dose (2-4 capsules/day) and titrated to achieve a therapeutic effect. Laboratory studies should be performed weekly until lipid and thyroid functions are stable, and then intermittently during therapy.

Histone Deacetylase Inhibitors

Histone deacetylase (HDAC) inhibitors modulate gene expression by inhibiting the deacetylation of histone proteins associated with DNA, thereby permitting expression of a number of genes. HDAC inhibition has been shown to induce histone acetylation, cell cycle arrest, and apoptosis in leukemia and lymphoma cell lines. Depsipeptide was the first HDAC inhibitor tested in clinical trials at the NCI, and responses were seen in patients with T-cell lymphomas who received 14 mg/m^2 given intravenously on days 1, 8, and 15 of a 21-day cycle. Two multicenter phase II trials of romidepsin have been completed and have led to U.S. Food and Drug Administration (FDA) approval for romidepsin in CTCL. In both studies, the dose was 14 mg/m^2 given by a 4-hour intravenous infusion weekly × 3 on a 4-week schedule. The overall response rate in 167 patients with advanced or refractory CTCL was 35% with 6% achieving a clinical complete response. The median response duration was 11 and 14 months in the NCI and the sponsor phase II studies, respectively. The most frequent adverse events (all grades) were nausea, constitutional symptoms, and thrombocytopenia. Reversible ST-T segment changes and QT prolongation were seen on electrocardiograms but returned to baseline within 24 hours and there were no clinically relevant sequelae.

Vorinostat (Zolinza, suberoylanilide hydroxamic acid), an orally bioavailable HDAC inhibitor, has also been FDA approved for advanced or refractory CTCL. In a phase II single-agent study, oral vorinostat was administered at doses of 400 mg daily, 300 mg twice a day for 3 days with 4 days' rest, or 300 mg twice daily for 14 days with 7 days' rest, followed by 200 mg twice daily. The overall response rate in this heavily pretreated population was 24%. The 400-mg-daily schedule had the most favorable response rate and was subsequently evaluated in a phase II study that led to the approval of the drug. In this study of 74 patients with refractory CTCL, including 61 with stage IIB or higher disease, the response rate was 29%, with a median time to response of 56 days and a median response duration ranging from 34 to 441+ days. The recommended dose of vorinostat is 400 mg/day. The most common side effects are gastrointestinal (diarrhea in 49%, nausea in 43%, anorexia in 26%), fatigue, and mild thrombocytopenia, which is reversible on discontinuation of the drug. Dehydration may occur because of anorexia, and patients should be encouraged to remain well hydrated and to use antiemetics if needed.

Denileukin Diftitox

Denileukin diftitox (Ontak) is a fusion protein consisting of the *IL-2* gene joined to the active and membrane-translocating domains of diphtheria toxin. Denileukin diftitox intoxicates cells expressing both intermediate- and high-affinity IL-2 receptors by inhibiting protein synthesis. The expression of the IL-2 receptor on MF/SS cells and on other T- and B-cell lymphomas has been defined by immunohistochemistry. In the clinical trials of denileukin diftitox, expression of the CD25 subunit of the receptor on at least 20% of the tumor cells was required for entry.

In the pivotal trial that led to FDA approval of denileukin diftitox, the drug was administered at a dose of either 9 mg/kg or 18 mg/kg for 5 days every 21 days in 71 patients with relapsed or refractory CTCL (Table 17-4). The median number of prior therapies in this study was five. The overall response rate was similar for both dose groups and was 30% overall, with 10% complete responses (7 patients) and 20% partial responses (14 patients). Most of the responses occurred in the first four cycles of therapy, and the median response duration was approximately 6.9 months. The major toxicities included a reversible elevation of hepatic transaminases, a hypersensitivity syndrome associated with drug infusion, and a mild vascular leak syndrome that occurred in 29% of patients. A subsequent study combining corticosteroid pretreatment with denileukin diftitox in a less heavily pretreated group of patients demonstrated a response rate of 70% with a significantly reduced incidence of hypersensitivity reactions and clinically significant vascular leak.

TABLE 17-4   Approved Agents for Cutaneous T-Cell Lymphoma

Agent (Class)	Indication	Efficacy Data			
		Study	N	ORR (%)	DOR (Mo)
Romidepsin (HDAC inhibitor)	Patients with CTCL who have received systemic therapy	Pivotal	96	34	15
		Supportive	71	35	11
Denileukin diftitox (fusion protein)	Tumors that express CD25	Pivotal	71	30	4
Bexarotene (retinoid x-receptor activator)	Cutaneous manifestations	Pivotal	62	32	≥5
Vorinostat (HDAC inhibitor)	Cutaneous manifestations	Pivotal	74	30	≥6
		Supportive	33	24	4

CTCL, cutaneous T-cell lymphoma; DOR, duration of response; ORR overall response rate, HDAC, histone deacetylase.

A randomized, placebo-controlled phase III trial has been completed comparing denileukin diftitox at doses of 9 and 18 µg/kg daily for 5 days on a 21-day schedule in patients with earlier stage CTCL who have had fewer prior therapies. Of 144 patients treated, 67% had stages I-IIA disease. The overall response rates were 46%, 37%, and 15% for the 18-µg, 9-µg, and placebo arms, respectively. A combination study of bexarotene and denileukin diftitox was initiated based on the observation that bexarotene up-regulates expression of IL-2 receptor on lymphoma cells and enhances the susceptibility of these cells to undergo apoptosis in the presence of denileukin diftitox. Fourteen patients with refractory CTCL received escalating daily doses of bexarotene (75-300 mg) and denileukin diftitox (18 µg/kg for 3 days every 21 days). The overall response rate for all evaluable patients was 70%, with 4 complete responses (35%) and 4 partial responses (35%). This study demonstrated that doses of bexarotene greater than 150 mg/day were capable of in vivo up-regulation of CD25 (IL-2) expression and may enhance the efficacy of denileukin diftitox.

Monoclonal Antibodies

Alemtuzumab, a humanized monoclonal antibody that targets the CD52 antigen, has been shown to be active in relapsed or refractory T-cell lymphomas. Because of its profound effects on immune effector cells, alemtuzumab treatment has been associated with significant immunosuppression and a high incidence of opportunistic infections. Studies with lower doses of alemtuzumab (10 mg three times/wk) have reported responses in 6 of 10 patients, including 2 complete responses and 4 partial responses, with minimal immunosuppression. Zanolimumab a high-affinity, fully humanized monoclonal antibody that targets the CD4 receptor, has shown promising results in 49 patients with biopsy-proven CD4+ CTCL, including 23 patients with advanced stage disease. Patients were initially treated with intravenous zanolimumab at a dose of 280 mg/wk, which was increased to 560 mg/wk in early stage patients and 980 mg/wk in patients with advanced disease. Partial remissions were reported in 16 of 36 (44%) evaluable patients overall, including 3 of 6 with advanced disease at 980 mg/wk.

A novel antibody targeting the CCR4 chemokine receptor has recently demonstrated activity in patients with CTCL and in adult T-cell leukemia. The antibody KW0761 was engineered to have enhanced antibody-dependent cellular cytotoxicity activity owing to defucosylation. The antibody was administered intravenously once a week for 4 weeks, at a dose of 0.1, 0.3, or 1 mg followed by a 2-week observation period and then every other week to 38 patients with CTCL. The most frequent adverse events were chills, headache, nausea, pyrexia, infusion-related reactions, and back pain. Of the 38 patients (23 with MF, 15 with SS), the response rate was 33% in MF and 47% in SS. Remarkably, 53% of patients with SS had a complete response in their blood. Further studies are planned for this antibody in patients with advanced MF/SS.

Cytotoxic Chemotherapy

A number of conventional cytotoxic agents have demonstrated activity in CTCL, including cyclophosphamide, chlorambucil and prednisone, etoposide, and methotrexate. Although combination chemotherapy regimens have produced higher responses in patients with advanced refractory CTCL, these responses have not been durable. A study of infusional EPOCH (etoposide, vincristine, doxorubicin, bolus cyclophosphamide, and oral prednisone) in advanced refractory CTCL demonstrated an overall response rate of 80% (12 patients), with 4 (27%) complete responses. However, the median response duration was just 8 months (range 3-22 mo) and the median survival was 13.5 months. Treatment-related toxicity was significant, with 61% of the patients experiencing grade 3/4 myelosuppression. Because of the high risk of infection and myelosuppression and modest response durations with combination chemotherapy, single-agent therapies are preferred except in patients who are refractory or who present with extensive adenopathy and/or visceral involvement and require immediate palliation. Other aggressive regimens, such as hyperfractionated cyclophosphamide, vincristine, doxorubicin, and dexamethasone (hyper-CVAD) and ESHAP, Etoposide, methylprednisone, cytarabine, cisplatin have demonstrated similar activity and toxicity.

Purine Analogues

The nucleoside analogues have demonstrated significant activity in CTCL, with a response rate of 56% for dose-escalated pentostatin (3-5 mg/m^2/day for 3 days on a 21-day schedule) in 42 patients with CTCL. The incidence of infectious complications with pentostatin was initially high but was subsequently reduced by prophylactic trimethoprim and antiviral therapies. In a combination study of pentostatin at 4 mg/m^2/day for 3 days with intermediate-dose IFN-α, the overall response rate was similar, but the median progression-free survival was improved to 13.1 months.

Fludarabine and cladribine have demonstrated more modest single-agent activity in MF/SS. The combination of fludarabine with IFN-α had greater efficacy with an overall response rate of 51% (4 complete responses, 14 partial responses) with a median progression-free survival of 5.9 months and an overall survival of 19.6 months; however, hematologic toxicity was significant, with 62% of patients experiencing grade 3/4 neutropenia. Similarly, a combination of fludarabine (18 mg/m^2) and cyclophosphamide (250 mg/m^2) for 3 days monthly was associated with a duration of response (DOR) of 10 months but with significant hematologic toxicity.

Gemcitabine has demonstrated impressive clinical activity in advanced and refractory CTCL, with a 70% response rate when administered on days 1, 8, and 15 of a 28-day schedule at doses of 1000 to 1200 mg/m^2. The incidence of grade 3 neutropenia with this regimen was 25%, and the median response duration was 8 months. In a study of chemotherapy-naïve patients treated with 1200 mg/m^2, the response rate was 70%, with 5 complete responders.

Liposomal Doxorubicin

Pegylated liposomal doxorubicin has been associated with response rates of up to 80% in several small clinical trials in relapsed CTCL. In one study at a dose of 40 mg/m^2 every 28 days, the response rate was 56%. In another trial of dose-escalated liposomal doxorubicin, the response rate was 88% with a response duration of 14+ months. In a study of stage IVB patients who received 20 mg/m^2 every 28 days, the overall response rate was only 30% with no complete responders, suggesting that doses of 30 to 40 mg/m^2 are most efficacious. With the exception of infusion-related events, liposomal doxorubicin was well tolerated.

Pralatrexate

Pralatrexate (Folotyn) is a promising new folate antagonist with activity in patients with T-cell lymphoma and has been approved for patients with aggressive peripheral T-cell lymphoma. Pralatrexate has a high affinity for the reduced folate carrier and is an efficient substrate for polyglutamylation by the enzyme folylpolyglutamyl synthetase (FPGS), resulting in extensive internalization and accumulation within tumor cells. Pralatrexate inhibits dihydrofolate reductase (DHFR), resulting in disruption of DNA synthesis and subsequent tumor cell death.

Pralatrexate was granted accelerated approval by the FDA for patients with relapsed or refractory peripheral T-cell lymphoma (PTCL) at a dose of 30 mg/m^2 weekly by intravenous push for 6/7 weeks, based on the results of the PROPEL Prospective study of pralatrexate in relapsed peripheral T-cell lymphoma study. In the PROPEL study, 12 patients with transformed MF were treated and responses were seen in over 25% of patients, many of whom had been refractory to a cyclophosphamide, hydroxydaunoimycin, Oncovin, prednisone (CHOP)–like regimen. A subsequent phase I study was conducted in advanced and refractory CTCL that explored different doses and schedules, including doses of 10 to 30 mg/m^2 for 2 of 3 or 3 of 4 weeks. The optimal schedule for safety and efficacy was 15 mg/m^2 weekly $\times$ 3 every 4 weeks. In the phase II cohort expansion at this dose, the overall response rate was 45%, and the median response duration had not been reached at the time of the report. Toxicities from pralatrexate included mucositis in 17% of patients and mild neutropenia; vitamin B$_{12}$ and folate supplementation are recommended to ameliorate the severity of mucocutaneous toxicity.

AUTOLOGOUS AND ALLOGENEIC BONE MARROW TRANSPLANTATION

Results with autologous stem cell transplantation have not been promising in patients with MF/SS. One major issue in many studies is eradication of disease prior to transplant, and most patients have undergone extensive prior therapy. Allogeneic stem cell transplantation has been shown to induce complete and durable remissions in a small number of patients with CTCL, with disappearance of the malignant clone from the peripheral blood. Reduced-intensity allogeneic transplantation has been developed to reduce the toxicity related to induction therapy and to increase graft-versus-lymphoma effect and has been shown to induce a graft-versus-host effect in a small number of patients with advanced refractory MF and transformed disease. The City of Hope has reported a 2-year progression-free survival of 45% and NRM Non-relapse mortality of 27% in 11 CTCL patients. M. D. Anderson has reported

results for 19 CTCL patients who received total skin irradiation followed by a reduced-intensity regimen. The complete response was 58%, but 4 patients died in complete remission from transplant complications. Of 8 patients who relapsed in the skin, 5 had a response to reduced immunosuppression or donor lymphocyte infusions. These results suggest that allogeneic transplantation is feasible and may be associated with a prolonged disease-free survival in patients with advanced or refractory CTCL and may be considered in selected patients in whom an appropriate donor is available.

SUGGESTED READINGS

Akpek G, Koh HK, Bogen S, O'Hara C, Foss FM. Chemotherapy with etoposide, vincristine, doxorubicin, bolus cyclophosphamide, and oral prednisone in patients with refractory cutaneous T-cell lymphoma. *Cancer.* 1999;86:1368–1376.

Berger CL, Xu AL, Hanlon D, Schechner J, Glusac E, Christensen I, et al. Induction of human tumor-loaded dendritic cells. *Int J Cancer.* 2001;91:438–447.

Bernengo MG, Novelli M, Quaglino P, Lisa F, De matteis A, Savois P, et al. The relevance of the CD4+ CD26– subset in the identification of circulating Sézary cells. *Br J Dermatol.* 2001;144:125–135.

Bunn PA Jr, Huberman MS, Whang-Peng J, Schechter GP, Guccion JG, Matthews MJ, et al. Prospective staging evaluation of patients with cutaneous T-cell lymphomas. Demonstration of a high frequency of extracutaneous dissemination. *Ann Intern Med.* 1980;93:223–230.

Bunn PA Jr, Lamberg SI. Report of the Committee on Staging and Classification of Cutaneous T-Cell Lymphomas. *Cancer Treat Rep.* 1979;63:725–728.

Diamandidou E, Colome-Grimmer M, Fayad L, Duvic M, Kurzrock R. Transformation of mycosis fungoides/Sézary syndrome: clinical characteristics and prognosis. *Blood.* 1998;92:1150–1159.

Diamandidou E, Colome M, Fayad L, Duvic M, Kurzrock R. Prognostic factor analysis in mycosis fungoides/Sézary syndrome. *J Am Acad Dermatol.* 1999;40:914–924.

Dmitrovsky E, Matthews MJ, Bunn PA, Schechter GP, Makuch RW, Winkler CF, et al. Cytologic transformation in cutaneous T cell lymphoma: a clinicopathologic entity associated with poor prognosis. *J Clin Oncol.* 1987;5:208–215.

Duvic M, Hymes K, Heald P, Breneman D, Martin AG, Myskowski P, et al. Bexarotene is effective and safe for treatment of refractory advanced-stage cutaneous T-cell lymphoma: multinational phase II-III trial results. *J Clin Oncol.* 2001;19:2456–2471.

Foss FM, Ihde DC, Breneman DL, Phelps RM, Fischmann AP, Schechter GP, et al. Phase II study of pentostatin and intermittent high-dose recombinant interferon alfa-2a in advanced mycosis fungoides/Sézary syndrome. *J Clin Oncol.* 1992;10:1907–1913.

Foss FM, Ihde DC, Linnoila IR, Fischmann AB, Schechter GP, Cotelingam JD, et al. Phase II trial of fludarabine phosphate and interferon alfa-2a in advanced mycosis fungoides/Sézary syndrome. *J Clin Oncol.* 1994;12:2051–2059.

Graham SJ, Sharpe RW, Steinberg SM, Cotelingam JD, Sausville EA, Foss FM. Prognostic implications of a bone marrow histopathologic classification system in mycosis fungoides and the Sézary syndrome. *Cancer.* 1993;72:726–734.

Harmon CB, Witzig TE, Katzmann JA, Pittelkow MR. Detection of circulating T cells with CD4+CD7– immunophenotype in patients with benign and malignant lymphoproliferative dermatoses. *J Am Acad Dermatol.* 1996;35:404–410.

Huberman MS, Bunn PA Jr, Matthews MJ, Ihde DC, Gazdar AF, Cohen HH, et al. Hepatic involvement in the cutaneous T-cell lymphomas: results of percutaneous biopsy and peritoneoscopy. *Cancer.* 1980;45:1683–1688.

Jones D, Dang NH, Duvic M, Washington LT, Huh YO. Absence of CD26 expression is a useful marker for diagnosis of T-cell lymphoma in peripheral blood. *Am J Clin Pathol.* 2001;115:885–892.

Kim YH, Bishop K, Varghese A, Hoppe RT. Prognostic factors in erythrodermic mycosis fungoides and the Sézary syndrome. *Arch Dermatol.* 1995;131:1003–1008.

Kurzrock R, Pilat S, Duvic M. Pentostatin therapy of T-cell lymphomas with cutaneous manifestations. *J Clin Oncol.* 1999;17:3117–3121.

Lynch JW Jr, Linoilla I, Sausville EA, Steinberg SM, Ghosh BC, Nguyen DT, et al. Prognostic implications of evaluation for lymph node involvement by T-cell antigen receptor gene rearrangement in mycosis fungoides. *Blood.* 1992;79:3293–3299.

Olsen EA, Bunn PA. Interferon in the treatment of cutaneous T-cell lymphoma. *Hematol Oncol Clin North Am.* 1995;9:1089–1107.

Olsen E, Duvic M, Frankel A, Kim Y, Martin A, Vonderheid E, et al. Pivotal phase III trial of two dose levels of denileukin diftitox for the treatment of cutaneous T-cell lymphoma. *J Clin Oncol.* 2001;19:376–388.

Piekarz RL, Robey R, Sandor V, Bakke S, Wilson WH, Dahmoush L, et al. Inhibitor of histone deacetylation, depsipeptide (FR901228), in the treatment of peripheral and cutaneous T-cell lymphoma: a case report. *Blood.* 2001;98:2865–2868.

Salhany KE, Greer JP, Cousar JB, Collins RD. Marrow involvement in cutaneous T-cell lymphoma. A clinicopathologic study of 60 cases. *Am J Clin Pathol.* 1989;92:747–754.

Sausville EA, Eddy JL, Makuch RW, Fischmann AB, Schechter GP, Matthews M, et al. Histopathologic staging at initial diagnosis of mycosis fungoides and the Sézary syndrome. Definition of three distinctive prognostic groups. *Ann Intern Med.* 1988;109:372–382.

Sausville EA, Worsham GF, Matthews MJ, Makuch RW, Fischmann AB, Schechter GP, et al. Histologic assessment of lymph nodes in mycosis fungoides/Sézary syndrome (cutaneous T-cell lymphoma): clinical correlations and prognostic import of a new classification system. *Hum Pathol.* 1985;16:1098–1109.

Scarisbrick JJ, Child FJ, Clift A, Sabroe R, Whittaker SJ, Spittle M, et al. A trial of fludarabine and cyclophosphamide combination chemotherapy in the treatment of advanced refractory primary cutaneous T-cell lymphoma. *Br J Dermatol.* 2001;144:1010–1015.

Scheffer E, Meijer CJ, Van Vloten WA. Dermatopathic lymphadenopathy and lymph node involvement in mycosis fungoides. *Cancer.* 1980;45:137–148.

Talpur R, Ward S, Apisarnthanarax N, Breuer-Mcham J, Duvic M. Optimizing bexarotene therapy for cutaneous T-cell lymphoma. *J Am Acad Dermatol.* 2002;47:672–684.

Toro JR, Stoll HL Jr, Stomper PC, Oseroff AR. Prognostic factors and evaluation of mycosis fungoides and Sézary syndrome. *J Am Acad Dermatol.* 1997;37:58–67.

Vonderheid EC, Bernengo MG, Burg G, Duvic M, Heald P, Laroche L, et al. Update on erythrodermic cutaneous T-cell lymphoma: report of the International Society for Cutaneous Lymphomas. *J Am Acad Dermatol.* 2002;46:95–106.

Zinzani PL, Baliva G, Magagnoli M, Bendandi M, Modugno G, Gherlinzoni F, et al. Gemcitabine treatment in pretreated cutaneous T-cell lymphoma: experience in 44 patients. *J Clin Oncol.* 2000;18:2603–2606.

MOLECULAR GENETICS OF CUTANEOUS LYMPHOMAS

Derek V. Chan, MD, PhD, and Henry K. Wong, MD, PhD

INTRODUCTION

Cutaneous lymphomas are a clinically heterogeneous group of lymphoid neoplasms with diverse pathologies and clinical courses. Because the skin is a major immune organ and plays a critical role in immune surveillance and defense against pathogens, the normal role is for B and T cells to traffic through the skin to carry out host defense. When defects arise in the regulation of proliferation of B and T cells, progression to malignancy can develop in the skin. Both cutaneous B-cell lymphomas (CBCLs) and cutaneous T-cell lymphomas (CTCLs) can present primarily on the skin, with diverse clinical manifestations. Cutaneous lymphomas in general have a better prognosis than their systemic counterparts, and histologic and molecular genetic characterization is important for diagnosis, treatment, and determining prognosis. B cells show more consistent molecular characterization than T cells, but molecular characterization of the latter with relation to new biomarkers may lead to improved markers for diagnosis and classification.

In the past several years, a joint World Health Organization—European Organization for Research and Treatment of Cancer (WHO/EORTC) effort in 2005 categorized known variants of cutaneous lymphoma, with attention to biologic profiles, clinical presentations, and prognoses. Additional revisions were undertaken in consensus criteria that were integrated in the 2008 WHO classification for nodal and extranodal lymphomas, which captures the full clinical, pathologic, and molecular spectra of these neoplasms and the features most important in diagnosis, prognosis, and treatment.

In general, cutaneous lymphomas can originate from lymphocytes of either the B or the T lineage. In this chapter, we outline the major genetic changes that have been identified from recent studies of CBCLs and CTCLs in the context of diagnosis and treatment.

CUTANEOUS B-CELL LYMPHOMAS

Primary CBCLs are considered extranodal lymphomas and do not show any involvement of systemic or other extracutaneous sites. In general, CBCLs are indolent and show slow growth. Confirmation of cutaneous involvement is important in treatment and prognosis. The differentiation of the subtype is difficult to make based on clinical presentation, but the affected location can be helpful. In general, such cutaneous lymphomas affect the upper body, with the exception of large B-cell lymphoma of the leg type. For differentiation of the subtype, biopsy of the lesion with histologic and molecular immunologic characterization is important.

As progress in the understanding of lymphomas advances, genetic characterization can provide additional insights into B-cell lymphomas of the skin. In general, B-cell lymphomas of the skin show changes that can be commonly seen in B-cell skin malignancies. The pathogenetic basis of these changes is unclear, but studies have identified recurrent signature genetic changes associated with specific B-cell malignancies. CBCLs represent approximately 30% of all primary cutaneous lymphomas. There are three major cutaneous presentations, marginal zone, follicular, and diffuse large cell lymphoma of the leg. Generally, they have relatively favorable prognoses with 5-year survivals greater than 90%. The exception is diffuse large cell lymphoma of the leg, the most aggressive type, with a more guarded prognosis with 5 year survivals of 20% to 25%. For this clinical variant, more aggressive systemic treatment is required. For CBCLs, primary lesions in general do not show chromosomal translocations, unlike with their systemic counterparts.

In general, monoclonality can be used to detect malignant populations in primary cutaneous marginal zone lymphoma (PCMZL), primary cutaneous diffuse large B-cell lymphoma, leg type (PCDLBCL,LT), and primary cutaneous follicular center lymphoma (PCFCL). One recent study using the BIOMED-2 protocol to detect B-cell clonality via immunoglobulin heavy chain (IGH), immunoglobulin kappa chain (IGκ, and immunoglobulin lambda chain (IGκ) rearrangements found the following results: 100% of PCFCLs ($n = 5$), 83.3% of PCMZLs ($n = 6$), and 100% of PCDLBCL, LTs ($n = 6$) had monoclonality. In contrast, only 22.2% of benign lymphocytic infiltrates had monoclonality. Despite these findings, the authors of this study noted that it might be most useful in cases of indolent PCBCLs and for `differentiating possible benign lymphocytic infiltrates. Additional studies have shown that the atypical cells in PCFCL are derived from the germinal center whereas those of PCMZL are derived from B cells in the marginal zone of the spleen.

Primary Cutaneous Marginal Zone B-Cell Lymphomas

PCMZLs make up between 2% and 16% of all cutaneous lymphomas. Lesions have been reported to present as papules (3 cases), plaques (17 cases), nodules (21 cases), or tumors (18 cases) and have been reported to be more often multifocal (36 cases), as opposed to solitary (11 cases) or localized (3 cases) in one study of 50 patients with this disease. Of note, 8 patients had multiple types of primary lesions. The trunk has been reported to be the most common site of presentation (30 cases), followed by the arms and legs (17 cases each), and the head and neck (6 cases). In a study of 62 patients with PCMZLs, the mean and median ages of patients were 51.3 and 55.5 years, respectively, with a range of ages 17 to 86 years, and the male-to-female ratio was 1.69:1. The estimated 5-year survival rate was 98%.

The clinical presentation is of enlarging skin nodules. These lesions are not generally symptomatic. Histologically, the atypical cells are small and may be comprised of the following types of B cells: marginal zone, monocytoid, or plasmacytoid. In addition, plasma cells may also contribute to PCMZLs. A possible link between *Borellia burgdorferi* infection and this lymphoma has been noted in Europe, although this has not been reported in the United States or Asia. However, in a recent study, evidence of

B. bugdorferi infection via polymerase chain reaction (PCR) DNA analysis was not detected in any of 60 cases from Germany, the United States, and Asia. In addition, it has been suggested that a translocation of chromosomes 11 and 18, resulting in an *API2-MALT1* fusion protein, might be relevant in PCMZLs because it is found in other mucosal-associated lymphoid tissue (MALT) lymphomas. The t(11:18) translocation has been detected in 4 of 51 cases of skin lymphomas. However, in the aforementioned study of 60 patients with PCMZL, *Borrelia* DNA and the *API-MALT1* fusion transcript were *not* found in cases from Asia, Germany, or the United States. Furthermore, in another study of 12 specimens of PCMZLs, none of the specimens had an *API-MALT1* fusion transcript detectable by PCR. However, DNA methylation of the *DAPK* gene *was* detected in 43% of cases compared with 8% of controls. The *p16* gene was methylated in 49% of cases, compared with 14% of controls. Differential cytosine-phosphate-guanine (CpG) DNA methylation of *p14, MGMT, TIMP3, CDH1,* and *RARB* was found when comparing PCMZL patients with controls. Furthermore, 2 out of 5 patients with PCMZL were found to have plasmacytoid differentiation, and of these 2, both were found to have downregulation of CD19, CD20, bcl6, and PAX5. Such changes have been confirmed by prior studies. In addition, 2 of 5 cases of PCMZL were also noted to express XBP-1, a transcription factor that plays a role in plasma cell differentiation, and this was expressed in normal tonsils also.

Primary Cutaneous Follicle Center Lymphomas

PCFCLs are the most common primary CBCL and comprise approximately 57% of such lymphomas, according to one study. The location, age, and sex of patients affected can be variable. In one study, the male-to-female ratio was 1.69:1, and the mean and median ages of the affected individuals was 51.3 years and 55.5 years, respectively, with an age range of 17 to 86 years. The estimated 5-year survival rate in this study was 98%. In another study, the ratio of males to females was 7:9, the mean age was 64 years, and the age range was 33 to 83 years. In this study, head and neck lesions predominated (12 cases), followed by trunk lesions

(6 cases), and then extremity lesions (1 case). In a recent study, the male-to-female ratio was 19:5, and the mean and median ages were 58.3 years and 57 years, respectively, with an age range of 33 to 87 years. In this study, the majority of patients had lesions on the trunk (20 cases), 2 patients had lesions on the extremities, and 1 patient had a lesion on the head. Primary lesions are typically either single or small clustered erythematous nodules or papules that are nonpruritic.

In a gene expression profile analysis, PCFCL and secondary follicular center lymphoma were both found to have CD79a, CD79b, syk, BLNK, CD19, CD20, PAX5, TCL1, Oct-2, Bob-1, CD21, BCL-6, ICOS, CXCR5, CXCL13, RGS13, BCL7A, BCL11A, and LMO2. With respect to chromosomal translocations, a t(14:18) resulting in bcl-2 expression has only been reported in a single case of PCFCL. In contrast, bcl-2 expression has been widely reported in nodal follicular center cell lymphomas. Furthermore, in a gene array study involving cDNA microarrays containing at least 40,000 genes, primary and secondary cutaneous follicular lymphomas did express up-regulation of typical B-cell receptor markers and B-cell development–associated transcription factors, compared with tonsil, normal skin, and CTCL controls (i.e., CD79a, CD79b, syk, BLNK, PAX5, TCL1, and Oct-2). These tumors, in addition to the tonsil specimens, also expressed germinal center B-cell–associated genes (*Oct-2, Bob-1, CD21, bcl-6, ICOS, CXCR5, CXCL13, RGS13, BCL7A, BCL11A,* and *LMO2*).

Primary Cutaneous Large B-Cell Lymphomas, Leg Type

PCDLBCL,LTs, have a markedly worse prognosis than other primary CBCLs because the 5-year survival rate for these lymphomas has been estimated to be 58%. In general, this subtype typically affects older patients because the mean and median ages were 70.6 years and 72 years, respectively, with a age range of 43 to 86 years. With respect to molecular markers, FoxP1 has been preferentially identified in PDCLBCL,LT compared with primary cutaneous large B-cell lymphoma (PCDLBCL), non-leg type.

Other molecular changes have been shown to be helpful in diagnosis. In a study of 29 patients

with PCDLBCLs, 11 of 14 of the PCDLBCL,LTs, exhibited breakpoints by fluorescence in situ hybridization (FISH) in at least one of the following loci: *IGH, MYC, BCL-6, and MLT1*. Six of these 11 cases had translocations at the *MYC* locus, and 5 of these 6 involved translocations involving the *IGH* locus. Five of these 11 cases had rearrangements involving the *BCL6* locus, and 2 of these 5 also involved the *IGH* locus. In contrast, PCFCL and PCMZL did not exhibit these translocations. In another study, amplification of a region containing the *BCL-2* and *MALT-1* genes, 18q21.31-q21.33, was found in 8 of 12 patients with PCDLBCL,LT. Deletion of portions of 9p21.3, a region containing *CDKN2A, CDKN2B,* and *NSG-x* was found in 5 of 12 patients, and deletion of 9p21.3 was found on both chromosomes in 5 of 12 patients with PCDLBCL,LT, compared with none of the 19 patients with PCFCL. In addition, all 7 patients with PCDLBCL,LT, and a deletion of 9p21.3 and/or complete methylation of CDKN2A died as a result of the lymphoma. In another study, 43 of 64 patients had homozygous loss of the *CDKN2A* locus, responsible for encoding *p16* and *p14ARF*. Hypermethylation of the *p16* promoter was found in 6 cases, but none of the *p14ARF* cases had detectable promoter hypermethylation. In patients with genetic alterations at the *CDKN2A* locus, survival was markedly worse compared with patients without detectable genetic alterations because the reported 5-year survival rates between those with alterations and those without alterations were 43% and 70%, respectively. Hence, *CDKN2A* inactivation is associated with a worse prognosis in patients with PCDLBCL,LT.

CUTANEOUS T-CELL LYMPHOMAS

Mycosis fungoides (MF) is the most common variant of the CTCLs, accounting for approximately 44% of all cutaneous lymphomas. In general, the survival rate for the early stages of MF is excellent and it typically shows an indolent course. The 5-year survival when the lymphoma is restricted to the skin is 88%. As the clinical stage of diagnosis worsens, with plaques affecting greater than 10% of the body surface area, tumors, or associated with lymph node involvement, the prognosis is worse and the long-term survival decreases. Sézary's syndrome (SS), differentiated by MF with generalized erythroderma, clonal leukemic blood involvement, lymphadenopathy, is more aggressive and accounts for approximately 3% of cutaneous lymphomas and has a correspondingly lower 5-year survival rate at 24%. MF typically affects older individuals, and there is a slight bias toward the male sex, as the median age at diagnosis is usually between 55 and 60 years of age. Up to twice as many males as females are diagnosed with the disease.

On histology, the biopsy of lesions of MF shows lymphocytic epidermotropism and intraepidermal aggregates of atypical cells (Pautrier's microabscesses). Pautrier's microabscesses are highly specific to CTCL; however, these are not always detected, and hence, their presence is not necessary for the diagnosis to be made. The nuclei of atypical cells may resemble the brain and, hence, have been termed *cerebriform cells*. With respect to the surface markers, atypical cells in MF are typically CD3+, CD4+, CD8–, and CD45RO+. However, reduced expression of CD3, CD26, CD5, and/or CD7 has been reported. Additional surface markers have been analyzed such as CCR4 and CTLA-4, and these show consistent expression. Although these markers reveal properties of the malignant cell, these markers have not been adapted for routine diagnosis.

With respect to the molecular genetics of mycosis fungoides, T-cell receptor rearrangement studies often show evidence of monoclonality. Results from the BIOMED-2 study have resulted in many laboratories utilizing the InVivoScribe primers for detection of T-cell receptor gene clonality for clinical use.

To further understand the pathogenesis of CTCL, a number of groups have performed genetic studies using a variety of arrays to map defects. From preliminary studies, several groups have reported numerous chromosomal abnormalities in MF, including chromosomes 1, 6, 7, 8, 9, 10, and 17, especially in advanced MF. However, consistent chromosomal translocations that correlate with prognosis or biologic behavior have not been reported, complicating their use in the diagnosis of MF. Despite this difficulty, however, a frequent reproducible chromosome loss on 10q and abnormalities in tumor suppressor genes

such as p15, p16, and p53, has been reported. These changes are seen commonly in cancers and may contribute to the proliferative nature of this cancer. Nevertheless, the presence of these changes suggest that there may be additional genetic markers that may be used to aid in the diagnosis of MF.

With respect to SS, increased frequency of changes in chromosomes 1, 2, 6, 7, 12, and 14 have been reported. A t(14;14)(q12;q31) translocation has been reported, as well as a del(8)(p21) in patients with SS. Table 18-1 outlines a listing of chromosomal abnormalities in SS.

Comparative genomic hybridization (CGH) has been utilized to find changes in DNA copy numbers. Losses of DNA in SS have been greater than those chromosome regions gained. Losses have been greatest at 1p, 10q25-26 and 13q21-q22, and chromosome 19 whereas gains have been greatest at 4q, 8/8q, 17q21-q25, and chromosome 18. Using single nucleotide polymorphism (SNP) arrays in conjunction with array CGH, copy number losses were most often found at 17p13.2-p11.2, 10p12.1-q26.3, and 9q13-q21.33. Copy number gains were most often found at 17p11.2-q25.3, 8p23.2-q24.3, and 10p15.3-p12.2. From these data, it appears that area of chromosomes 10 and 17 play an integral role in SS, although one review has noted that chromosomes 10, 13, 8, and 18 are the key chromosomes for which there are common abnormalities.

Differential expression of genes in SS has also been observed. Some genes of interest that are more highly expressed in SS include *BAG4, BTRC, NKIRAS2, PSMD3, TRAF2, BUB3, SET, TWIST, EphA4, Her2/neu, JUNB,* and *cMYC.* Interestingly, decreased levels of MXI1 and MNT, antagonists to cMYC, have been reported to be decreased in SS. The loss of *TP53* (p53 tumor suppressor) has been reported in SS and may correlate with a loss of apoptosis in neoplastic cells. In addition, loss of additional tumor suppressor genes such as those coding for p15, p16, and Fas (CD95) have been reported, and the loss of the latter has been reported in both blood and lesional skin. In addition, up-regulation of STAT3 and STAT5 on 17q21.31 correlates with a T helper 2 (Th2) phenotype and interleukin-2 (IL-2) downstream events, in accordance with cellular proliferation.

Epigenetic changes have also been reported in cancers, and CTCL does not appear to be different

TABLE 18-1   T-Cell Lymphomas

Chromosomal Location and/or Abnormality	References
Chromosome 1	Solé et al. (1994); Johnson, Dewald, Strand, Winkelmann (1985)
Chromosome 1—Loss of material—1p33-36	Thangavelu et al. (1997)
Chromosome 2	Solé et al. (1994)
Chromosome 4	Solé et al. (1994)
Chromosome 6	Solé et al. (1994); Johnson, Dewald, Strand, Winkelmann (1985); Thangavelu et al. (1997)
Chromosome 8—Loss of material	Thangavelu et al. (1997)
Chromosome 8—Deletion [Del(8)(p21)]	Izykowska & Przybylski (2011)
Chromosomes 8 & 17—Translocation t(8;17) (q11;p11)	Thangavelu et al. (1997)
Chromosome 10—Monosomy	Solé et al. (1994)
Chromosome 10	Thangavelu et al. (1997)
Chromosome 10—10q22-24	Izykowska & Przybylski (2011)
Chromosome 12—12p11-12	Izykowska & Przybylski (2011)
Chromosome 14	Solé et al. (1994); Berger & Bernheim (1987)
Chromosome 14—Translocation [t(14;14) (q12;q31)]	Shah-Reddy, Mirchandani, & Koppitch (1982)
Chromosome 14—14q11	Izykowska & Przybylski (2011)
Chromosome 14—14q32	Izykowska & Przybylski (2011)
Chromosome 17	Thangavelu et al. (1997)
Chromosome 17—17p	Izykowska & Przybylski (2011)

in this regard. For instance, hypermethylation of the tumor suppressor genes *HIC1, BCL7a, PTPRG, THBS4, p73, p16, CHRR, TNS1*, and *p16(INK4a)* has been reported. Promoter hypermethylation of the *Fas* gene has also been reported, and this may contribute to the relative resistance of CTCL cells to apoptosis. Because epigenetic changes to tumor suppressor or apoptosis-inducing genes have been noted in CTCLs, this likely explains why histone deacetylase (HDAC) inhibitors such as romidepsin and vorinostat have been found to be effective in the therapy of these lymphomas. Such drugs may reverse the expression of such genes and restore tumor suppression or induce the ability of neoplastic cells to undergo apoptosis. With respect to promoter hypomethylation, this phenomenon has been described in multiple other cancers, including prostate and colorectal cancer. To date, the concept of promoter hypomethylation in CTCLs has not been well described. It is likely that promoter hypomethylation, perhaps of genes affecting cell growth, may also be described in CTCLs.

SUMMARY

Genetic changes play critical roles in the pathogenesis of cancer. With the discovery and the application of molecular techniques that permit high-resolution interrogation of the genome, studies of cutaneous lymphomas have uncovered numerous novel genetic changes. These changes may be associated with altered gene expression associated with the deregulated proliferative nature of these malignancies and further studies are warranted to elucidate the specific role in oncogenesis. Nevertheless, the development of novel therapies that alter gene expression, such as the HDAC inhibitors vorinostat and romidepsin, and demethylating drugs, such as deazacytidine, indicate that targeting genetic mechanisms is effective in the treatment of cutaneous lymphomas. Continued characterization of genetic changes may lead to the identification of critical deregulated pathways associated with the development of cutaneous lymphomas and to the development of specific treatments.

SUGGESTED READINGS

Aguilera NSI, Tomaszewski MM, Moad JC, Bauer FA, Taubenberger JK, Abbondanzo SL. Cutaneous follicle center lymphoma: a clinicopathologic study of 19 cases. *Mod Pathol.* 2001;14:828–835.

Berger R, Bernheim A. Cytogenetic studies of Sézary cells. *Cancer Genet Cytogenet.* 1987;27:79–87.

Bosga-Bouwer AG, van Imhoff GW, Boonstra R, van der Veen A, Haralambieva E, van den Berg A, et al. Follicular lymphoma grade 3B includes 3 cytogenetically defined subgroups with primary t(14;18), 3q27, or other translocations: t(14;18) and 3q27 are mutually exclusive. *Blood.* 2003;101:1149–1154.

Brito-Babapulle V, Hamoudi R, Matutes E, Watson S, Kaczmarek P, Maljaie H, et al. p53 allele deletion and protein accumulation occurs in the absence of p53 gene mutation in T-prolymphocytic leukaemia and Sézary syndrome. *Br J Haematol.* 2000;110: 180–187.

Calame KL. Plasma cells: finding new light at the end of B cell development. *Nat Immunol.* 2001;2:1103–1108.

Cerroni L, Volkenandt M, Rieger E, Soyer HP, Kerl H. bcl-2 protein expression and correlation with the interchromosomal 14;18 translocation in cutaneous lymphomas and pseudolymphomas. *J Invest Dermatol.* 1994;102:231–235.

Dereure O, Portales P, Clot J, Guilhou JJ. Decreased expression of Fas (APO-1/CD95) on peripheral blood CD4+ T lymphocytes in cutaneous T-cell lymphomas. *Br J Dermatol.* 2000;143:1205–1210.

Dereure O, Portales P, Clot J, Guilhou JJ. Decreased expression of fas (APO-1/CD95) on lesional CD4+ T lymphocytes in cutaneous T cell lymphomas: correlations with blood data. *Br J Dermatol.* 2001;145: 1031–1032.

Fink-Puches R, Zenahlik P, Bäck B, Smolle J, Kerl H, Cerroni L. Primary cutaneous lymphomas: applicability of current classification schemes (European Organization for Research and Treatment of Cancer, World Health Organization) based on clinicopathologic features observed in a large group of patients. *Blood.* 2002;99:800–805.

Hallermann C, Kaune KM, Gesk S, Martin-Subero JI, Gunawan B, Griesinger F, et al. Molecular cytogenetic analysis of chromosomal breakpoints in the IGH, MYC, BCL6, and MALT1 gene loci in primary cutaneous B-cell lymphomas. *J Invest Dermatol.* 2003;123:213–219.

Johnson GA, Dewald GW, Strand WR, Winkelmann RK. Chromosome studies in 17 patients with the Sézary syndrome. *Cancer.* 1985;55:2426–2433.

Karenko L, Hyytinen E, Sarna S, Ranki A. Chromosomal abnormalities in cutaneous T-cell lymphoma and in its premalignant conditions as detected by G-banding and interphase cytogenetic methods. *J Invest Dermatol.* 1997;108:22–29.

Karenko L, Kähkönen M, Hyytinen ER, Lindlof M, Ranki A. Notable losses at specific regions of chromosomes 10q and 13q in the Sézary syndrome detected by comparative genomic hybridization. J Invest Dermatol. 1999;112:392–395.

Li C. Inagaki H, Kuo TT. Primary cutaneous marginal zone B-cell lymphoma: a molecular and clinicopathologic study of 24 Asian cases. *Am J Surg Pathol.* 2003;27:1061–1069.

Limon J, Nedoszytko B, Brozek I, Hellmann A, Zajaczek S, Lubinski J, et al. Chromosome aberrations, spontaneous SCE, and growth kinetics in PHA-stimulated lymphocytes of five cases with Sézary syndrome. *Cancer Genet Cytogenet.* 1995;83:75–81.

Mao X, Lillington DM, Czepulkowski B, Russell-Jones R, Young BD, Whittaker S. Molecular cytogenetic analysis of cutaneous T-cell lymphomas: identification of common genetic alterations in Sézary syndrome and mycosis fungoides. *Br J Dermatol.* 2002;147:464–475.

Mao X, Orchard G, Lillington DM, Russell-Jones R, Young BD, Whittaker SJ. Amplification and overexpression of JUNB is associated with primary cutaneous T-cell lymphomas. *Blood.* 2003;101:1513–1519.

Mohr B, Illmer T, Oelschlägel U, Nowak R, Hölig K, Paaz U, et al. Complex cytogenetic and immunophenotypic aberrations in a patient with Sézary syndrome. *Cancer Genet Cytogenet.* 1996;90:33–36.

Navas IC, Ortiz-Romero PL, Villuendas R, Martínez P, García C, Gómez E, et al. p16(INK4a) gene alterations are frequent in lesions of mycosis fungoides. *Am J Pathol.* 2000;156:1565–1572.

Pandolfino TL, Siegel RS, Kuzel TM, Rosen ST, Guitart J. Primary cutaneous B-cell lymphoma: review and current concepts. *J Clin Oncol.* 2000;18:2152–2168.

Scarisbrick JJ, Woolford AJ, Russell-Jones R, Whittaker SJ. Allelotyping in mycosis fungoides and Sézary syndrome: common regions of allelic loss identified on 9p, 10q, and 17p. *J Invest Dermatol.* 2001;117:663–670.

Shah-Reddy I, Mirchandani I, Koppitch FC. Sézary syndrome with a 14:14 (q12:q31) translocation. *Cancer.* 1982;49:75–79.

Shapiro PE, Warburton D, Berger CL, Edelson RL. Clonal chromosomal abnormalities in cutaneous T-cell lymphoma. *Cancer Genet Cytogenet.* 1987;28: 267–276.

Skinnider BF, Horsman DE, Dupuis B, Gascoyne RD. Bcl-6 and Bcl-2 protein expression in diffuse large B-cell lymphoma and follicular lymphoma: correlation with 3q27 and 18q21 chromosomal abnormalities. *Hum Pathol.* 1999;30:803–808.

Smoller BR, Santucci M, Wood GS, Whittaker SJ. Histopathology and genetics of cutaneous T-cell lymphoma. *Hematol Oncol Clin North Am.* 2003;17: 1277–1311.

Solé F, Woessner S, Vallespi T, Pérez Losada A, Florensa L, Irriguible D, et al. Cytogenetic studies in five patients with Sézary syndrome. *Cancer Genet Cytogenet.* 1994;75:130–132.

Storz, MN, van de Rijn M, Kim YH, Mraz-Gernhard S, Hoppe RT, Kohler S. Gene expression profiles of cutaneous B cell lymphoma. *J Invest Dermatol.* 2003;120:865–870.

Thangavelu M, Finn WG, Yelavarthi KK, Roenigk HH Jr, Samuelson E, Peterson L, et al. Recurring structural chromosome abnormalities in peripheral blood lymphocytes of patients with mycosis fungoides/Sézary syndrome. *Blood.* 1997;89:3371–3377.

Willemze R, Kerl H, Sterry W, Berti E, Cerroni L, Chimenti S, et al. EORTC classification for primary cutaneous lymphomas: a proposal from the Cutaneous Lymphoma Study Group of the European Organization for Research and Treatment of Cancer. *Blood.* 1997;90:354–371.

Wood GS, Kamath NV, Guitart J. Absence of *Borrelia burgdorferi* DNA in cutaneous B-cell lymphomas from the United States. *J Cutan Pathol.* 2001;28:502–507.

FUTURE STRATEGIES IN DIAGNOSIS AND TREATMENT OF CUTANEOUS LYMPHOMAS

Lauren C. Pinter Brown, MD

DIAGNOSIS

From 1979, when the term "cutaneous T-cell lymphoma" (CTCL) was used during a historic meeting of the Mycosis Fungoides (MF) Cooperative Group at the National Cancer Institute of the United States to the 2005 World Health Organization—European Organization for Research and Treatment of Cancer (WHO/EORTC) Classification for Cutaneous Lymphomas, to the current WHO Classification of Tumours of Haematopoietic and Lymphoid Tissues, our classification of cutaneous lymphomas reflects our growing knowledge of differences in either cell of origin, histopathologic appearance, clinical presentation, and/or natural history of the separate entities that we now know as *cutaneous lymphomas.* This elucidation of distinct entities that will continue has allowed us to be more accurately informed about the natural history of these disorders and how this may be changed by appropriate and tailored therapies. Clearly, this dissection of known diagnostic entities will continue in the future and will allow us to focus more keenly on how to best design treatments and improve the prognosis of our patients.

Two good examples of this evolving knowledge can be found in the study of the differences between the cells of patients who present with *Sézary's syndrome (SS),* in the past considered an erythrodermic, leukemic subtype of MF, and those who present with more classic patch/plaque MF and in the study of CD30+ cutaneous lymphoproliferations forming de novo and in the context of a previous diagnosis of MF.

Studying the clonal malignant cells from blood of patients with SS and T cells isolated from skin of patients with more classic MF, Campbell and coworkers found these two populations of cells varied dramatically in their expression of CCR7-selectin and CD27. Sézary cells were found to strongly express these antigens as well as CCR4 with variable common leukocyte antigen (CLA) expression, and T cells from the skin of patients with classic MF were found to be lacking such expression and instead demonstrated expression of CCR4 and CLA consistently. It was concluded that Sézary cells exhibited antigens most consistent with a "central memory T-cell"; MF cells exhibited antigens most like a "skin resident effector memory T cell." This work demonstrating that SS may be a different condition, not a subtype of MF, is further corroborated by the knowledge of the clinical presentation of these two entities that, in the majority of the cases, appear to have distinct clinical presentations, with rare evolution from one entity to the other, and by genomic differences that have been demonstrated between the two entities.

Clearly as a distinction between these two entities evolves and we obtain a better understanding of how these entities interrelate, this will have a profound effect on the staging and the implied prognosis of these patient groups. Moreover, the different therapeutic needs of these two patient groups may be further emphasized. Futher work on the expression of CD158k (KIR3D2L), a killer cell immunoglobulin-like cell surface receptor, on Sézary cells and the detection of its transcript in the erythrodermatous skin of patients with SS may also assist in the more precise diagnosis of this condition.

Current pathologic criteria cannot reliably distinguish between primary cutaneous anaplastic large cell lymphoma (C-ALCL) and the other CD 30+ lymphoproliferations, lymphomatoid papulosis and transformed mycosis fungoides (T-MF). Therefore, current diagnostic practices require collaboration between pathologist and clinician to establish a definitive diagnosis. Furthermore, at the present time, the development of a skin lesion with the appearance of C-ALCL pathologically and perhaps clinically found in the setting of a previous diagnosis of MF must be considered transformation of MF to tumor stage. Histologic T-MF, for many a turning point in the natural history of their disease with a dire prognosis, may be defined by the presence of more than 25% of large cells in dermal infiltrates, either CD30+ or CD30–, thus creating a conundrum. Do all skin lesions resembling C-ALCL developing in the milieu of previously diagnosed MF carry with them a poor prognosis or is it possible for P-ALCL to develop in a patient independently of their MF, thus leaving the patient's prognosis unchanged?

Wada and colleagues studied the detection of interferon regulatory factor-4 (IRF-4) translocations by florescence in situ hybridization techniques (FISH) in skin biopsies representing a variety of CD30+ cutaneous T-cell lymphoproliferations and found that such testing had a statistically significant specificity and positive predictive value of 99% and 90%, respectively, in the ability to distinguish C-ALCL from other CD30+ lymphoproliferative disorders. Using similar techniques, Pham-Ledard and associates found that IRF-4 rearrangements could define a subgroup of C-ALCL and T-MF, suggesting that the development of C-ALCL in the setting of MF may not correspond to large cell transformation of MF. Such distinctions between C-ALCL and T-MF are not merely semantic but also guide our discussions with patients regarding their prognosis and the selection of treatments. The further ability to clarify these conditions may make a major impact on how the treatment of some patients is approached.

TREATMENT

As the incidence of all non-Hodgkin's lymphomas continues to increase, for example, by 20% in the past two decades in the United States, and the cutaneous lymphomas are largely incurable and chronic conditions, the necessity for finding new and better methods of treatment continues to be a priority.

Primary Cutaneous B-Cell Lymphoma

The primary cutaneous B-cell lymphomas (CBCLs) can broadly be divided into those that behave in a biologically indolent fashion—primary cutaneous follicle center lymphoma and extranodal marginal zone lymphoma—and a more aggressive entity, primary cutaneous diffuse large B-cell lymphoma (PCDLBCL), leg type. The last entity, PCDLBCL, may behave in a clinical fashion that that could best be described as between the two furthest ends of the spectrum of primary CBCL.

PCDLBCL, leg type, has a gene expression profile of activated B-cell–like diffuse large B-cell lymphoma (DLBCL), carrying a worse prognosis with increasing numbers of skin lesions. Cyclophosphamide, hydroxydaunoimycin, Oncovin, prednisone (CHOP) chemotherapy remains of unclear benefit in this patient group. In the future, pending randomized trials now ongoing for DLBCL and specifically for DLBCL, with nongerminal center, or activated B-cell–like phenotype, we may be able to extrapolate from these data to the treatment of PCDLBCL, leg type, and consider alternative therapies such as CHOP with the addition of bortezomib, or dose-adjusted rituxan-EPOCH (etoposide, vincristine, doxorubicin, bolus cyclophosphamide, and oral prednisone) infusional therapy.

The indolent primary CBCLs have an excellent prognosis with a 5-year survival over 95% and require systemic therapies only in the minority of patients with extensive cutaneous disease or those who develop extracutaneous disease. Although it is unlikely that large clinical trials will be performed in this small patient population, we may look at the extensive research activity now occurring in the area of treatment of systemic indolent B-cell lymphomas for possible future treatment options. Here, two major areas of research are pertinent: (1) the development of novel antibodies to expand the activity of rituximab and the radioimmunotherapeutic extensions of this antibody (2) and the development of novel targeted therapies.

An example of a novel anti-CD20 antibody with different methods of cell kill than rituximab is GA-101, a humanized antibody that may have improved antibody-dependent cell-mediated cytotoxicity (ADCC). As a type II antibody, although it lacks the ability to trigger complement-dependent cytotoxicity (CDC), it has demonstrated improved direct induction of cell death. Clinical trials in various B-cell malignancies are ongoing and results are anticipated.

Novel targeted agents such as those targeting the microenvironment, the immunomodulatory

(IMiD) agents, such as lenalidomide or pomalidomide, that have been derived from the parent compound thalidomide may be useful oral agents in the treatment of indolent B-cell lymphomas.

Further examples of targeted therapies that can inhibit a specific signaling pathway that are important to B-cell lymphoma cell growth and survival include Bruton tyrosine kinase inhibitors, such as PCI-32765; inhibitors of the PI3/AKT/mTOR pathway, such as CAL-101 (a PI3 inhibitor); perifosine (an AKT inhibitor); and temsirolimus and everolimus (RAD001), intravenous and oral targets of mammalian target of rapamycin (mTOR).

An additional rational therapeutic target, bcl-2, can be inhibited by such agents as ABT-263. Results from phase II clinical trials of these agents are awaited. The reader is referred to the excellent review of these targets and drugs by Reeder and coworkers.

Cutaneous T-Cell Lymphomas

CTCL is a heterogeneous group of disorders, some of which may be appropriately treated topically in their early stages and some may require systemic treatment at diagnosis. In the realm of future topical treatments, current research is limited to improving and possibly shortening the delivery of total body electron beam for patients with MF and improving the formulation of nitrogen mustard to allow for easier access and a more consistent product.

The area of systemic treatments, particularly the study of new antibodies or antibody drug conjugates, is possibly the most exciting one in terms of advancement of treatment for future patients with CTCL. With respect to systemic treatments, we look to trials in T-cell lymphomas mostly of the aggressive types to yield clues for future treatments in CTCL.

Antibody and Antibody Drug Conjugates to Treat T-Cell Lymphomas

Given the phenomenal practice-changing effect of rituximab, an antibody that targets CD20+ B cells, a priority in the area of clinical research that addresses optimizing treatment for T-cell malignancies has been the search for an efficacious and safe antibody. Initial attempts with sipilizumab, an anti-CD2 antibody for use in T-cell malignancies, showed it to be efficacious, but with an unacceptable occurrence of Ebstein-Barr virus–positive (EBV+) lymphoproliferative disorder in 14% of patients. These patients were characterized by a lower natural killer and CD2 count. A second, more targeted antibody, zanolimumab (HuMax-CD4), an anti-CD4 antibody, was evaluated in a phase I trial for patients with MF and SS. With the exception of depression of total CD4 counts, the drug showed an overall response rate of 56%, with a median duration of response of 81 weeks after 17 weekly infusions. The overall response rate was slightly higher in MF than SS (34% vs. 22%); however, only 9 patients with SS participated in the trial.

More recently, other targeted antibodies, such as KW-0761, an anti-chemoreceptor 4 (CCR4) antibody, and brentuximab vedotin (SGN-35), an anti-CD30 antibody (SGN-30) conjugated with a chemotherapeutic agent, monomethyl auristatin E (MMAE) have been evaluated.

KW-0761 is a defucosylated humanized anti-CCR4 antibody that was first studied in patients in Japan with relapsed or refractory adult T-cell leukemia/lymphoma (ATLL), a relatively chemoresistant disease. In the phase I study, 30% of such patients attained a response, 13% of these complete. No maximal tolerated dose was identified. Reporting on the subsequent phase II trial, 27 patients with relapsed or refractory ATLL were shown to have an overall response of 54% and 27% of patients demonstrating a complete response.

In a phase I/II study in the United States of patients with relapsed or refractory MF, SS, or T-MF, an overall response of 39% was seen with patients with SS appearing to respond at a higher rate than patients with MF (47% vs. 35%). Focusing on the blood compartment of patients with SS, 80% of patients responded in blood with 47% of these being complete responses by flow cytometry. Further studies with this promising agent are ongoing.

The CD30+ lymphoproliferative disorders in the skin include lymphomatoid papulosis (LyP), primary cutaneous anaplastic large cell lymphoma (PCALCL), and T-MF. A chimeric antibody directed to CD30, a member of the tumor necrosis factor receptors, SGN-30 was utilized to treat such patients who required systemic treatment with promising results in the majority of patients; a response rate of 70% and a 43% complete response rate. The same antibody, however, when utilized for patients with systemic lymphoproliferative disorders that express CD30, Hodgkin's lymphoma (HL), and systemic anaplastic large cell lymphoma (S-ALCL) was not as efficacious, producing 29% stable disease with no responders among patients with HL and 17% overall response in S-ALCL.

In an effort to improve efficacy and maintain an acceptable toxicity profile, SGN-30 was conjugated to MMAE, a tubulin inhibitor, to produce SGN-35. Initial phase I studies with patients who had relapsed or refractory HL or S-ALCL were promising, showing an 86% tumor regression and an overall response rate of 38%. This study was followed by phase II trials in relapsed or refractory HL and S-ALCL with astounding results. In S-ALCL, SGN-35 was reported to produce an overall response of 87%, with 57% complete responses by investigator assessment. In relapsed or refractory HL, relapsing after high-dose therapy with autologous stem cell rescue, a 95% tumor shrinkage was seen, with an 83% reduction in B symptoms of fever, night sweats, or weight loss. The salient toxicity was peripheral neuropathy, which was mild and believed to be manageable. A global study of SGN-35 in the treatment of CD30+ skin lymphomas is being planned.

Novel Therapeutic Drugs

Finally, we can examine some novel drugs that have been studied in CTCL, primarily MF and SS, and some preliminary information regarding drugs that may have activity in T-cell malignancies. Clearly, knowledge of the unique metabolism of the T lymphocyte is much less than in the more common B-cell lymphomas, lending a somewhat chaotic pattern to research efforts in T-cell malignancies.

Bortezomib is a proteasome inhibitor delivered conventionally via a biweekly intravenous route. Zinzani and colleagues reported on 12 patients, most with relapsed or refractory CTCL, but some with peripheral T-cell lymphoma (PTCL) in skin only, who were treated with conventional doses of bortezomib and experienced an overall response of 67%, with 17% complete response.

Lenalidomide, discussed previously in the setting of B-cell lymphomas, was studied in eight patients with MF or SS and found to produce a response rate of 38%.

Forodesine (BCX-1777), a purine nucleoside phosphorylase inhibitor (an enzyme in the purine salvage pathway), is orally bioavailable and was studied in 36 patients with relapsed or refractory MF or SS. An overall response rate of 39% with a median duration of response of 127 days and median time to response of 42 days was seen. Forty-five percent of patients with SS had a partial response in blood.

PF-3512676 (formerly CpG 7909) is a Toll-like receptor 9 agonist that is injected subcutaneously weekly for 24 weeks. This interesting agent was studied in patients with relapsed or refractory MF and SS. Data on 28 patients revealed a 32% response rate with 3 complete responses with a well-tolerated treatment.

Tipifarnib, an oral farnesyl transferase inhibitor, was administered to 12 patients with PTCL or CTCL with a resultant response rate of 50%, half of these being complete responses.

The activity of both bendamustine and desatinib, drugs that are accepted treatment for B-cell malignancies and chronic myelogenous leukemia, respectively, in relapsed or refractory PTCL was described. Bendamustine was studied in the BENTL trial of the GOELAMS group. Thirty-eight patients with relapsed or refractory PTCL or CTCL were treated. The majority of the patients were diagnosed with PTCL, with only 2 having CTCL, tumor phase. In this study, the overall response rate was 47% with 29% complete remissions and a median duration of response of 157 days after six cycles of treatment. Desatinib was studied in phase I for relapsed or refractory non-Hodgkin's lymphoma. Interestingly, two patients with PTCL experienced sustained complete remissions (lasting over 2 years from initiation of drug) and a third experienced a partial response.

CONCLUSIONS

Clearly, phase III or larger phase II trials are difficult in this patient population because the broad areas of CBCLs or CTCLs contain many heterogeneous entities, and each condition is relatively uncommon, leaving small numbers of patients at each institution or country to participate in clinical trials. We now have more agreement on diagnosis and classification, staging and staging procedures, and how to best assess response in clinical trials, as well as appropriate clinical trial endpoints. To best accomplish the goals of the completion of larger phase II and phase III trials in this population to advance our knowledge of these entities and how they can best be treated and to expand treatment options, consortiums of interested parties/institutions will need to be formed and need to cooperate globally with similar interested groups. This is an achievable goal.

SUGGESTED READINGS

Campbell JJ, Clark RA, Watanabe R, Kupper TS. Sézary syndrome and mycosis fungoides arise from distinct T-cell subsets: a biologic rationale for their distinct clinical behaviors. *Blood.* 2010;116:767–771.

Chen R, et al. *Blood.* 2010;116: abstract 283.

Dumaj G, et al. *Ann Oncol.* 2011: abstract 126.

Duvic M, et al, Blood 2007, 110(11), abstract 122.

Duvic M, et al. *Blood.* 2010;116: abstract 962.

Duvic M, Reddy SA, Pinter-Brown L, Korman NJ, Zic J, Kennedy DA, et al. A phase II study of SGN-30 in cutaneous anaplastic large cell lymphoma and related lymphoproliferative disorders. *Clin Cancer Res.* 2009;15:6217–6224.

Forero-Torres A, Leonard JP, Younes A, Rosenblatt JD, Brice P, Bartlett NL, et al. A Phase II study of SGN-30 (anti-CD30 mAb) in Hodgkin lymphoma or systemic anaplastic large cell lymphoma. *Br J Haematol.* 2009;146:171–179.

Ishida T, et al. *Blood.* 2010;116: abstract 285.

Kim YH, Duvic M, Obitz E, Gniadecki R, Iversen L, Osterborg A, et al. Clinical efficacy of zanolimumab (HuMax-CD4): two phase 2 studies in refractory cutaneous T-cell lymphoma. *Blood.* 2007;109:4655–4662.

Kim YH, Girardi M, Duvic M, Kuzel T, Link BK, Pinter-Brown L, et al. Phase I trial of a Toll-like receptor 9 agonist, PF-3512676 (CPG 7909), in patients with treatment-refractory, cutaneous T-cell lymphoma.*J Am Acad Dermatol.* 2010;63:975–983.

NPham-Ledard A, Prochazkova-Carlotti M, Laharanne E, Vergier B, Jouary T, Beylot-Barry M, et al. IRF4 gene rearrangements define a subgroup of CD30-positive cutaneous T-cell lymphoma: a study of 54 cases. *J Invest Dermatol.* 2010;130:816–825.

O'Mahony D, Morris JC, Stetler-Stevenson M, Matthews H, Brown MR, Fleisher T, et al. EBV-related lymphoproliferative disease complicating therapy with the anti-CD2 monoclonal antibody, siplizumab, in patients with T-cell malignancies. *Clin Cancer Res.* 2009;15:2514–2522.

Querfeld C, et al. *Blood.* 2005;106: abstract 3351.

Reeder CB, Ansell SM. Novel therapeutic agents for B-cell lymphoma: developing rational combinations. *Blood.* 2011;117:1453–1462.

Shustov A, et al. *Blood.* 2010;116: abstract 961.

van Doorn R, van Kester MS, Dijkman R, Vermeer MH, Mulder AA, Szuhai K, et al. Oncogenomic analysis of mycosis fungoides reveals major differences with Sézary syndrome. *Blood.* 2009;113:127–136.

Wada DA, Law ME, Hsi ED, Dicaudo DJ, Ma L, Lim MS, et al. Specificity of IRF4 translocations for primary cutaneous anaplastic large cell lymphoma: a multicenter study of 204 skin biopsies. *Mod Pathol.* 2011;24:596–605.

William BM, et al. *Blood.* 2010;116: abstract 288.

Witzig TE, et al. *Blood.* 2010;116: abstract 267.

Yamamoto K, Utsunomiya A, Tobinai K, Tsukasaki K, Uike N, Uozumi K, et al. Phase I study of KW-0761, a defucosylated humanized anti-CCR4 antibody, in relapsed patients with adult T-cell leukemia-lymphoma and peripheral T-cell lymphoma. *J Clin Oncol.* 2010;28:1591–1598.

Younes A, Bartlett NL, Leonard JP, Kennedy DA, Lynch CM, Sievers EL, et al. Brentuximab vedotin (SGN-35) for relapsed CD30-positive lymphomas. *N Engl J Med.* 2010;363:1812–1821.

Zinzani PL, Musuraca G, Tani M, Stefoni V, Marché E, Fina M, et al. Phase II trial of proteasome inhibitor bortezomib in patients with relapsed or refractory cutaneous T-cell lymphoma. *J Clin Oncol.* 2007;25:4293–4297.

INDEX